# International Health Worker Migration and Recruitment

This book is the first comprehensive study of international health worker-migration and -recruitment from the perspective of global governance, policy and politics.

Covering 70 years of history of the development of this global policy field, this book presents new and previously unpublished data, based on primary research, to reveal for the first time that international health worker-migration-and -recruitment have been major concerns of global policy-making going back to the foundations of post-war international cooperation. The authors analyse the policies and programmes of a wide range of international organisations, from WHO, ILO and UNESCO to the IOM, World Bank and OECD, and feature extended analysis of bilateral agreements to manage health worker migration and recruitment, critiquing the claim that they work in the interests of all countries. Yeates' and Pillinger's ground-breaking analysis of global governance presents an assiduously researched study showing how the interplay and intersections of several global institutional regimes – spanning labour, migration, health, social protection, trade and business, equality and human rights – shape global policy responses to this major health care issue that affects all countries worldwide. It discusses the growing challenges to public health as a result of the globalisation of health labour markets, and highlights how global and national policy can realise the health and health-related Sustainable Development Goals for all by 2030.

This research monograph will be of key interest to students and scholars of Global Governance, Global Public Policy, Global Health, Global Politics, Migration Studies, Health and Social Care, Social Policy and Development Studies. Policy makers and campaign activists, nationally and globally, will appreciate the practical relevance and applications of the research findings.

**Nicola Yeates** is Professor of Social Policy in the Department of Social Policy and Criminology at The Open University, UK. Notable books include *Globalizing Care Economies and Migrant Workers* (2009), *Understanding Global Social Policy* (2014), *The Global Social Policy Reader* (2009), *World-regional Social Policy and Global Governance* (2010), *Social Justice* (2008) and *Globalization and Social Policy* (2001).

**Jane Pillinger** is an independent social policy researcher and policy advisor working in the areas of migration, employment and gender equality. She has carried out research and policy advice for global unions, social partner organisations, international organisations such as ILO, IOM and UNWomen, as well as national and European organisations and advocacy movements. She is a Visiting Research Fellow in the Department of Social Policy and Criminology at The Open University, UK.

# Routledge Studies in Governance and Public Policy

For more information about this series, please visit: www.routledge.com/Routledge-Studies-in-Governance-and-Public-Policy/book-series/GPP

# International Health Worker Migration and Recruitment

Global Governance, Politics and Policy

**Nicola Yeates and Jane Pillinger**

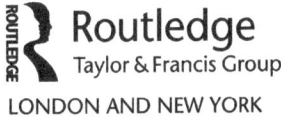

Routledge
Taylor & Francis Group

LONDON AND NEW YORK

First published 2019 by Routledge

2 Park Square, Milton Park, Abingdon, Oxon OX14 4RN
605 Third Avenue, New York, NY 10017

*Routledge is an imprint of the Taylor & Francis Group, an informa business*

First issued in paperback 2021

Publisher's Note

The publisher has gone to great lengths to ensure the quality of this reprint but points out that some imperfections in the original copies may be apparent.

*British Library Cataloguing-in-Publication Data*
A catalogue record for this book is available from the British Library

*Library of Congress Cataloging-in-Publication Data*
A catalog record has been requested for this book

ISBN: 978-1-138-93330-9 (hbk)
ISBN: 978-1-03-217816-5 (pbk)
DOI: 10.4324/9781315678641

Typeset in Times New Roman
by Wearset Ltd, Boldon, Tyne and Wear

# Contents

## 3 Elaborating the global policy field: the 1977 Nursing Personnel Recommendation

56

## 4 The rise of 'ethical recruitment': momentum without enforcement

85

# Tables

# Appendices

# Acknowledgements

This book has had an extraordinarily long gestation period. It is inspired by the longer lineages of academic and policy research on the health workforce, international migration and social policy in which the authors have been immersed for at least two decades. The idea for this joint book specifically dates back about five years or so, when we undertook a joint project to track international policy responses on human resources for health migration (Yeates and Pillinger 2013) as part of a Canadian Institutes for Health Research/University of Ottawa grant awarded to Nicola Yeates at The Open University. The depth and breadth of analysis we have aimed to offer in this book goes way beyond that project and what it was possible to do at the time.

Works such as this are invariably best undertaken in the context of unstinting support gained from immersion in conducive institutional and intellectual environments. It has undoubtedly benefited from support over the years by The Open University where Nicola Yeates is Professor of Social Policy and Jane Pillinger is a Research Fellow in the Department of Social Policy and Criminology. We would like to thank the OU's Faculty's Centre for Innovation, Knowledge and Development, the Citizenship and Governance network and the Migration network for enabling stimulating and collegiate exchanges. We especially thank the International Development and Inclusive Innovation Research Area for providing financial support for aspects of this work, and the Faculty more broadly for funding Nicola Yeates to participate in academic conferences in the UK and internationally at which aspects of this book have been presented and discussed. These include the conferences of the Historical Materialism collective (School of Oriental and African Studies), the Global Labour Studies group (University of Illinois), and the Global Dynamics of Social Policy Collaborative Research Centre (University of Bremen), together with those of the UK Social Policy Association, the East Asian Social Policy Network, and the International Sociological Association.

No book is ever truly the work of the authors alone. In this, we were supported by a small army of experts and allies. We would like to acknowledge the unstinting and amazing support from UN libraries staff who responded rapidly, helpfully and with good grace to numerous requests for help in locating documentation and tracking various sources in the UN archives. We thank in particular staff at the Dag Hammarskjöld Library and the ILO library to whom we are eternally grateful. We are also thankful for the excellent library facilities at The Open University and the library staff there in ensuring that academic researchers are supported in our work. We also thank the local independent bookshops to which we turned to access vital materials for this project and which were able to source and access them for us much more quickly and cheaply than any tax-avoiding corporate online retailer could.

We have individually and jointly greatly benefited from discussions with and feedback from numerous colleagues from different academic disciplines and from myriad intellectual and political perspectives within the academy and outside of it. Many colleagues have provided feedback on at least some parts of the manuscript. Others offered us useful advice, ideas and leads to follow up. Others simply encouraged us or sparked connections we had not previously made. There are way too many to name individually, but we wish to acknowledge and thank (in alphabetical order) in particular: Baba Aye, Tuba Agartan, Adele Blackett, Cristina Behrendt, Gary Browning, Ross Fergusson, Genevieve Gencianos, Chris Holden, Alexandra Kaasch, Meri Koivusalo, Rianne Mahon, Remco Van de Pas, Ito Peng, Theo Papadopoulos, Nicola Piper, Raia Prokhovnik, Gaby Ramia, and Dave Wield. They variously listened, encouraged, read, commented, asked questions, challenged us, and reflected back insights from their own work. They are a source of inspiration and their own work informs this one in different ways. They stimulated our thinking, encouraged us to be sharper in our analysis, spurred us to dig more deeply and widely, and helped us progress this work to its thankful conclusion. The book is all the better for it, and we thank them for their generosity, collegiality and personal warmth. The usual disclaimer applies: they bear no responsibility for any of the contents of the book, the arguments we advance, or any mistakes or omissions that we may have made.

We thank all at Routledge who have responded with good grace to all our requests and queries, and who have provided excellent editorial and production support. We have benefited from the guidance of our commissioning editors, Andrew Taylor and Sophie Iddamalgoda, and Paul Whittle, Allie Hargreaves and Pip Clubbs at Wearset for the support during the production process. We are particularly indebted to Paul Whittle for reading our manuscript and for his patience in helping us improve our argument and clarity of communication throughout the copyediting process.

We are thankful for our intellectual partnership and personal friendship, which has been a source of mutual inspiration and support. Our biggest gratitude goes to our families who have been amazingly supportive during the whole project. Nicola wishes to thank Ross, Charlie and Daisy, and Jane wishes to thank Veronique de Boysson, for their unstinting support and love during the hard graft of writing of the book. In our respective households, Veronique and Ross shouldered much of the domestic labour and forfeited an unreasonable amount of quality leisure time in the name of this project.

Finally, we dedicate this book to all the health workers around the world, migrant or otherwise. They are the cornerstone of high-quality health services available for all on a universal basis and are fundamental to any aspiration to realise public health goals and socially just societies. We wholeheartedly concur with the universal truth articulated by the Global Health Workers' Alliance: there is no health without a workforce. Without their expertise, and their availability in sufficient numbers, at the right time in the right place, with the right equipment, at least one of us would not be alive today.

Nicola Yeates and Jane Pillinger

# Acronyms and abbreviations

| | |
|---|---|
| AAAH | Asia Pacific Action Alliance on Human Resources for Health |
| ADBI | Asian Development Bank Institute |
| ASEAN | Association of Southeast Asian Nations |
| AU | African Union |
| BLA | Bilateral Labour Agreement |
| BWI | Building and Woodworkers International |
| CARICOM | Caribbean Community |
| CEC | Commission of the European Communities |
| CGFNS | Commission on Graduates of Foreign Nursing Schools |
| CHS | Commission on Human Security |
| CIETT | International Confederation of Private Employment Agencies |
| COMISCA | Council of Health Ministers of Central America |
| COSECSA | College of Surgeons of East, Central and Southern Africa |
| CSOs | Civil Society Organisations |
| DfID | Department for International Development |
| DNA | Designated National Authority |
| ECOSOC | United Nations Economic and Social Council |
| EPSU | European Federation of Public Service Unions |
| ESA | Eastern and Southern Africa region |
| EU | European Union |
| GATS | General Agreement on Trade in Services |
| GFMD | Global Forum on Migration and Development |
| GHWA | Global Health Workforce Alliance |
| GHWN | Global Health Workforce Network |
| GSPs | Global Skills Partnerships |
| HI | Historical institutionalism |
| HM | Historical materialism |
| HOSPEEN | European Hospital and Health care Employers' Association |
| HRH | Human Resources for Health |
| HSE | Health and Safety Executive (UK) |
| HW4All | Health workers for all and all for health workers |
| IGOs | International Governmental Organisations |
| ILC | International Labour Conference |

| | |
|---|---|
| ILO | International Labour Organization |
| IMF | International Monetary Fund |
| INGOs | International Non-Governmental Organisations |
| IOE | International Organisation of Employers |
| IOM | International Organization for Migration |
| IOs | International Organisations |
| ISRI | Independent Stakeholders Reporting Instrument |
| ITU | International Telecommunications Union |
| ITUC | International Trade Union Confederation |
| JPEPA | Japan–Philippines Economic Partnership Agreement |
| LMICs | Low- and medium-income countries |
| MDGs | Millennium Development Goals |
| MoA | Memorandum of agreement |
| MoU | Memoranda of understanding |
| MRA | Mutual recognition agreement |
| NGOs | Non-governmental organisations |
| NHWA | National Health Workforce Accounts |
| NIEO | New International Economic Order (UN) |
| OECD | Organization for Economic Cooperation and Development |
| OSCE | Organization for Security and Cooperation in Europe |
| PAHO | Pan-American Health Organization |
| PPPs | Public Private Partnerships |
| PSI | Public Services International |
| RCSI | Royal College of Surgeons Ireland |
| SADC | Southern African Development Community |
| SDGs | Sustainable Development Goals |
| SEGIB | Ibero-American General Secretariat |
| TISA | Trade in Services Agreement |
| UHC | Universal Health Coverage |
| UN | United Nations |
| UNCfSD | United Nations Commission for Social Development |
| UNCSTD | United Nations Conference on Science and Technology for Development |
| UNCTAD | United Nations Commission on Trade and Development |
| UNDP | United Nations Development Programme |
| UNECE | United Nations Economic Commission for Europe |
| UNESCAP | United Nations Economic and Social Commission for Asia and the Pacific |
| UNESCO | United Nations Educational, Scientific, and Cultural Organization |
| UNFAO | United Nations Food and Agriculture Organisation |
| UNFPA | United Nations Population Fund |
| UNGA | United Nations General Assembly |
| UNGMG | Global Migration Group |
| UNGP | United Nations Guiding Principles (for business and human rights) |

| | |
|---|---|
| UNHCR | United Nations High Commissioner for Refugees |
| UNHEEG | UN High-Level Commission on Health, Employment and Economic Growth |
| UNHLD-MD | United Nations High Level Dialogue on Migration and Development |
| UNHRC | United Nations Human Right Council |
| UNICEF | United Nations Children's Fund |
| UNITAR | The United Nations Institute for Training and Research |
| UNSG | United Nations Secretary General |
| US DHEW | United States Department of Health, Education and Welfare |
| WANA | West Asia–North Africa Institute |
| WB | World Bank |
| WHA | World Health Assembly |
| WHO | World Health Organization |
| WHO DG | WHO Director-General |
| WHO-EAG | WHO's Expert Advisory Group on the Relevance and Effectiveness of the WHO Global Code of Practice |
| WHO-AFRO | WHO Regional Office for Africa |
| WHO-AMRO | WHO Regional Office for the Americas |
| WHO-EMRO | WHO Regional Office for the Eastern Mediterranean |
| WHO-EURO | WHO Regional Office for Europe |
| WHO-SEARO | WHO South East Asia Regional Office |
| WMO | World Meteorological Organisation |
| WONCA | International Council of Nurses and World Organization of National Colleges, Academies and Academic Associations of General Practitioners/Family Physicians |
| WHO-WPRO | WHO Regional Office for the Western Pacific |
| WTO | World Trade Organization |

# 1 The global dynamics of international health worker-migration and -recruitment policy

## 1 Global governance, social policy and a new lens on health worker-migration

The last two decades have witnessed a resurgence of academic and policy research on international health worker-migration. Thanks to the cumulative efforts of myriad research projects and programmes to elucidate international trends in the international mobility of health professionals – physicians, nurses, midwives, dentists, occupational therapists, surgeons, pharmacists, pharmacologists, psychiatrists and health administrators – and to chart and assess the diverse measures to manage such flows, we now have a reasonably comprehensive picture of the scale, drivers, dynamics and consequences at the national level of this major social phenomenon affecting most, if not all, countries worldwide.

Yet for all the advances in the state of knowledge in this field there remains a significant void in the otherwise rich literatures that abound on this subject. With nearly all studies focusing on trends in relation to specific countries worldwide and the national measures they put in place to manage health workforce mobility, the main concern of research and analysis has been domestic spheres of policy-making and governance. Thus, it is the *national* ideational drivers, regulatory institutions, policy actors, processes of policy-making, and the content of *national* policy and its outcomes that command the overwhelming share of attention. This 'methodologically nationalist' orientation has dominated the research field on this topic (as so many others in the social and political sciences) to such an extent that questions about how the governance, politics and policy of this major social phenomenon play out on a transnational scale in cross-border spheres of governance have not been the dedicated focus of extensive research. None of the otherwise rich research literatures on global migration governance, global health governance or global social governance considering the role of cross-border spheres of governance in policy formation policy have attended to international health worker-migration or -recruitment as a field of global governance and policy formation in its own right or as an issue within those wider fields. Nor have studies on national policy initiatives and responses tended to wholly engage with the now-extensive literature on transnational actors as major organisational features in policy formation (Yeates 2018a).

Although this is a significant gap that this book aims to fill, we are not working from a totally 'blank canvas'. Global institutions have not been the explicit subject of extended research in relation to this issue, though the little analysis of this that does exist has been written from a health planning perspective which is concerned with the practicalities of health workforce organisation, planning and management (hence that literature's use of the term *human resources* for health). Moreover, it focuses on just one global initiative – the World Health Organisation (WHO) Code of Practice on the International Recruitment of Health Personnel (WHO 2010a) (e.g. Bourgeault *et al.* 2016; Buchan *et al.* 2016; Campbell *et al.* 2013; Dhillon 2016). This has elicited rich data and analysis which we draw on in the book. Even so, the focus of those studies is very much from a global health perspective, and the wider social and public policy contexts of health workforces as a vital development resource and global issue is largely absent from them. Compared with other areas of social or public policy concerning comparably important 'global challenges', this is a notable and lamentable gap in the research field.

As a result, we know far less than we should – or could – about the 'shape', nature and characteristics of international health worker-migration and -recruitment from a global governance and policy perspective. The state of knowledge about how state and non-state actors act 'outwardly' in spheres of cross-border governance of different kinds to influence or pursue goals and objectives on this issue is all too rudimentary, as is understanding of how different global institutional regimes intersect and what their impacts are. Because of these analytical and data gaps, we do not yet have a full picture of the global dynamics of global policy and governance. Empirically and analytically, these are significant omissions which this book aims to help fill. Because of the salience of health worker-migration as a key contemporary social issue, the dearth of research into these global governance aspects of its dynamics significantly limits in turn our understanding of how the globalisation of health care economies, social reproduction and social development more broadly are unfolding. This means that there are unfulfilled opportunities for theory development in relation to the contemporary condition of the global governance of health, the welfare state, and social restructuring, including the conditions lending weight to certain policy ideas in particular settings becoming dominant or changing. Of significance are the implications of this gap for policy as political practice. Not having a fuller understanding of cross-border spheres of governance as active sites of policy formation and resource mobilisation also means that we do not have a clear picture of the implications of the full force of globalising dynamics in all their varied forms for realising the right to health as a universal and indivisible human right as well as a global development goal. This limits understanding of what opportunities do actually exist to realise those rights and goals.

This state of affairs is *even more* anomalous because this is a highly active policy field. In 2013 we undertook a short survey of contemporary international initiatives in the field of 'human resources for health' (Yeates and Pillinger 2013). We identified a rich, dynamic and complex terrain. It was one that we found to be actively 'populated' by numerous social actors, multiple policy spaces and myriad initiatives. We found at least eight multilateral organisations, two global campaign coalitions, and five global forums, partaking in policy-making, standard-setting, technical assistance, data systems, and research on international health worker-migration. We found numerous initiatives of different sorts: normative frameworks for rights-based approaches to migration; voluntary codes on the ethical recruitment of health workers; diasporic initiatives aimed at 'brain gain' and development for source countries; data and forecasting on future health workforce requirements; measures aimed at scaling up health workforce capacity, and international partnerships revolving around health worker-migration.

Our finding that there were multiple modes of international cooperation, coordination and integration at work also suggested there is a wider story to be told beyond one of an ever-growing list of actions and projects by international organisations (IOs).[1] Numerous global initiatives were regularly issued and renewed, and followed common identifiable logics, in ways suggestive of sys-tematised knowledge production and resourcing, pointing to the existence of a highly-institutionalised sphere of governance and policy. Such activity was recurrent, even if the forms it took were diverse, over time and across organisa-tions. Moreover, a critical density of activity in the form of projects, partner-ships, and policies spanning multiple organisations was apparent. In addition, this highly active, yet complex, terrain was underpinned by a set of universally shared norms that transcended any one country. The right to migrate, to health and to decent work, together with international human rights and trade con-siderations, shaped myriad policies and initiatives emanating from cross-border spheres of governance. In short, this was more than a set of ad hoc activities: it was a rules-based field shaped by social norms, laws, political and financial resources that were mobilised in various ways, and which cohered, stabilised and gave meaning to the multiple initiatives underway.

Furthermore, the governance structures and policy approaches involved were marked less by overall agreement or unification than by multiplicity, fragmen-tation and variance. IOs as diverse as the United Nations (UN), World Bank (WB), Organisation for Economic Cooperation and Development (OECD), and International Organization for Migration (IOM) were all active participants in this field. Just as each brought their own approach to social and economic policy so too they brought their own approach and agendas to bear on the question of the international migration of health workers. It is not just that these approaches could be readily identified but that they vied with each other, such that it seemed to matter which organisation is involved in what initiative – not least because it was a guide to what were to become the dominant discourses and approaches in the evolving field. At the time, we looked at a restricted set of organisations and their responses in this field, but we were already aware that more extensive research – both in terms of covering a wider range of organisations and over a longer period of time – would have uncovered a greater number and range of social actors. We were also aware that it would also have brought to the fore the multiplicity of structures and modes of governance shaping health worker-migration. Extended research would, we felt, have identified a far more complex, and ultimately more interesting, way into what was evidently a major global social formation and a 'new' realm of global governance, with its own material, ideational, institutional foundations, dynamics, consequences and impacts. In all, the range of initiatives and organisations we found in our initial research provoked our intellectual curiosity to understand better the institutional frameworks in which they were negotiated and the multiplicity of actors, ideas and resources involved. The findings of that short study suggested the additional extensive, in-depth research that has become this book.

Since that time, the global policy field has become if anything increasingly dynamic and 'busy'. Besides the WHO Global Code (2010a), health workforce availability, universal health care and labour migration issues are all the subject of major global initiatives. The health workforce, including its migration, is anchored into the Sustainable Development Goals (SDGs) (UNGA 2015),[2] reflecting the now-widely accepted precepts that it is a cornerstone of effective health systems and sustainable development. This 'mainstreaming' has supported calls for greater accountability in policy-making at all levels for health impacts on the basis that there are significant public policy consequences of weak health systems for population health and well-being.[3] Such global initiatives intersect with on-going global campaigns for universal health coverage (UHC) that are also multifarious in their organisational composition. As the complexity of the initiatives has grown, so too has understanding of the nature of the issues at stake. By way of illustration of this, we invoke the titles of three recent publications which cogently encapsulate understanding of the significance of health worker-migration as one of the foremost global social issues of our time. One report, jointly commissioned by the Global Health Workers' Alliance (GHWA) and WHO aptly states *No Health Without Health Workers* (Campbell *et al.* 2013). The second and third are editorials from *The Lancet*: *No health workforce, no global security* (The Lancet 2016) and *Health-care workers as agents of sustainable development* (The Lancet Global Health 2015). Collectively, these titles convey how international health worker-migration is increasingly understood as a matter of the utmost strategic significance for public health, for human security and for social and economic development for all countries, at whatever their 'level' of development, worldwide.

In short, health worker-migration has become the subject of active policy making at the global level and in cross-border spheres of governance involving myriad institutions, actors, ideas and campaigns, but it has not been the direct focus of academic or policy analysis. In this first major study of this issue from this perspective, we elucidate the contours, dynamics and impacts of global governance and policy with regard to highly skilled health worker-migration. The remainder of the chapter introduces the subject of the book at further length. Section 2 sets out the overall aims of the book and defines its scope. Section 3 discusses the salience of our study of international health worker-migration and -recruitment in terms of theory and policy. Section 4 describes the sources of research data underpinning the study and the methods used to construct it. Section 5 explains how the research materials are organised and key elements of the argument on a chapter-by-chapter basis. Section 6 provides a brief note about the terminology used throughout the book and statement about the social values underpinning it.

## 2  Aims and scope of the book

Our book aims to contribute to filling major analytical and empirical gaps in research on health worker-migration and -recruitment governance, politics and policy with a view to contributing to the research literatures on global social governance and policy more widely. Based on rigorous original research, it presents the results of a comprehensive social policy study from the perspective of its global governance and the social politics of global policy formation. In this, we offer the first *extensive and sustained* academic global policy analysis of international health worker-migration and -recruitment. We examine in depth the origins, initiation and development of the global governance of international health worker-migration and -recruitment as seen through the lens of the global policy field as it has unfolded over the last seven decades. To this end, we examine:

- the diverse institutions, actors, norms, discourses, policies and practices that constitute global governance and policy in respect of international health worker-migration and -recruitment;
- how this issue is framed and taken up by diverse social actors within institutions of global governance and global policy-making;
- the material, ideational and normative foundations and drivers of the global politics, policy and governance of international health worker-migration, in historical and contemporary settings; including how (and why) these have changed over time;
- how global policy initiatives are addressing (or are attempting to address) the causes and consequences of health worker-migration in source and destination countries worldwide – and their effectiveness in doing so; and
- key issues and priorities for global policies in the light of the SDGs, with a particular focus on diverse and interlocking commitments on health, labour, social protection, human rights and equality, and socio-economic development.

Our study seeks to elucidate answers to questions such as: How and why have cross-border spheres of governance become such important sites of action on international health worker-migration? What kinds of policy approaches and solutions are taken up by global organisations and how have they become instituted in key global initiatives? What are the implications of the overall trajectories we see in this global policy field for the policy space and creative opportunities for transformative solutions to emerge?

As a *Social Policy* study of the globalisation of international health worker-migration and -recruitment policy, we contest the idea that this phenomenon can be comprehensively understood only from the perspective of health workforce planning or a 'human resources for health' perspective. This statement may initially seem counter-intuitive but, we contend, it is only by situating the creation and reproduction of this global policy field within a broader landscape in which questions of power, social justice and social development feature prominently that the structural and institutional features of the global governance of health worker-migration can be fully revealed. Furthermore, just as the roots of health workforce availability and international migration reside outside of the health sector, so we look at global health regimes in relation to other regimes operating in different sectors. Thus, we deploy a multi-sectoral analysis of the global policy field that is cognisant of myriad intersecting socio-institutional regimes that include the health sector but extend way beyond it. Indeed, we argue that it is *only* possible to comprehend the global governance of this phenomenon using such an approach. It is precisely the intersections among multiple global institutional regimes spanning health and migration, as well as social protection, equality, trade, business and human rights governance, structuring the dynamics of global policy formation in this area in which we are interested. In doing so, we 'rescue' analysis of the phenomenon solely as a matter of and for health, to emphasise its wider significance for social provision and as a matter of direct concern to international economic and social development more broadly. In a context where the causes of high levels of health worker-migration that we see today lie in long-term trajectories of uneven and differentiated development, the 'institutional intersectionalism' that we show is a central feature of global governance in this area also helps understand the complex and often contradictory pressures on individual health workers to emigrate for work abroad as well as on policy-makers at global, regional and national levels.

Before elaborating the analytical tenets of the study, it is important to clarify what lies within and what outside the scope of the book. Falling squarely *within* its scope is the sphere of multilateral (cross-border) governance and policy-making as seen through the ideas, norms, laws, rules, and initiatives emanating from IOs such as the UN, WB, OECD and World Trade Organization (WTO). We consider these organisations in depth: they are prominent global policy actors whose role in shaping the contours of this global policy field has never before been mapped. We also include bilateral modes of governance because of the close relationship between bilateral and multilateral modes of governance in migration, trade and development policies. Indeed, bilateral agreements are a prevalent mode of this global policy field, and they have been promoted by major global policy actors over many decades. Such agreements are highly significant in the discursive and institutional rise of 'circular' and 'return' migration approaches, and they are inseparable from wider currents that are eroding the right of migrants to permanent settlement and the emergence of differentiated (and unequal) migration rights. Our inclusion of bilateral modes of governance allows us to further elaborate on a major theme in this global policy field.

Falling *outside* the scope of this study are multilateral governance on a *world–regional* scale. Regional organisations such as the European Union (EU), Association for South-East Asian Nations (ASEAN) and the Caribbean Community (CARICOM), amongst others, are becoming increasingly active and 'vocal' in this domain (Yeates 2014a, 2018a; Yeates and Pillinger 2013, 2018). However, they cannot be accommodated within the confines of the book. For the same reason, we do not cover the impacts of global policies on national policy-making other than as explored through the lens of bilateral agreements. At the same time, we recognise that the boundaries between global and sub-global (world–regional, domestic) political and governance spheres, and between national and international actors, influences and ideas, are blurred. The task of analysing the intersections between different scales and spheres of governance (private as well as public), each with different institutional and socio-political 'logics', must fall to a future book.[4]

## 3 Why international health worker-migration and -recruitment? Evidence, theory and policy

### 3.1 International migration and recruitment, health workforce availability and universal health coverage

Of all the factors that determine access to health care and the health and welfare of populations, there is no doubt that the international migration of health workers has received a very significant share of the attention. There is good reason for this. Emigration significantly impacts upon the overall availability of health workers in any given country, and the health workforce shortages that it can lead to in the source country adversely compromise the quality and efficacy of health services there. This is a set of connections that are by now well understood. Indeed, it has long been recognised that effective health care services depend on sufficient numbers of suitably skilled, qualified and experienced health workers being available to staff the full range of primary health, preventative, diagnostic, treatment and rehabilitative services necessary for everyone in any given country. Thus there is a clear link between the availability of health workers and the provision of high quality health care, access to which is a major (albeit not the only) determinant of health outcomes. As GHWA, a major global advocacy coalition in the health field, rightly proclaims: there is no health without a workforce.

This insight derives from research studies examining what happens when the health workforce is insufficiently numerous to provide health services capable of meeting even essential health needs. Africa has the highest burden of disease of any continent, but has only 3 per cent of the world's health workers, and less than 1 per cent of the world's financial resources. Scholars have repeatedly highlighted how sub-Saharan Africa has been adversely affected by health worker shortages, especially in disadvantaged and rural areas (Adepoju 2007; Dovlo 2007; Awases *et al.* 2004), to the extent that these have severe (fatal) impacts on health outcomes (Chen and Boufford 2005). In Malawi, for example, where 64 per cent of nursing posts are unfilled, the high maternal mortality rates and an inability to expand antiretroviral (ARV) therapy are attributed to nurse emigration (Muula *et al.* 2006). This is in a context where the country is already very heavily dependent on medical aid (25–30 per cent of medical staff working in Malawi are doing so under the auspices of charitable projects) (ibid.). The Botswana government has also raised how health worker emigration gives rise to workforce shortages, constraining capacity to expand HIV services.

The lack of available medical and nursing staff linked to higher rates of disability, morbidity and death is an issue also experienced elsewhere in the world. South-East Asia is among the populous regions of the world with a very high disease burden and high rates of emigration, and has consistently experienced critical shortages of health workers (Yeates and Pillinger 2018). The Caribbean, which bears a high disease burden and a long history of high levels of health worker emigration, has three times as many trained nurses who qualified in the region practising in countries outside of it than in it (Tomblin-Murphy 2016). Even countries in high-income parts of the world are not immune from emigration-induced health workforce depletion. The incorporation of countries in the south and east of Europe into the EU has been a major driver of health worker-migration out of the public health sector and emigration overseas, while post-communist restructuring in central and east Europe has been accompanied by emigration and a deterioration in population health (Hardy *et al.* 2016). Across different development contexts, studies have underscored time and time again the salience of health workforce availability and international migration of health workers as interconnected issues and critical factors affecting the quality of health care and health outcomes. Indeed, the benefits of technological advances in diagnostics and (life-saving) medicines will remain a theoretical possibility if there are not enough qualified and skilled health workers to diagnose cases, dispense medicines and provide effective on-going care for all those affected.

Further vivid illustration of this point is provided by the experience of the outbreak of the Ebola virus in West Africa in 2014. At the time of the outbreak, Sierra Leone had only 119 doctors serving a population of nearly six million people (a ratio of 50,000 : 1) and in Liberia and Guinea there was only one doctor for every 100,000 people. This compares to 100 : 1 in the UK. These ratios fall well below WHO's recommended minimum of at least 23 doctors, nurses and midwives per 10,000 of the population. In Liberia, there were only 3,352 hospital beds for a population of nearly 4.5 million and in Guinea there were a similar number of beds (3,435) for a population of nearly 11.5 million. These are also countries that have seen significant levels of health worker-migration. For example, it is estimated that 10 per cent of Sierra Leone's trained nurses are working in the UK health system, largely because of a lack of resources and low pay. The lack of health workers in these countries coupled with weak health systems were undoubtedly major factors contributing to the spread of the virus throughout populations there.

However, evaluative evidence shows that measures to retain health workers once they are in the workforce can be effective in helping to boost the health workforce. Malawi's comprehensive Emergency Human Resources Programme, which includes gross-salary increases and a period of compulsory public-health service for nurses trained at public expense, is reported to be effective in retaining existing nurses and enticing those that have left nursing to return to the profession (Little and Buchan 2007). Zambia has also seen a decline in health worker-migration as a result of health care workers receiving an extra 25 per cent recruitment and retention allowance on top of their basic salary. Additional rural and hardship payments are given to nurses in rural and remote areas (GHWA 2013). Combining wage and non-wage measures to support recruitment and retention tend to produce the best outcomes (Khaliq *et al.* 2009; Padarath *et al.* 2003).

Understandably, research literatures have largely been oriented towards (and preoccupied with) the relationship between the rise of a global health workforce numbering in the region of 40–50 million people, adversity faced by the many hundreds of millions of people who cannot access health care services, and depletion of resources for development, including resources that could be used to extend health services on a universal basis. To be sure, international migration of health workers is not in itself the only factor determining the availability of a health workforce or the quality of health care services and health systems. Aside from international migration, other types of mobility of health workers, for example from rural to urban areas or from public to private sectors, and from health to other sectors, affect whether sufficient numbers of health workers with the right skills, in the right place at the right time are available to provide services (Buchan 2010; Campbell *et al.* 2013). Practising a profession in a country other than the one in which education and training was completed, especially when the source country is globally poor and experiences combinations of high disease burdens, health worker shortages and health work vacancies, is just one aspect of geographical maldistribution, which, in turn, is one factor in the complex mix of factors determining health workforce availability. In this, it has been constantly emphasised that difficulties in attracting and retaining health workers are principal causes of shortages (Campbell *et al.* 2013; WHO 2016c), while the size and composition of the health workforce is affected by multiple factors such as the rate at which health workers enter into and complete training, overall labour force participation rates, early retirement from the health sector and outflow to other sectors, migration from rural to urban areas, unemployment and the structure of employment generally, including the balance between full-time and part-time work and pay and working conditions in the health sector more widely (Yeates and Pillinger 2018).

Buchan (2010) argues that because international migration plays one part in health worker shortages, focusing on international migration alone deals with a symptom of shortages rather than the root causes of health workforce (un)availability which include limited funding, low pay, limited career opportunities, geographical maldistribution, inadequate infrastructure, and economic and political instability. These causes, he argues, need to be squarely in the overall picture of health workforce policy and planning, which should be primarily preoccupied with ensuring there are adequate resources to train and retain health workers where they are needed (ibid.). It is indeed the case that health worker shortages are not solely attributable to international migration: such shortages can co-exist with a substantial pool of skilled medical and nursing labour who have not emigrated but who are not practising their professions. This is the case for Australia, for example, a major recruiting country where permanent inward migration of overseas registered nurses has increased six-fold since 1990 (Pillinger 2012), as well as for the Philippines, a major health worker 'donor' country internationally, where there are an estimated 200,000 unemployed and underemployed nurses (Lorenzo *et al.* 2007; Pillinger 2013).

As these examples show, the relationship between health worker-migration and health worker shortages is far from straightforward. Some countries would have a 'shortage' of health workers even if all those who were trained stayed to work in their home countries. In the Philippines, aggregate production is adequate but many nurses train with the expectation of emigrating (and actually do so) while a sizeable proportion of trained nurses who do not emigrate do not practise their profession. In Bangladesh, aggregate nurse production is a key factor in its shortages, as it does not train sufficient nurses per capita (Yeates and Pillinger 2018). At the same time, it is clear that export-oriented health workforce strategies and cultural expectations favouring medical or nurse training as a route to emigration can overwhelm efforts to increase aggregate supply in the domestic health workforce to address shortages, such that there is an increased supply of 'ready-made' health workers available in the global labour market.

It is clear, then, that the relationship between international migration of health workers, health workforce shortages, health care quality and health outcomes is complex and context-specific. Nevertheless, it is also palpably clear that international migration *is* a determinant of whether there are enough health workers in any given country who are suitably skilled and qualified to provide the requisite range of services in the right places and at the right time. By insisting on this point, we emphasise that we do not assign blame to health workers for underlying causes of health workforce unavailability or argue that preventing them from migrating will solve labour shortages in the health sector. The freedom to migrate is enshrined in international law as a fundamental human right, and we neither believe nor argue that health workers should be deterred or prevented from living or working in countries other than those in which they were born and/or qualified. There are certainly significant benefits to individuals, families and their communities from emigrating to practise abroad, even if the net benefits to them are not as significant as is often proclaimed. At the same time, it is vital that the right to migrate needs to be seen alongside the right to health and to development. In this respect, it is important that the issues are framed not just as ones of international migration (whether as household survival, labour or social reproduction strategies) but also as international *recruitment* (strategies principally of higher-income countries). Indeed, international recruitment (particularly ethical recruitment) is a significant feature of the social and institutional order in which health worker-migration occurs. Hence the inclusion of recruitment alongside migration in the title of this book.

### 3.2 Global(ising) dynamics of health and social policy: interdependencies among unequal partners

International health worker-migration affects most countries worldwide but it does so unevenly, and the impacts are experienced very differently around the world. There is a major difference between nurses or doctors emigrating from Canada or Ireland to practise their profession in Australia or the UK and those emigrating from India or Ghana to do similarly. Indeed, this is a global issue not so much for the fact that health workforce availability is an issue for all countries (although it is) or that many countries have long histories of health worker emigration (they do) but *precisely* because international migration and recruitment dynamics are so embroiled in global structural inequalities and dependencies that they rebound beyond territories of individual nation-states to draw entire economies and systems of health and welfare into relations of interdependency among unequal 'partners'. In this sense, international migration of health workers cannot simply be seen in terms of individual preferences and choices, devoid of reference to these structural inequalities and histories of uneven development that underpin that migration.

In other words, the meaning and significance of the phenomenon is varied. Global processes are at once universal (they draw in all countries worldwide, generating structural, systemic links, ties and connections between them) *and* particular (they 'touch down', or manifest themselves, in context-specific ways, mediating how universalising processes unfold and their consequences) (Yeates 2001, 2018a). In the same way, there are universal commonalities and context-specificities when it comes to our topic. Place remains an important determinant of the propensity to recruit overseas, emigration or access health care. Thus, many low- and middle-income countries provide a growing pool of health workers migrating to higher-income countries facing health worker shortages, yet they are unable to meet the global goal of 4.45 (midwives, nurses, physicians) per 1,000 population and are often the countries that have the greatest difficulty in achieving universal health coverage (UHC). Reliance on overseas health workers drawn from such countries has significantly increased in high-income countries, such as the UK, Germany, USA, Canada and Australia, which increasingly face shortages of health workers. In the last decade, there has been a 60 per cent rise (from just over a million to nearly two million) in the number of migrant doctors and nurses working in OECD countries (OECD 2015). In the UK there is a workforce shortage of 100,000 doctors and nurses, which is expected to rise to between 250,000 and 350,000 by 2030 (King's Fund, Health Foundation and Nuffield Trust 2018). Unless major destination countries like the UK adopt radically different strategies than those they have pursued to date, then they will continue to be reliant on enticing sufficient numbers of overseas health workers to migrate there to work in order to fill vacancies.

However salient all of these issues are for global health, they are *social policy and development* issues of the first order. This is because health is not *only* a goal in its own right: it is a determinant of the overall welfare of populations and of social protection systems more generally that constitute vital means of social participation. Health is, moreover, a critical factor in social and economic development. In terms of the financial costs alone of bearing high disease burdens which there is insufficient capacity to address, even in terms of providing essential health services, the costs of the widening of the population health gap run into trillions, whether calculated in terms of lost earnings, reduced productivity, lower economic investment, or the collective costs of sustaining people of working age who are unable to work (Ahmad 2005; Buchan, Dhillon and Campbell 2017). Increasingly, health is viewed as an economic and social resource and a public good capable of stimulating economic growth and development, with the economic arguments playing a significant role in turning the attention of heads of key global organisations to the importance of tackling global health worker shortages, particularly in low- and middle-income countries (Buchan, Dhillon and Campbell 2017). Lack of access to health care can, as we know from African experiences of not being able to scale up promising treatments for HIV/AIDs, TB and malaria due to a lack of staff, alter the trajectory of societal development. The contemporary political struggles over health worker-migration and -recruitment are, then, struggles over social provision and the meaning of 'development'. Struggles over global health worker-migration and -recruitment policy are essentially ones about different patterns of social policy, provision and development that produce very different distributive outcomes.

If international migration and recruitment strategies are key elements of a wider picture in which global uneven development is a principal structural determinant, then they are also integral to the globalisation of health and welfare more generally. Unfolding over an extended period, globalisations of many different sorts have markedly shaped development conditions 'at home' and 'abroad', and the services sector has been integral to these processes of global economic and social restructuring. Seen as a structural feature of the globalising world order and, in particular, through the lens of the *transnational scales and modes* by which health and welfare is organised, regulated, funded and delivered (Yeates 2009b, 2012), a vista is opened up onto a major global social phenomenon of our time. It is a landscape in which there has been a significant expansion of the range of cross-border health and social care services as part of the ongoing restructuring of the global economy (Yeates 2009b, 2014b). Reproductive services economies, including health, have been at the foreground of this restructuring, not just as a 'handmaiden' to economic restructuring but as a major feature, indeed driver, of that restructuring in its own right (Truong 1996; Yeates 2009b, 2012, 2014b).

Transnational circuits of capital and labour are significant features of the contemporary global health care economy. The restructuring and rescaling of the social organisation of social provision have seen public services and health care at the forefront of marketisation, commercialisation and privatisation with transnational capital intersecting the production and consumption of health care (Hardy *et al.* 2016) in ways that bear directly upon health workforces and the provision of quality health services. Increasing numbers of highly skilled workers are being drawn into international migration streams, of which health workers form a significant share. One in three international migrants work in the health sector and the global health workforce numbers 40–50 million people worldwide. Most of these are women. Thus, such cross-border labour streams are now also comprised of women seeking work in overseas marketised segments of domestic, social and health care economies, often travelling alone, unaccompanied by a male partner (Sassen 2000; Yeates 2004a, 2004b, 2005b, 2009b, 2012; Kofman and Raghuram 2010).

Although these circuits are by no means historically new (Yeates 2009b) they have nonetheless evolved and changed in a number of important respects (Yeates 2014b). First, they have proliferated and extended in geographic scale, drawing in more countries of the world as well as increasing numbers of households and workers worldwide. Second, they have been commodified, becoming a major site of wealth accumulation and profit generation. Closely related to this is their corporatisation, in the sense of being intersected by commercial interests that are organised on national and transnational scales, and have global reach. Third, they have become institutionalised in normative frameworks and legal rules structuring and protecting (albeit unequally) the rights of participants and have given rise to the development of public- and private- sector health care infrastructures (Yeates 2014b: 189, and passim). These normative frameworks are agreed multilaterally through cross-border spheres of governance and implemented nationally as much as they are decided unilaterally within domestic spheres. Multilateral frameworks, we contend, are a vital part of the ongoing multilateralisation of transnational circuits of capital and labour. Yet, emphasising an earlier point, these frameworks have not received their rightful share of attention in research and policy literatures and therefore, accordingly, they constitute the principal subject of this book. We now set out our approach to researching and analysing these frameworks.

### 3.3 Analytics of global governance and policy

Our Social Policy study of global governance and policy is underpinned by transnationalist, institutionalist, labourist and historical analytics. Methodological transnationalism, to begin with, provides a productive approach, oriented as it is to the social links, ties, activities and processes cutting across countries in ways that focus on the transactions involved in 'cross-bordering' (of governance, policy formation) including the interactions between social actors in the making and remaking of global policy (Yeates 2012, 2018a). Because transnationalist analytics assigns a greater role to agency power than permitted by many structuralist accounts of globalising phenomena, it overcomes the overwhelming and fatalism-inducing constraints of universalistic systemic forces that many see in 'strong' globalisation 'scripts' (Khagram and Levitt, 2005; Yeates 2002). This is especially helpful when it comes to our study of the emergence and development of a global policy field, since political economy analyses tend not to be fine-tuned enough to explain such transactions in the form of, for example, the inter-play between institutions, actors and ideas in concrete contexts over time, and how these produce change or sustain inertia.

The concept of global governance, which anchors our study, is most associ-ated with the academic disciplines of political science (and its specialist fields of comparative politics and international relations) and sociology (political and organisational). It contains many different theoretical traditions, but three important features characterise this scholarship overall. First, all attend to the macro formal and informal 'rules' (values, norms and laws) structuring political, social, and economic organisation, relationships between and among individuals and social groups, and outcomes. Second, they emphasise that these 'rules' are created and exercised across a range of levels or 'scales' including in cross-border spheres of governance as well as in national ones. Just as governance is pluralistic and differentiated, so is global governance. Power and authority are dispersed across many sites, across different scales and among myriad actors. These sites, scales and actors do not exist independently of one another but inter-sect such that the outcomes of global governance are in effect co-produced (Yeates 2018a). Third, global governance is a *contested* process. The definition of norms and rules of conduct, decision-making and policy formation is a key terrain of political struggle among social actors. The global 'rules' that become institutionalised reflect the balance of power between social forces embodied in policy actors as well as consensus among (often highly) disparate such actors with different identities, values, preferences, strategies and tactics. The channels of contestation and action that are available to them to determine, for example, the nature of health and social provision, or the extent and nature of regulation, are in turn structured by interactions between institutions and processes. They shape the range of social actors able to influence policy formation in any mean-ingful way. They enable certain ideas to flourish and take hold. They structure how policy ideas proceed through institutional processes into concrete policies and programmes. At the same time, this is not an immutable field: institutions evolve; organisational fields are not fixed; policy actors prove more influential at certain times than others; campaign coalitions emerge, dissipate and re-form.

How (global) social policies emerge, are maintained, transformed, or remain unchanged requires an appreciation of the interplay of institutions, actors and ideas. Institutions, defined as 'more or less coherent, interconnected set of rou-tines, organisational practices, conventions, rules, sanctioning mechanisms, and practices that govern more or less specific domains of action' (Moulaert *et al.* 2016: 3), are essential to understanding the conditions, constraints and creative opportunities shaping global policy formation, including the work of social actors in bringing about change in institutional 'regimes' and/or specific policies. From the perspective of our book, we identify seven principal global institutional 'regimes' making up the institutional architecture of global health worker-migration and -recruitment governance. Most obviously, this global policy field straddles intersections of global health and global migration, the contours and characteristics of which are remade over time. In addition, global institutional regimes on international trade and business, international development aid, labour, social protection, and equality and human rights all also come into play. We show that consideration of all of these, together with their interaction effects, is necessary for a comprehensive picture of global governance in this field, including how these shape the set of actors 'at the table', their preferences and strategies, and the policy options that become 'most favoured'.

We furthermore argue that institutional regimes are neither unified nor 'belong' to any single global organisation. For example, the global 'rules' on international labour migration are differentiated according to whether they concern 'highly skilled' or 'unskilled' labour, regular or irregular migration and so on. Similarly, global labour governance inheres multiple dimensions spanning decent work, social protection, health services, education, training most commonly associated with the International Labour Organization (ILO), the World Health Organization (WHO), the UN Children's Fund (UNICEF), the WB and UNESCO, as well as the social regulation of public and private employers and intermediary migration agents through human rights and business governance mechanisms and instruments within the UN, WTO and OECD. In global health worker-migration policy, a wide range of multilateral organisations participate in specific initiatives that bear the hallmarks of intersections of global institutional regimes. The organisational features of this global policy field share many of the characteristics of migration governance more generally. While the WTO oversees trade negotiations, and the International Monetary Fund (IMF), along with the Financial Stability Board, manages capital mobility, there is no single international organisation regulating migration. WHO approaches issues of migration from a health needs and 'human resources for health' perspective, while ILO focuses on labour and social protection issues affecting all categories of labour, migrant or not. UNICEF has an interest from the perspective of children's rights to health. The WB has an interest in migration as one factor in wider economic development. Only the IOM has a sole focus on migration issues, but it has no regulatory or standard-setting role, and in keeping with its main emphasis on lower-skilled migration, displacement and returns, its remit rarely covers skilled health worker-migration other than through diaspora programmes. There are various other consultative global fora within and outside of the UN, such as the High-Level Dialogue on Migration and Development (UNHLD-MD), the Global Migration Group (UN-GMG); the Global Forum on Migration and Development (GFMD) promoting multilateral dialogue but they have no role in the development of multilateral policies or standards. Most of these organisations now attend to the issue of health worker-migration and -recruitment in some way.

As we previously signalled, the most expansive approach to global governance would go beyond the realm of cross-border governance and the policies that multilateral organisations promulgate to consider the multiple levels or scales of governance and how the intersection of these are played out in diverse contexts across the world. Such an approach is beyond the scope of this book and we restrict our focus on IOs (governmental and non-governmental) in the making of this global policy field over time. This decision reflects the fact that we take seriously the idea that transnational and non-state global actors are relatively autonomous from states and that there has been no previous comprehensive or in-depth study of them in relation to global health worker-migration.[5] In this, we build on a long tradition of theoretical and applied scholarship in this realm which shows they have a great deal of control over their own agendas: they have the authority to develop their own proposals and institute programmes of social action within a common framework, and they do so across a range of public policy issues and sectors (Barnett and Finnemore 2004; Deacon 2007, 2013; Haas 1990; Orenstein 2008; Orenstein and Schmitz 2006; Reinecke 1998; Yeates 2018a). The governance and politics of policy-framing and decision-making of these organisations, and the interplay between them *matter* and they constitute the proper subjects of enquiry in their own right in any study of governance, regulation and policy formation. IGOs are 'elite', highly institutionalised, and in many ways the most visible global policy actors in global governance. By dedicating our focus on these, we channel attention towards concrete organisational settings and the work of bureaucrats, politicians and others involved in long-term processes of interstate cooperation, coordination and integration to identify common political programmes revolving around practical social problems. As sites of, and actors in, cross-border policy-making, they shape the pace, course, timing and effects of globalising trends on health and welfare institutions and the course of social policy change (Yeates 2001, 2018a; Deacon 2007; Orenstein 2008).

Seeing global governance in pluralistic terms, as a multi-actor process unfolding within defined institutional contexts and involving consensus rather than just coercion, opens up a panorama onto the emergence and development of the global health worker-migration policy field in which many questions arise: which social actors 'make' global policy? What kinds of ideas underpin the policy options and solutions they propose? How do they influence it – through what mechanisms, and with what kinds of resources? How are their ideas and strategies shaped by the institutional contexts in which they work? Why do global policies arise and change over time in given areas, and in response to what combination of circumstances? How is it that some policy approaches and options become dominant and prevail and others don't? These are all questions that are the stock of social policy analysis in general, but our study is particularly informed by key tenets of historical institutionalism (HI) and historical materialism (HM). Both theoretical traditions encompass multiple approaches and inflections within them. Below we identify those we find especially relevant in this context.

The influence of historical institutionalism is seen in our focus on macro contexts of governance and our concrete approach to the combined effects of institutions and processes shaping the global policy field in defined contexts, in different configurations and under historical circumstances that change over time

(Skocpol and Pierson 2002; Mahoney and Rueschemeyer 2003; Rueschemeyer and Stephens 1997; Pierson 2000). With much of the health worker-migration literature on this focusing on health workforce-management and -planning from the perspective of essential health needs and human resources, and which centres almost exclusively on WHO, we are attuned to *multiplicities* – of relevant sectors, policy domains, social actors, social and institutional contexts and processes, ideas and initiatives. In this, we focus not on a single institutional regime (e.g. health) or organisational site (e.g. WHO) of contestation, but on how *sets* of organisations and institutions evolve and interact with each other to shape the definition of global policy. We highlighted earlier in this section that we identified seven principal institutional regimes and a score of principal IOs which form these sets, and this is a tangible example of the kinds of multiplicities we invoke. We employ historical institutionalism's ideas about 'critical junctures' and 'formative episodes' throughout the book, seeking to explain the constraints and opportunities structuring what it is possible to achieve in terms of policy development and reform at particular points in time.

The influence of HI in our study is also seen in our temporal arguments and our approach to history. Solely focusing on the few years leading up to and following the adoption of the WHO Global Code omits the long historical antecedents of that instrument, including the effects of past global policy campaigns in this field that were won or lost, and of political conflicts that were resolved or which remained undecided and therefore contestable. Taking a long-range perspective, spanning 70 years from the mid-1940s to the present day, enables us to look more deeply into the long-term development of the policy field, including how past histories shape contemporary trajectories. In this, we take history seriously, using it to illustrate prior responses and contexts, show that many of the current concerns about the global dynamics of health worker-migration governance and global responses to it are institutionally embedded, and analyse socio-institutional processes unfolding over a substantial stretch of time.

Our study sits within a theoretical tradition that is also broadly inspired by historical materialism (HM) that in its 'transnational form' is concerned with the global modes and dynamics of economic production and social reproduction (see Section 3.2). Thus, we are not only concerned with the combined effects of institutions' interactions and configurations of organisations, actors and ideas, but also with their interplay with material contexts in which they operate and their material capabilities for promoting progressive social development. In this, our study is rooted in a broadly global materialist analytics of global governance that makes visible the array of social forces grounded in capitalist social structures (in all their profound political and economic diversity worldwide) that are globalis*ing* (and thus contested and incomplete) (Yeates 2001, 2009b, 2014b). We emphasise the plurality of historical circumstance*s* and contexts shaping global policy, notably the materialities of social organisation and development resources that, for all the alleged unifying effects of 'globalisation' remain variegated and highly uneven across different zones and territories of the world (Abu Sharkh and Gough 2010; Yeates 2018a). We do not offer a unified theory of global governance and its relationship to globalisation processes or to the many different 'worlds' of capitalism that exist, but our study is generally informed by theoretical propositions about the nature of global governance (as seen through the arena of interstate forums of cooperation in the making of global policy) that are anchored in broader environments of capitalist development and historical processes unfolding over time. This materialist analytics sustains focus on the structural embeddedness of global governance and policy formation in the globalising health services economies. It also opens a vista onto ways of understanding that the multilateralisation of governance and policy that we document in this book has taken place alongside the multilateralisation of health worker-migration itself. Our focus is on the former of these, but return to discuss this relationship in the concluding chapter.

An important feature of our materialist analytics of global governance and policy is the corresponding labourist perspective. We emphasise that labour is a major historic actor in the globalising dynamics of health economies. Cognisance of how labour generally and health workers particularly are selectively incorporated into global labour forces helps retain a sense of place – it matters immensely where in the world you 'become' a health care worker just as it matters from where and to where you emigrate. It also focuses attention on the structural forces and drivers underpinning that migration (including international recruitment strategies enabled or undertaken by states) and reminds us that labour is not unified or 'free floating' (dis-emplaced) but embedded in socio-institutional contexts that vary across time and place. This emphasis on simultaneous embeddedness and structural differentiation of labour (Hardy *et al.* 2016) is applicable to the health workforce as it is to labour more generally (see also Yeates' review of intersectionality in nursing workforces (Yeates 2012)).

It is also applicable, we contend, to theoretical analytics of global governance. Assigning significant weight to the agency of workers and their trade unions as historic social actors, we aim to rescue the social conditions of work and the agency power of labour from being marginalised in explanations of global policy and governance. In this, we reject the relegation of labour to the status of passive victims of ineluctable globalising forces otherwise steered principally by states and capital, instead highlighting labour as a principal driver of global policy. In so doing, we build on myriad studies demonstrating persuasively that labour's participation in globalising processes has been vibrant and robust, and that it has shaped the nature, pace, timing and effects of socio-economic restructuring across a broad range of sectors (Munck 2002; Munck and Waterman 1999; Sigler 2010; O'Brien 2000; Yeates 2008, 2009b) – including in relation to health care. Our study extends these insights to a domain of global governance that has not previously been considered by global labour studies, global health policy or global social policy. Thus, we examine how global labour struggles are played out in global governance, showing that (health) labour plays a strategically significant, formative role in several global institutional regimes (e.g. decent pay and general working conditions, including freedom of association and social dialogue, social protection, access to health care provision, amongst others).

We foreground the role of labour and other civil society associations more widely as major social forces and strategic actors in global governance, advocacy and policy making on international health worker-migration. For example, just as many national unions are affiliated to global union federations, so specialised branches of global unions have emerged. The global union federation for public services, Public Services International (PSI), has been active in health workforce issues and health worker-migration, pressing for rights-based approaches to migration, ethical recruitment, and decent work and social protection for migrant health and social care workers. Trade unions were also members and partners of the Global Health Workforce Alliance, a multi-sectoral association that was integral to realising the WHO Global Code and which became the Global Health Workforce Network of WHO in 2016. Indeed, labour has continually (re)shaped the normative and legal foundations of global health worker-migration policy since its outset, principally through ILO and the UN system in general and latterly through WHO. Rejecting framings of health workforces as 'human resources' to be managed, we show the extent to which labour advocacy movements are major transnational policy actors in this global field, pressing for more robust labour standards, advancing fundamental rights at work within global health policy, defending quality public services, promoting equality-based social protection, advocating universal health care in the collective interest, and monitoring country compliance with global health worker-migration and -recruitment policy.

## 4 Method and evidence

Our study undertakes an in-depth exploration of the initiatives of multiple multilateral organisations over an extended period of time spanning seven decades since the foundation of the UN system in the mid-1940s. As such, a comparative dimension is structured into the study, as we track the key developments over time and among different IOs. We elaborate on our periodisation of time in Section 6 of this chapter. For now, we focus on methods and evidence underpinning the study.

We bring substantial original evidence and analysis based on primary research and secondary analysis of diverse sources of international data. Our analysis of the development of the global policy field of health worker-migration governance traced over six chapters (2 to 7) is based on original archival research going back to 1946 and stretching forward to the present day. We undertook a systematic search for UN official documentation pertaining to its initiatives on cross-border health worker-migration. We used extensively the UN libraries system for this, notably the Dag Hammarskjöld Library, the Library of the UN Office in Geneva (UNOG), the United Nations Information Service (UNIS) Library, the ILO Library (including its online database, Labordoc), and the WHO Library and Information Services (WHOLIS) and its Institutional Repository for Information Sharing (IRIS). We also consulted the e-libraries of the OECD, the World Bank, the IOM and the Global Forum on Migration and Development.

We concentrated on the official documentation emanating from the UN bodies and agencies in New York and Geneva, and did not include UN regional commissions or UN agencies' regional offices in systematic analysis. Nor did we include the regional offices of multilateral organisations such as the World Bank. Our aim is to uncover how the global policy field developed over time and that justifies restricting the scope of our focus to the central UN bodies. It has not been possible to cover variance within these complex UN and other multilateral systems and organisations in terms of (whether and) how their overall commitments are played out in practice on a regional or national scale.

These resources were systematically searched on a year by year basis to track the number and evolution global policy initiatives on or pertaining to international migration and recruitment of health workers. Search terms 'international migration', 'international recruitment', 'health personnel', 'health professionals', 'health workforce', 'shortage', 'brain drain', 'brain circulation', 'health care', and 'health services' were used in combination to sift significant quantities of resolutions, policy initiatives, meeting notes, and studies spanning seven decades. This was a mammoth task. Constructing the UNGA's activity since its earliest days entailed searching about 18,000 documents on the UN database. Ascertaining WHO's history involved systematic searches of seven decades' worth of WHA documentation at two major volumes per year each consisting of 100–300 pages. Similar searches were undertaken for ILO over the decades, and for other international organisations and bodies. In each case, documentation was sifted to check relevance and analysed to identify instances of intervention, connections and thematic threads using manual coding techniques. The results of this research exercise were used to construct a 'timeline' of principal UN activity (decisions, resolutions, recommendations) in relation to international health worker-migration, taken by organs and bodies of the UN and by its specialised agencies. The timelines are set out in Appendices 1–3. The full bibliographic specifics of all the research and reports we consulted that are actively used and cited in the text are listed in the References.

In addition to the primary (archival) research, the chapters are underpinned by extensive secondary analysis of international datasets and/or significant re-interpretation of literatures. Notably, Chapter 4 presents original analysis of the passage of the WHO Global Code based on re-interpretation of academic, policy and 'grey' literatures on this topic. Chapters 5 and 6 present our findings from our own analysis of WHO's Independent Stakeholders' Reporting Initiative database. Chapters 4 and 6 do similarly in relation to the self-assessment returns ('National Reporting Instrument' (NRI)) submitted by governments as part of their obligations to report every three years on progress they have made in implementing the WHO Global Code, including arrangements that take account of the needs of developing countries and economies in transition. NRIs were introduced in Second Round reporting (2015–2016) to monitor progress in implementing the WHO Global Code and the most recent data available is from 2015. To date, only WHO staff have undertaken such detailed analysis of the NRIs in the Reporting Rounds. We undertook our own in-depth analysis of the

NRI return for each WHO member state. We scrutinised the returns of all countries reporting over the two rounds.

There are some limitations to the NRI database as not all countries make returns and while there is a standard template that each country needs to complete, it is ultimately the decision of each country to decide what information is to be entered and what is to be excluded from its own return. We do not claim that it is a highly comprehensive global database of international agreements on international health worker-migration. That said, it is the most comprehensive accessible dataset on the various initiatives, including bilateral labour agreements (BLAs), pertaining to health worker-migration. We undertook further quality checks on the data, especially where there seemed to be prima facia inconsistencies in governments' responses as reported in their country's NRI return. The results of this 'data cleaning' exercise are incorporated into the data tables and the chapters.

Chapter 7 draws on a range of contemporary data and policy developments on international health worker-migration inspired in part by the ambitious agenda set out in the 2030 Sustainable Development Agenda, as well as the ever-present yet growing concerns about health worker shortages. We draw on a diverse set of academic, official policy and 'grey' literature sources relating to migration, human rights, economic restructuring, global advocacy and contemporary debates about economic and sustainable development. This also extended to published data from WHO, ILO and OECD, amongst others. The data in Tables 7.1 and 7.2, for example, are re-worked and compiled by us using ILO and OECD data sources.

## 5 Outline and structure of the book

The following six chapters (2 to 7) constitute the empirical 'heart' of the book, in that they present original research evidence and analysis of the global governance, politics and policy on international health worker-migration and -recruitment spanning seven decades. The research materials are broadly organised around key historical episodes. The chapters elaborate three discernible major phases in the overall development of this field over time.

The first phase, from the immediate post-War period of the mid-1940s until the late 1970s, corresponds with Chapters 2 and 3. These chapters examine the longer historical antecedents to the contemporary global policy field that are the subject of Chapter 5 onwards. During this first phase the global policy field was initiated and underwent relatively rapid institutionalisation. It is one in which the UN was an active and dominant global policy actor, enjoying near hegemonic status in this area (as it did across many social policy sectors). Its initiatives elaborated the normative framework underpinning the policy field which was embedded in the post-war global institutional regime and reflected its liberal economic and social values. Many of the initiatives undertaken during the 1960s defined the 'institutional topography' of the policy field and set it on a course that was to endure over the coming decades. Because of the UN's centrality in global governance at this time, Chapters 2 and 3 focus on it, tracing in some detail the processes by which international health worker-migration and -recruitment was taken up as a major global development issue.

Chapter 2 focuses on the growing involvement of an ever-wider range of UN agencies that during the 1950s and 1960s established highly skilled medical migration as a major global policy issue. This arose, we argue, from growing attention to the international migration of highly skilled labour more generally ('brain drain') as well as to the expansion of health, social protection, education, training and employment provision more generally. UNESCO, ILO and the United Nations Conference on Trade and Development (UNCTAD) were the principal actors at this time, supported by the United Nations Secretary General (UNSG). They defined the terrain, identifying with a high degree of clarity the *global* policy issues at stake, the foundational principles of the global policy field, and an array of well worked-up global policy options. We trace the intellectual and political lineages of, and linkages between, UNESCO, ILO, UNCTAD, and locate the roots of global policy radicalism in this field to this time and the efforts of these agencies to strengthen arguments for radical approaches to highly skilled migration and recruitment founded on redistribution and regulation.

Chapter 3 spotlights the role of WHO and ILO during this first phase in their focus on health worker-migration and -recruitment. In particular, it focuses on the mid-1970s when a series of initiatives by them culminated in the first ever global policy instrument to regulate international migration and recruitment of highly skilled health workers – the ILO Nursing Personnel Recommendation (ILO 1977c). Although this was 'only' a Recommendation and had no legal force, it was nevertheless a landmark in global policy as it formally elaborated global policy principles and guidance spelling out the conditions under which countries should *not* recruit nurses from each other. We consider the institutional, political and social forces that gave rise to the ILO instrument at this point in time. We argue that although ILO and WHO were in different ways both instrumental to this multilateral agreement, the Recommendation's migration and recruitment provisions bear the hallmark of the foundational principles and ideas elaborated within the UN but *outside* of WHO, whose 'position' on the regulation of nurse migration and recruitment was weakly imprinted. At the same time, the Recommendation was not without its limitations, and we pinpoint ILO's institutional failure to monitor its implementation as a major problem in that it contributed to the closure of policy space precisely at a time when it should have done the opposite.

The second phase in the history of global policy making in this field is taken up by Chapters 4 and 5 which discuss how 'ethical recruitment' became the dominant approach in global health worker-migration policy during the opening decade of the 21st century. The chapters trace the rise of ethical recruitment initiatives in this context and their multilateralisation over the course of the decade when they culminated in a second multilateral agreement – the WHO Global Code of Practice on the International Recruitment of Health Personnel (WHO 2010a). We assess the efficacy of these initiatives in terms of whether they embody policy approaches and mechanisms capable of instituting a more robust form of regulatory control on international recruitment and migration in the interests of health and social protection more widely. Global policy had needed to address considerable challenges: not only had the scale of health worker-recruitment and -migration grown to levels way in excess of those evident during the 1960s and 1970s, but the UN was partially marginalised within the neo-liberalising global political economy of global policy making. Indeed, it became just one among many global agencies whose policy approaches vied with the UN normative framework. At the same time, the 'new' (neo-liberal) economic and political priorities constituted a 'hostile' environment for those seeking to strengthen and expand global regulation of the thriving global health care economy. Not only were the social and economic scars from two decades of global neo-liberal restructuring evident but there was a retreat from most forms of binding regulation for all social sectors, except for international trade where international law was strengthening corporate rights to access overseas markets. Feeding into this was evidence of the serious depletion of developing countries' economic resources, and the often-fatal effects of the mal-distribution of health workers worldwide especially in the poorest countries.

Chapter 4 sets out how the large-scale political, ideological and institutional shifts across trade, health, labour and migration during the 1980s and 1990s gave rise to voluntary 'ethical' recruitment initiatives during the first decade of the 21st century. It traces how such initiatives proliferated and multilateralised over the course of the 2000s, culminating in the WHO Global Code. The chapter discusses the diverse actors, ideas, and drivers of the Global Code, from its initial proposal through negotiations to the final agreement. We show the range and nature of alliances of non-state advocacy actors working on concert with developing and (some) developed country governments. We argue that WHO had a keen interest in a successful outcome to demonstrate its relevance as a prime global health actor addressing matters of global health through global policy even though considerable institutional and political constraints limited what it could (and did) achieve.

Chapter 5 discusses the efficacy of the WHO Global Code through the lens of its implementation. Implementation failures undermined the ILO Nursing Personnel Recommendation so it is important to know whether this second landmark agreement has fared any better in that respect. We review multiple sources of evidence pertaining to the track record of the Global Code's efficacy in this respect, and show that its achievements to date are tempered by significant weaknesses. We argue that many of these problems derive from the design of the Code itself. We identify the restricted scope and inaccessibility of the implementation mechanism as key issues, alongside a lack of resources to support countries' take-up of the Code's provisions. Part of our critique of the WHO Global Code centres on the restriction to governments as its only 'legal' subjects. This, we argue, is a major issue given the significance of private (commercial) sector organisations in the dynamics of international health worker-recruitment. We feature original analysis and discussion of the issues pertaining to the private commercial sector in health workforce-migration and consider their implications for the Global Code. Doing so extends the scope of our 'investigative gaze' beyond the condition of national states to also encompass a consideration of the extent to which private commercial sector actors are – and should be – the direct subjects of global regulation in this area. In this context, we consider whether global provisions and initiatives calling for the regulation of private enterprises – through binding business and human rights initiatives – that were developed outside of the WHO Global Code could provide a basis, or source of inspiration, for future global policy development in relation to health worker-recruitment.

Chapter 6 discusses how inter-governmental bilateral agreements have become increasingly significant in the global governance of health worker-migration over the past two decades. We argue that IOs have been a propelling force behind the expansion of bilateral modes of cross-border governance, ranging from bilateral trade and labour agreements to diaspora and knowledge exchange programmes. Drawing on examples from across the world and presenting original analysis of the content and effectiveness of key agreements, we discuss the extent to which they promote ethical recruitment and reciprocal arrangements, particularly in mitigating some of the harmful effects of outward migration on developing countries. We argue that bilateral agreements are increasingly significant as means of promoting circular and temporary migration and we consider the implications of this for rights-based approaches to migration. We conclude that extant bilateral agreements principally benefit advanced industrialised recruiting countries to the detriment of developing source countries, and that such agreements are, in their present form, generally unhelpful as means of achieving global universal health coverage and decent work.

Chapter 7 turns to the third and latest phase in the history of this global policy field. This phase started in the middle of the second decade (*c.*2015–2016) with the global agreement for the 2030 Sustainable Development Agenda and is still unfolding. We trace the global political and policy dynamics that 'mainstreamed' health workforce and migration issues in global policy and the challenges inherent in that, as well as the intersections between these debates and those concerning the role of migration for development and shared global responsibility for tackling poverty and under-development. We particularly consider the extent to which there can now be said to be an integrated, coherent global policy on international health worker-migration and -recruitment and identify greater multi-stakeholderism and the increasing engagement of organisations outside of the UN normative system as major challenges. We consider how the enhanced role of the private sector in global health may impact on the realisation of global goals on health worker-migration and UHC.

The final chapter (Chapter 8) concludes the book. It draws together the arguments and evidence presented throughout the book and highlights the insights that our study brings to knowledge and understanding of the global governance, politics and policy dynamics of international health worker-migration and -recruitment. We reflect upon the book's contributions to academic research literatures on health and welfare as well as its insights for global social policy as a political practice of policy-making. The chapter discusses emerging global policy issues and questions arising from this study for strategies to realise socially-equitable and inclusive health care during the third decade of the 21st century.

## 6 A note on terminology and values

There is various terminology on the international migration of health workers. For the purposes of this book we refer to 'source countries' (encompassing 'countries of origin' and 'sending countries'); 'countries of destination' (covering 'recruiting countries' and 'countries of employment' of migrant health workers), and 'health workers' (to encapsulate the varying terms 'health professionals', 'highly skilled health workers', 'human resources for health' and 'health personnel'). The types of migration and recruitment we refer to in future chapters are exclusively those which take place on an international (cross-border) basis, unless we specify otherwise. We refer to health worker-migration and -recruitment in relation to the global policy field as this encapsulates its content, and we spell this out in full each time to spare ourselves and readers a further acronym. It is also worth clarifying that we use the term 'international organisation' as an umbrella term to encompass international governmental organisations (IGOs) (e.g. ILO, WB) and international non-governmental organisations (INGOs) (e.g. GHWA) where relevant. However, we use IGO or INGO where we specifically refer to one rather than the other.

Our normative standpoint is that the right to health requires comprehensive, well-resourced and socially-inclusive health and welfare systems that are underpinned by egalitarian and cohesive social structures. From the vantage point of this study, this translates into a global governance and policy agenda rooted in human rights, social justice and supportive of promoting even economic and social development within and between countries. Working towards the development of a coherent vision for a reformed framework for global health worker-migration governance needs to be based on these principles.

Finally, it is perhaps also a reflection of the contemporary politics of international migration that we feel it necessary to reiterate our strong support for core UN principles which hold that voluntary migration is a fundamental human right which is universal and indivisible and that international migration should be governed on the basis of equality of treatment, non-discrimination, fundamental rights at work and respect for human rights at all stages of the migration process.

## Notes

1 See Section 6 for clarification about how we use this term.
2 Health workforce migration straddles the health and migration goals. SDG Goal 3 aims to '[s]ubstantially increase health financing and *the recruitment, development, training and retention of the health workforce* in developing countries, especially in least developed countries and small island developing States' (authors' emphasis). SDG

Goal 10 aims to '[f]acilitate orderly, safe, regular and responsible migration and mobility of people, including through the implementation of planned and well-managed migration policies'. See Appendix 4.

3 As well as being a global goal in its own right, health workforces underpin many of the other goals in health that aim to reduce preventable causes of mortality and morbidity, end epidemics of key communicable diseases, and achieve universal health coverage and universal access to health care services. They also underpin goals outside of the health sector, notably those relating to poverty, gender equality, sanitation, access to safe drinking water, nutrition, sexual and reproductive health, and reproductive rights (Appendix 4). We discuss this further in Chapter 7.

4 See Yeates 2018a for this idea of 'co-production' and Orenstein (2008) for 'co-determination'. We started this analysis in Yeates and Pillinger (2018) in relation to governance of health worker-migration in Asia Pacific in which we argued that it may be less useful to think of global, regional and bilateral forms of international policy as existing at different 'levels' since these different modes of governance 'are co-present and co-operate within the same policy "space"' (Yeates and Pillinger 2018: 102).

5 However, we do not assume that IOs sit at the apex of an institutional or normative hierarchy of levels, or that they are necessarily more powerful than states.

# 2 Initiating the global policy field

## The role of the UN

## 1 Introduction

This is the first of two chapters that examine the long historical antecedents to the contemporary global policy field of health worker-migration and -recruitment. This chapter, together with Chapter 3, focuses on the rise and early development of these issues as a key agenda within the UN system and the ascendance of the UN-led global policy field of health worker-migration and -recruitment. The chapters trace the development of myriad global initiatives back to the earliest days of the UN system, examining four decades of such initiatives from the 1940s to the early 1980s. Across these two chapters we chart the growing involvement of multiple UN agencies in the early definition of the global policy field and the issues to which they responded through their programmes of action. We attend to the institutional and geo-political dynamics that at once enabled and constrained the scope for global regulation, the multiple actors involved (and the nature of cooperation and contestation among them), and the key ideas and discourses that framed and shaped their responses. The chapter's long historical perspective sets the scene for subsequent chapters' focus on the twenty-first century.

The present chapter focuses on the 1960s and 1970s. It traces a series of key developments arising from the activism of a widening range of UN agencies that cumulatively established health worker-migration as a global policy issue in the context of the international recruitment and migration of highly skilled labour more generally ('brain drain'). UNESCO, ILO and UNCTAD spearheaded this campaign, defining the global policy issues at stake and elaborating the foundational principles of the global policy field. Chapter 3 continues this analysis with a specific focus on how WHO and ILO galvanised global action on health worker-recruitment and -migration, leading to the elaboration of specific global 'rules' through the first-ever global instrument in this field.

Through detailed analysis of the origins of this global policy field based on primary archival research, these two chapters jointly provide an expansive historical perspective. First, we show that the origins of this policy field reside firmly in the UN system, which implanted global liberal principles deep into it. As we show later, these principles have endured, even if the structural organisational features of the field are now very different. From a contemporary vantage point, reminded of the marginalisation of the UN over three decades of neo-liberal globalisation, the evidence we bring to bear is a useful reminder of the UN's historic boldness of vision and its global leadership. Second, this historical research fundamentally challenges narratives of global policy in this field that start with the WHO 2010 Global Code of Practice on the International Recruitment of Health Personnel (WHO 2010a) and which gravitate around WHO as the only international organisation in this field. We show that the originating forces in this field by no means started with WHO. Rather, the principal protagonists were UNESCO, ILO and UNCTAD. WHO was, at best, a late-arriving UN agency, and one amongst many. Third, the global policy field was characterised from the outset not only by the involvement of many UN specialised agencies, but also by multiple global initiatives that reflected a clear understanding of the significance of highly skilled labour migration and recruitment for countries' capacities (and capabilities) for social and economic development.

This chapter shows that the issues that the scale and dynamics of health worker-migration raised for countries' economic and social development strategies were being regularly monitored by the UN from its earliest days. It was from 1960, during the first UN development decade, that the global policy field had 'life' breathed into it thanks to the initiatives of the UN General Assembly (UNGA) and the United Nations Economic and Social Council (ECOSOC). These first *global* policy responses centred on the 'brain drain' and thus incorporated highly skilled health workers under a broader rubric also covering other highly skilled workers such as scientists. UNGA and ECOSOC were not only principal UN forums, but principal protagonists. The numerous scientific studies and technical assistance measures they initiated under this rubric scoped the significance of the problem in terms of its characteristics, scale and dynamics, and defined it as a major issue for economic and social development to be addressed as a priority by the UN system as a whole as well as by individual governments. These early initiatives paved the way for a more systematic focus on highly skilled health workers.

This chapter therefore charts the very beginnings of the definition of health worker-migration and -recruitment as a global issue and as a matter for global governance, regulation and policy. It attends to the factors that gave rise to UNGA's first resolution on this matter in 1960 and the initial (though fragmented) responses this gave rise to. It traces the expansion of UN actions from the 1960s onwards, including the formative roles of UNESCO and UNCTAD. UNESCO was instrumental at this time in framing highly skilled international migration as a key international development issue and proposing global policy and regulation based on the principles of redistribution. UNCTAD was similarly instrumental in its linking of such migration to a trade agenda through its innovative redefinition of the 'brain drain' as the 'reverse transfer of technology'. It also led efforts to negotiate a multilateral agreement that would halt and even reverse labour resource transfers involved in migration and recruitment dynamics. Our interest in this negotiating process is the ideational content of the policy proposals that were elaborated at this time rather than the institutional passage of the (ultimately doomed) UNCTAD Global Code of Conduct.

## 2 Activating ILO and WHO mandates

Amongst the early priorities of the establishment of ILO (1946) and WHO (1948) as formal international organisations were matters that brought them into contact with international migration issues. Since the proclamation of the UN Universal Declaration on Human Rights in December 1948, which established the right of the individual to migrate (i.e. to leave any country, including their own and to return to their own country) (Article 13), ILO, for its part, established a body of norms from 1948 and through the 1950s regarding principles governing labour migration and the rights of migrant workers. The Migration for Employment Convention (Revised) (C97) and Recommendation (R86) (1949), the Social Security (Minimum Standards) Convention (1952) and the Discrimination (Employment and Occupation) Convention (C111) and Recommendation (R111) (1958) were all instrumental to standard-setting in areas impacting on migrant workers – including health workers. These regulatory instruments address matters such as regulating the recruitment, introduction and placing of migrant workers, providing accurate information relating to migration, stipulating minimum conditions during transit and arrival, the adoption of an active employment and social security policy, and international collaboration in all of these matters (see Appendix 3). ILO Convention No. 97 (1949) refers to the importance of bilateral agreements and provides a model agreement to regulate matters of common concern. ILO's advice to countries seeking to enter into bilateral agreements is based on this framework. The early adoption of Convention No. 97 proved significant when, from the 1960s, the UN began to recommend forms of international cooperation based on bilateral agreements (Chapter 6).

Collectively, these post-war instruments built on ILO's considerable pre-UN track record in setting international labour standards. Its expansion into labour migration under the auspices of the UN reflected its institutional mandate to protect 'the interests of workers when employed in countries other than their own' (Preamble, ILO Constitution 1944). This expansion legitimised ILO as a major UN actor in global migration policy, a development which proved critical in ensuing decades. Underpinning its migration mandate was an agenda concerned with promoting labour standards founded on non-discrimination (including on the basis of national origin) and human rights. ILO Conventions thus elaborate fundamental human rights to a high standard of employment for all workers, social protection, safe and healthy working conditions, non-discrimination, earnings, freedom of association and collective bargaining (Article III, Declaration of Philadelphia (ILO 1944)). ILO's tripartite governance structure (governments, employers, workers) and its institutional provisions for monitoring the implementation of its instruments have similarly proved important for propelling its mandate to codify global standards.

By contrast, WHO is governed by member states through health ministries.[1] This structure means that member governments alone have 'proposal rights'. It imposes no constitutional duty, mandate or mechanism for incorporating non-state actors in its policy-formation process.[2] Neither does its institutional design include means of monitoring the implementation of its instruments: implementation mechanisms are written into agreements on a case-by-case basis. The contrasting governance mechanisms of ILO and WHO differentially structure the participation of different actors (state, business and labour in ILO, states in WHO), producing quite different institutional dynamics. Sometimes dismissed as a consultative forum without 'bite', we argue that WHO's annual World Health Assemblies (WHAs) have nevertheless proved an important means by which developing country governments in particular have been able to raise issues of concern. They have used the WHAs to maintain a focus on health services resourcing, including the issue of staff shortages linked to international migration (Chapters 3 and 5).

Unlike ILO, WHO has no institutional mandate on migration. Nevertheless, it has routine encounters with health worker-migration by virtue of being tasked 'to promote improved standards of teaching and training in the health, medical and related professions' (Article 2) as part of its overarching objective for 'all peoples [to attain] the highest possible level of health' (Article 1). This objective is guided by the principle that '[u]nequal development in different countries in the promotion of health and control of disease, especially communicable disease, is a common danger' (WHO 1946). This, combined with the technical support it provided for member countries to fulfil their 'responsibility for the health of their peoples and the provision of adequate health and social measures' remains a key route through which (in)adequate staffing in health services and the consequences of emigration were brought onto WHO's agenda.

WHO's mandate in relation to training of health professionals was the principal route through which it addressed the issue of sufficiency of institutional infrastructure and programmes to train health professionals in adequate numbers. Its first priority was the education and training of physicians (its attention to nurses and midwives started much later (Chapters 3 and 5)) and this was reflected in WHO's work programme (WHO 1958). This work brought it into direct contact with severe staff shortages across the health sector, including shortages of teachers, and how this was entangled with international migration dynamics. These were all subjects on which it began to accumulate knowledge during the 1950s in particular.[3]

Much of this early knowledge came from WHO's Fellowships scheme. Fellowships made direct financial provision to students and teachers to obtain advanced training in medical specialities by studying abroad.[4] Fellowships awarded each year were eventually numbered in thousands, and recruitment was extraordinarily international. By 1966 fellows came from 159 countries and territories, and studied in 93 others (WHO 1968). In the Americas and Europe most recruitment was intra-regional, whereas for the four other WHO regions the reverse was true (WHO 1968). Although the numbers involved were modest in the context of domestic workforces, so extensive was the Fellowships scheme that it helped build capacity in health and medical workforces, particularly of developing countries.[5]

The Fellowships scheme brought WHO into direct encounters with the socially-structured nature of health worker-migration and -recruitment and its impacts upon developing countries' abilities to develop and retain health workforces. It commented that 'Europe has vast potential means to assist other areas [of the world]' and that although '[m]uch of this potential is being used' only a small 'fraction of it is channelled through the [WHO]' (WHO 1968: 25). Its understanding of these global dynamics is clarified by these statements:

> The medical schools and institutions of Europe are thronged with overseas students for advanced or basic studies. The [WHO] has provided considerable numbers of fellowships for post-graduate studies and some for undergraduate students from newly independent countries which do not yet have a medical school; the latter face the problem of adaptation to the needs and conditions in their own countries.... Approximately one half of all WHO fellows from all parts of the world study in the European Region during some of the period covered by their fellowships.
>
> (WHO 1968: 25–26)

> On the whole, WHO fellows, on conclusion of their studies, are assigned to work corresponding to their training abroad. There are some failures due to difficulties met by fellows on returning home when there has been insufficient planning of the fellowships programme or under-development of the health services; also, some countries have difficulty in selecting candidates really qualified to undertake the proposed studies.
>
> (WHO 1968: 88)

These statements capture the circumstances under which medical education and training were provided, and the drivers of international physician migration. First, they indicate the degree to which medical training and education was conditioned by uneven development in the colonial and post-colonial periods. Provision was highly internationalised as well as being overwhelmingly concentrated in Europe and North America and coincided with lack of medical education and training infrastructures in other regions. Second, they highlight that medical education curricula and training programmes were oriented to the needs of the (mostly advanced industrialised) providing countries, focusing mainly on western diseases and approaches to medicine rather than those of developing countries. This raised important questions about the suitability of the education and training that students from developing countries were receiving, given that they were expected to return to the source country after their studies to practice their profession. Third, the statements highlight some of the barriers faced by the fellows upon returning to the source country. Adaptation costs were compounded by a lack of provision to re-integrate them. WHO addressed these issues more fully during the First UN Development Decade in the 1960s, which saw the UN focus on the relationship between the development of skilled workforces, labour conditions, international migration and wider economic development.

## 3  Early UN action on the migration of highly skilled labour

### 3.1  UNGA and ECOSOC lead the call to action

The start of the UN First Development Decade witnessed major initiatives by UNGA and ECOSOC to establish sufficient numbers of 'highly trained personnel' as a UN priority area.[6] These emphasised the importance of ensuring adequate training of national technical personnel as an integral element of economic development strategies and urged that this be given greater priority by the UN system and member countries. The interventions of UNGA and ECOSOC initiated the beginnings of the first wave of the global policy field of health worker-migration and -recruitment. This was a period of intense attention to the issue of needing sufficient numbers of technical personnel necessary to expand public (including health) services and accelerate industrialisation. This period witnessed multiple UN specialised agencies and committees being drawn in, and substantial programmes of research. UNGA and ECOSOC thus set in train an expansionist trajectory that conditioned the pace, scale and nature of UN activity beyond the remainder of the decade in relation to highly skilled workers in general. This was instrumental in realising a dedicated focus on highly skilled health workers in the late 1960s.

Over the ensuing five years UNGA and ECOSOC successfully built up momentum, passing (often multiple) Resolutions almost annually on national technical personnel shortages. The Resolutions they passed, and the conclusions of reports they commissioned, highlighted needs: for systematic assessments of human resources as part of a wider strategy of planning for social and economic development[7]; for the UN to expand its scale and scope of international action; and for developing countries to build capacity to make provision to train their own sufficient personnel.[8] These initiatives identified the development of education and training infrastructures, especially in developing countries, as a key response to the problem of the shortages of technical (intermediate and higher) personnel they faced.

WHO was the first UN agency to respond. In 1961 WHA passed its first resolution on this matter. This linked the problem of known workforce shortages to the imperative of developing national health services in the context of decolonisation and the development of newly-independent nations more generally. It mandated WHO to address health and medical labour shortages:

> [t]he WHO has an important part to play in promoting the fundamental and inalienable right of colonial countries and peoples to freedom and independence through assistance in raising levels of physical and mental health … one of WHO's urgent tasks is to help newly independent countries, and

those preparing for independence, to overcome deficiencies in health programmes and serious shortages in trained medical and health personnel.

(WHA 1961, 24 February)

WHO's Resolution was quickly followed by the adoption of a number of ILO standard-setting instruments, including ILO Recommendation on vocational training (R117) (1962), a follow-up Programme of Human Resources (1963) on the planning, organisation and methods of training, and Conventions concerning the objectives and general principles of social policy (C117) (1962) and the application of equal treatment in relation to Social Security (C118) (1962). The 1962 Social Security Convention was instrumental in instituting a global 'equality regime' governing the treatment of labour: it prohibited discrimination on the basis of national origin (amongst other social characteristics). In 1964, the ILO Employment Policy Convention (C122) and Recommendation (R122) further built on this equality regime (UNSG 1964, and Appendix 3). UNESCO similarly took decisive action to establish its authority in matters of technical education, passing a UNESCO Recommendation concerning technical education in 1962[9] and initiating a programme of research and a series of 'policy dialogues'. By 1967 it had commissioned seven research studies and organised five major conferences (and published reports from them), one of which was in conjunction with UN Economic Commission for Latin America (UNESCO 1968a). Resolutions on vocational training were rolled out regionally following initiatives from ILO and UNESCO and helped to spur momentum.[10]

Further support for UNGA's and ECOSOC's calls to action came from the UN's Advisory Committee on the Application of Science and Technology to Development.[11] A UNSG report bolstered arguments to strengthen developing countries' capacities to train their own personnel which, it was held, would mitigate permanent emigration from developing countries to developed ones for such training (UNSG 1964).[12] Many of the report's conclusions regarding shortages of skilled workers, lack of training capacity, the role of developed countries in training developing country personnel, and the provision of training education programmes in developing countries based on industrialised countries' requirements, were directly applicable to the health sector. These were all issues that WHO and other UN bodies were starting to engage with.

From the perspective of our study, there are three notable aspects about the UNSG 1964 report. It estimated gaps in global labour needs for highly skilled labour in the industrial sector, pre-dating by decades modelling techniques used by WHO and ILO to quantify global health workforce needs (Chapters 5 and 7).[13] It recommended that 'occupational health and measures for providing effective assistance in medical education and training to meet priority needs of developing countries' (UNSG 1964: 117) be included in future research programmes – thereby establishing the availability of sufficient highly skilled health workers as an issue of industrialisation on the UN agenda. And it recommended the further expansion of UN work to establish international standards on training (UNSG 1964: 118).[14]

By the mid-1960s the question of highly skilled labour shortages as a factor impeding economic development was firmly established as one on which the UN had an authority, and was subsequently taken up by several UN bodies and agencies. Still, further action was required. Specialised UN agencies were requested to intensify and expand their programmes on human resources development.[15] The 1965 UNGA placed this matter on ECOSOC's agenda as a discussion item, with input from ILO, UNESCO, the Food and Agriculture Organization of the United Nations (FAO), the United Nations Institute for Training and Research (UNITAR), and WHO.[16] This was the first time WHO had been explicitly identified as a relevant agency in this area, and it reflected growing evidence that medical personnel constituted a major occupational group within the overall category of national technical personnel. Further impetus to the expansion of the UN's role in this field arose from a mid-term review of the First UN Development Decade which highlighted that 'the gap between the standards of living in the developed and developing countries has widened instead of narrowing' (UNGA Resolution 2084 (XX) 1965). Further, although developing countries had made progress in establishing national development plans with targets in social and economic fields 'this action [had] not yet been accompanied to an adequate extent by action at the international level'.

### 3.2 Towards a global 'brain drain' policy: the role of UNESCO and UNSG

The UN's actions regarding highly skilled labour shortages (including in the medical and health sector) took greater shape from this point. The 1960s' expansionist agenda set by UNGA and ECOSOC continued to be pressed forcefully and the work programmes of UN agencies were intensified, including in two landmark developments in the human rights regime. Article 12 of the 1966 International Covenant on Civil and Political Rights reaffirmed the right to migrate and to choose a place of residence as a foundational universal civil and political right. The International Covenant on Economic, Social and Cultural Rights recognised the right of all peoples to self-determination and the pursuit of their economic, social and cultural goals, including the right to health and to just and favourable working conditions. These treaties copper-fastened the work initiated during the first half of the 1960s and supported the programmes to gather pace, to such an extent that by the 1970s the UN had expanded its initial concern with 'shortages' of highly skilled personnel to identify 'outflows' of highly skilled personnel from developing countries as a major issue for the developing countries aiming to undertake 'accelerated industrialisation', and for global economic and social development more broadly.

UNESCO was the first UN agency to substantively respond to the 'anxiety' of governments that 'while developing countries badly needed qualified human resources for their development, significant numbers of their most dynamic and trained personnel were migrating to industrialised countries' (d'Oliveira e Sousa 1989: 200). Its 1966 Resolution on the Economic, Social and Cultural Problems of Newly-Independent Countries set out its intention to participate in the planning and organisation of scientific activities relating to the 'human factor' in the development of these countries, paying specific attention to the problem of 'brain drain' and urging UNESCO to spearhead a programme of work on it (UNESCO 1966: 211).[17] Of especial note was that recruiting countries should compensate source countries for their losses of highly skilled labour. This proposal built on UNESCO's work on higher education which had suggested 'the possibility of setting up an international compensation fund for the benefit of Member States suffering from the "brain drain"' (UNESCO 1966: 177). This proposal proved influential, if contested, over the longer term (see below and Chapters 3 and 4).

ILO later featured the 'brain drain' in a report on issues concerning professional workers (ILO 1967), while UNGA passed its first 'brain drain' resolution and also published a report (UNSG 1967). Both reports were concerned with international labour supply of highly skilled personnel. ILO gave prominent treatment to medical and health personnel, especially nurses and midwives:

> The medical and paramedical professions have also registered substantial increases in numbers, due in particular to general economic development, the growth of the population, the improved level of medical care and the advances in medicine. Apparently the greatest shortages are of the middle ranks – midwives, nursing staff – though the lack of physicians, dentists, pharmacists and others is also felt in varying degrees of urgency. In Latin America, the scarcity of nursing staff is regarded as the most serious anomaly that exists at the present time. While there are about 30 male or female nurses for every 10,000 inhabitants in North America, there are not even five in Central and less than 2.5 in South America. The shortages registered everywhere in this profession are largely explained by the unsatisfactory pay and working conditions. In the developing countries, the already great need for medical and paramedical workers may be expected to be aggravated as their governments implement birth-control programmes, for new medico-social machinery will have to be set up on a vast scale and a real army of doctors, midwives, educators and even volunteers will have to be recruited.
>
> (ILO 1967: 17–18)[18]

The UNSG report, *Development and Utilisation of Human Resources* (UNSG 1967), was the second such report on the issue.[19] Like its first report (UNSG 1964), this one was also significant because of its highly articulated identification of the 'brain drain', its attention to medical and health labour migration, and its urgent call for a stronger global policy to coordinate and steer actions by national governments. Recognising that '[t]he professions most affected by the "brain drain" appear to be engineering, medicine, nursing and science', it linked the increased visibility of the (medical) brain drain to a growing international focus on development planning, including 'manpower planning':

In recent years the competitive international market for trained talent has grown larger, more fluid and more broadly international than ever before, and has been accompanied by an increasing tendency for the wealthier societies to outbid developing countries for the use of high-quality human capital, wherever it may come from. The widespread tendency for trained and able people to leave rural areas and concentrate in urban centres now seems to be taking an international form, sweeping trained ability from all lower-income areas towards higher-income ones and from them to the highest concentrations known in the present world, notably in the United States, whose large expenditures on scientific research and development are a gigantic world magnet.

(UNSG 1967: 50)

The report reiterated the inextricable connection between transfers of highly skilled personnel and mobility to undertake advanced studies in that the latter result in the delayed or non-return of students to the source country after training. It also drew attention to the policies of destination countries that help recruit and retain students. Thus it highlighted how '[t]he immigration policy of developed countries may also stimulate the flow through the virtual removal of entry restrictions on foreigners with high-level skills.' (UNSG 1967: 54). It also drew attention to the benefits to source countries of such international migration, in that '[i]n the case of some developing countries, the loss from the so-called "brain drain" is to some extent compensated by an inflow of technical skills from abroad'. Otherwise, it clearly affirmed the regressive redistribution inherent in such migration:

[t]o the extent that migration of highly trained personnel enables developed countries to benefit by the investment of developing countries in the training of persons who subsequently emigrate or fail to return, the 'brain drain' is a serious example of the progressive shift of resources from developing to developed countries, and thus runs counter to the purposes of the United Nations Development Decade.

(UNSG 1967: 54)

Supporting this were illustrative examples comparing the scale of outflows of highly skilled personnel to the outputs of medical schools:

between 30 and 50 per cent of the annual output of medical schools emigrates to the United States from Greece, the Philippines, Iran, Turkey, the Republic of Korea and a number of Central American countries.... There are more Iranian medical doctors in New York than in all of Iran.

(UNSG 1967: 54–55)

Of particular interest is the inclusion of data on the net savings on training costs made by developed recruiting countries. For example, the report cites a study[20] estimating that:

85,000 foreign engineers, physicians and scientists settled permanently in the United States from 1949 to 1964: By 1967 the figure will be approximately 100,000, representing a net saving in training of at least $2,000 million, and possibly as much as $4,000 million. The share of these immigrants originating from developing countries has been on the increase in recent years and is now estimated to be nearly one-third of the total.

(UNSG 1967: 54)

Given 'the important implications of the "brain drain" for the resources of highly skilled personnel available to developing countries' the report could not be clearer in its recommendations that UN action should be extended and strengthened (UNSG 1967: 55). Although it ultimately shied away from anything stronger than recommending a series of studies into the problem,[21] it was clear that these were envisaged as a basis for concrete forms of action to be considered at a later date, with the aim of slowing down, if not ending, the 'brain drain'.[22] Emphasising that the outcome of the recommended studies is not a prerequisite for more immediate unilateral action by governments to 'promote better manpower planning' (UNSG 1967: 55), and reiterating that the answer to the 'brain drain' does not lie in restriction of migration but rather in the provision of incentives, adaptation of training content, and improved facilities in source countries, the report nevertheless emphasised that:

> ... the problem is not one for developing countries alone to solve. Developed countries must encourage scientists from the developing countries to return home after their period of training or experience abroad. They should take the responsibility for providing arrangements whereby scientists from developing countries can keep close personal contacts with work in the more advanced laboratories and scientific institutions.... If even a limited remedy is to be found, it may have to lie in new concepts of international discipline on the part of the countries that absorb most of the 'brain drain'.
>
> (UNSG 1967: 56)

ECOSOC took up the cause, urging even 'more vigorous concerted action by the UN, and specialised agencies' (including WHO) to intensify the training of specialised technical workers.[23] A year later, UNSG was again tasked by UNGA to 'formulate suggestions for ways of tackling the problems arising from the outflow of trained personnel at all levels from developing to developed countries'.[24] By now, UNGA was 'noting with concern' 'that highly trained personnel from the developing countries continue to emigrate at an increasing rate to certain developing countries, which in some cases may hinder the process of economic and social development in the developing countries'. It reaffirmed that 'there is a need to take appropriate interim action at both the national and international levels, until these gaps have been bridged, to tackle the problems resulting from the outflow of trained personnel from the developing countries'.[25]

### *3.3  UNESCO's radicalism: gaining ground?*

UNESCO's analytical clarity about the dynamics of the (medical) 'brain drain' and its implications for global policy was far in advance of those of ECOSOC, UNGA or other UN agencies. Its work pre-dated the arrival of WHO into this field by three years. The report on 'the problem of emigration of scientists and technologists' for the Advisory Committee of the Economic and Social Council on the Application of Science and Technology to Development (UNESCO 1968a) provides rich insights into its burgeoning radicalism. Its promulgations were underpinned by analytical connections between the maintenance of global inequality, the provision of international aid, human rights and international migration. It made a highly significant and innovative intervention to elaborate a set of *global* policy proposals aimed at reversing the 'brain drain'. This call for international action marked a step-change in the nature of global policy responses. The introduction of a Director of UNESCO in an address to an international development conference in 1968 was delivered in a new register:

> ... the good that donor nations are doing with one hand is being cancelled by the other, consciously or not ... [and] while millions of dollars and man-hours of aid effort are being devoted to helping developing countries train their specialised manpower and to build their own educational institutions, it would seem to be rather counter-productive to be hiring away some of their best people for use in the donor country.
>
> (UNESCO 1968a: 13)

Quantifying the effects of the 'brain drain' on developing countries as initiated by the UNSG (UNSG 1967), a UNESCO study stated that 'emigration costs annually some $14 million for the Latin American countries alone, calculated as the direct cost of training' (UNESCO 1968a: 17). In a UNSECO report, Richard Titmuss, Professor of Social Policy at the London School of Economics, calculated the value of the 'brain drain' to developed countries and argued that:

> ... during the post-war period the immigration into the United States of 100,000 foreign medical scientists and engineers represented the economic equivalent of a capital import of $4,000 million. It is calculated that the resulting gain to the United States – i.e. the loss sustained by the other countries – represents the output of several large universities.
>
> (UNESCO 1968a: 19)

The report insisted that this was a *global* issue requiring a *global* response from the UN and other international organisations (UNESCO 1968a: 36).[26] A dedicated discussion on international measures points to the scope, as UNESCO saw it, for more robust global policy to this end:

The brain drain is by its very nature an international phenomenon. Hence the search for solutions to the problem cannot be limited to the national measures; 'joint action at the international level must also be planned.

(Ibid.: 37)

If the issue was defined as one of the 'brain drain' helping to maintain international inequality, 'strengthening the dominant position held by certain countries at the expense of others' (UNESCO 1968a: 38), then the consequent question was whether 'the "brain drain" [can] form the subject of international agreements?' (ibid.: 37). UNESCO concluded:

The answer to this question should probably be in the affirmative, though exactly opposite views are found in publications on the 'brain drain'.... It is obvious that the migration of specialists must be regulated.

(Ibid.: 37)

The clarity of this message was unrivalled at the time and it remains the clearest (although not necessarily the most eloquent or elaborate) expression of this position since. The report also elaborated path-breaking principles guiding a prospective global policy capable of not just halting but reversing the 'brain drain'. It considered a range of policy approaches to addressing this global social phenomenon: compensation from the 'winner countries' to the 'loser' countries; improving the organisation and coordination of the training of qualified scientists and technicians for the developing countries; protection of the professional, economic and social rights of qualified personnel as part of measures to stabilise conditions at home for those who would otherwise emigrate; the elaboration of international migration instruments for highly skilled personnel (such as bilateral agreements, measures prohibiting countries from recruiting from others through 'propaganda or measures which might disorient the people involved' (ibid.: 42); general measures to secure reciprocal advantages (e.g. assist developing countries to recruit personnel from developed countries'), and 'the preparation of a special international declaration condemning the "brain drain"' (ibid.: 43). The report dismissed the compensatory approach as impracticable, and found most merit in the international declaration idea which would sensitise and raise awareness among national public opinion of the catastrophic consequences of brain drain and create an atmosphere conducive to a solution to the problem of the freedom of movement of highly skilled personnel, 'in accordance with the Universal Declaration of Human Rights' (ibid.: 43).

Much of the report's vision lay in a range of policy approaches and options it set out. However, it was badged as 'preliminary' and UNESCO declined to make concrete proposals for action even though it expressed impatience with the fact that such measures as would be needed were up to now considered as matters of domestic action and unilateral measures by developing countries. Regrettably, much of this vision dissipated over time and UNESCO backed away from proposals for a strengthened *global* policy as well as from the idea that a just response to the 'brain drain' might be based on financial restitution to source countries. Following the recommendation of UNESCO's Executive Board that its General Conference confine itself to 'study[ing] suggestions which might contribute to lessening the impact of the 'brain drain' on science and technology in developing countries' (UNESCO 1968), a draft resolution was tabled in support of continuing this work – albeit along a different track. This did not meet with universal approval, and some (unnamed) delegates were unhappy that UNESCO should rescind on progressing further work along the lines set out in its report of 1968. One delegate suggested 'a moral charter for the skilled and talented who might migrate temporarily or permanently from their home countries'. Another delegate asserted that nothing new would be learnt from more studies of the 'brain drain' since 'it is an aspect of what occurs when two unequal economic systems meet', and urged more robust policy responses:

> Multilateral and bilateral arrangements which would regulate the flow and return of manpower, contribute towards the cost of training or increase local output of skills in developed countries so that they would no longer attract foreign talent, might be a more rewarding approach [than a moral charter].
>
> (UNESCO 1968b: 234)

Despite attempts to rescue what could be salvaged from the report, the battle was lost. UNESCO Resolution 3.25 mandated the Director-General 'to pursue studies on the economic, social and cultural causes and consequences of the international migration of talent as it affects the educational and scientific development of Member States'. The scope of these studies would focus on 'the problem of brain drain and the associated problem of reincorporation of fellows in their homeland after residence abroad'. They would explore how such reincorporation would be made easier for fellows in accordance with their qualifications and needs of development in their countries.[27]

This was a clear signal that UNESCO, at least, would go no further in pursuing a global policy to regulate (or indeed reverse) the international migration of highly skilled workers. Indeed, despite the consistent exhortations of UNGA, ECOSOC, UNESCO and UNSG throughout the 1960s, the Second UN Development Decade (1970–1979) failed to include any programme of action on migration whatsoever. The matter did not return to the UN development agenda until 1980.

Yet those voices calling for more robust global policy responses to the 'brain drain' would not quite disappear. Spurred by the UN Declaration on Social Progress and Development (UNGA 1969) which identified '[t]he formulation of national and international policies and measures to avoid the "brain drain" and obviate its adverse effects' (Article 21d), UNESCO's General Conference in 1970 passed a Resolution (1.243) calling upon member states to 'take appropriate measures to restrict encouraging of foreign scientists to leave or not to return to their countries'. It also requested that the Director-General report to the next General Conference on 'the answers of some member states concerning the 'anxiety' that brain drain caused them' and on 'the actions taken by other member states on the measures they have taken to prevent this migration'. The Director-General's report was duly considered at the 1972 General Conference which simply reiterated the known problem, albeit 'with concern' (UNESCO 1972). It did not return to the global policy proposals it made in 1966 or 1968, but neither did it waste an opportunity to point the finger at countries whose responsibility it was to institute measures to prevent the loss of skilled workers from developing countries:

> [T]he policy followed by certain industrialized countries of encouraging, through the offer of material and other advantages, scientists, engineers, technicians and other professionals from the developing countries to leave their own countries and not return, constitutes a factor that is detrimental to the efforts – in themselves limited by under-development – made by the countries concerned to ... adopt more effective measures to set up the requisite scientific infrastructure in the developing countries and, moreover, to check the policy of attracting scientists, engineers, technicians and other professionals followed by certain industrialized countries.
>
> (UNESCO 1972: 29–30)

By the following UNESCO conference there had been no follow-up action and the 'brain drain' was subsumed under other matters. A Recommendation on the Status of Scientific Researchers considered a whole range of measures of which international migration was just one element.[28]

## 4 UNCTAD reframes the debate: from 'brain drain' to resource drain

The UNESCO idea of a global policy capable of regulating flows of highly skilled personnel and affording a degree of protection and restitution to source countries might have seemed to be a dying, if not dead, ambition. But UNESCO's ambitions to develop a robust global policy in this area were kept alive by initiatives elsewhere in the UN. The World Population Conference (1974) considered the implications of international migration, particularly of skilled migration from developing to developed countries, for economic development. It endorsed the UN principle of voluntary migration but also warned that '[s]ince the outflow of qualified personnel from developing to developed countries seriously hampers the development of the former, there is an urgent need to formulate national and international policies to avoid the 'brain drain' and to obviate its adverse effects' (d'Oliveira e Sousa, 1989: 201). Many of the radical policy ideas developed under the auspices of UNESCO were taken up elsewhere in the UN (e.g. UNSG, UNCTAD, ILO). UNCTAD pushed in the direction of a global policy instrument in the form of a Code of Conduct on the Transfer of Technology. Although the proposed Code was not successfully concluded, protracted negotiations spanned more than a decade to the late 1980s, and kept the issue of outflows of highly skilled personnel prominent on the UN agenda. In this respect, it sustained the overall impetus around the need for global action to address such outflows, providing an enabling environment in which a focus on global migration governance and the migration of highly skilled workers could be sharpened.

Our discussion of these developments in the next section is less concerned with the institutional passage of the ill-fated Code of Conduct on the Transfer of Technology than with the ideas and policy approaches that it embodied and the accompanying programme of work underpinning their elaboration. The ideas circulated at that time broadened the range of global policy approaches beyond technical assistance, and helped shift attention away from unilateral approaches and emphases on developing countries' responsibilities – outside WHO, at least (Chapter 3). They continue to resonate in global policy research and initiatives on ethical recruitment (Chapters 4, 5 and 7). The negotiations also illuminate the 'limits' of what advanced industrialised recruiting countries would accept in a multilateral agreement, in ways that presage and provide important context for other attempts to progress a global agreement to regulate health worker-migration and -recruitment.

### 4.1 Bringing labour content into international capital flows

The UNSG, which since 1964 had been regularly reporting on 'outflows' of highly skilled personnel from developing to developed countries, continued to report on their causes and effects in relation to source and destination countries (UNSG 1972). This included the financial costs (losses) incurred by source countries. On this, the UNSG 1972 study was generally cautious in its calculations of how losses and gains were distributed between countries, but it nevertheless concluded that regarding health workers, 'the total gain for major receiving countries should be considered as being in the hundreds of millions of dollars' (UNSG/ECOSOC 1972, cited in d'Oliveira e Sousa 1989: 202). This gain, it was at pains to emphasise, 'is only the visible tip of the iceberg since the effects upon the process of development are as important, if not more so' (UNSG 1972).[29] This intervention signified an important shift in the conceptual and political bases of the debate, and informed the next round of work on global policy on highly skilled migration.

From the early 1970s this work progressed under the auspices of UNCTAD and ILO. In keeping with the UN focus on uneven development globally, particularly of the poorest countries, and the human right to migrate, these agencies once again took up the issue of 'brain drain' and articulated its relationship to development (ILO 1976a, 1976b; UNESCO 1974; UNCTAD 1971, 1973, 1974, 1975, 1977, 1979a, 1979b). Periodic research studies opened up space to discuss prospective policy action. In particular, they opened up a vista onto *global* policy to manage highly skilled international migration with a view to realising a better distribution of the share of risks, gains, and losses among the developed recruiting countries and developing source countries (UNESCO 1987; UNCTAD

1983b, 1983c, 1985a; UNSG 1980; Bhagwati 1976a, 1976b; Henderson 1970; Glaser 1978).

UNCTAD came to the issue from the perspective of trade and technology as significant factors of national development, and as part of its efforts to redress the weaker negotiating powers of developing countries in global fora.[30] Roffe (1985) argues that the impetus to UNCTAD's work in this area was shaped by a growing research base that enhanced understanding of the role of the transfer of technology in the development process of developing countries and the prevailing conditions in the flow of technology to these countries. The issues were twofold: the 'acute dependence of developing countries on the acquisition of technology from a limited number of suppliers' and 'the absence of scientific and technological infrastructure in the recipient countries, factors that hindered the adequate absorption and adaptation of the foreign technology' (Roffe 1985: 689–690). As a result, developing countries were faced with a problem of access to technology: they were 'unable to obtain the technology they need at the right price under the right terms and conditions and at the right time' (UNCTAD 1985c: 160).

Initially, the focus of intergovernmental agreements in the 1970s was on the legal and economic aspects of technology transfer, but this soon widened to incorporate other major elements including the adverse impacts of the reverse transfer of technology from developing countries, the measures to be taken to counteract it, and ways of promoting cooperative exchanges of skilled labour among developing countries, in a context of the overall goal to strengthen developing countries' capacity for collective self-reliance (UNCTAD 1985c: 165). Bringing labour mobility into these discussions and conceptualising highly skilled labour migration as a problem of 'reverse transfer of technology' (UNCTAD 1975) was an innovative step. Such migration was framed as a 'reverse' transfer because the international migration of highly skilled personnel constitutes a one-sided transfer of productive resources embodying technology in human skills, and the outflow of such resources from developing to developed countries (UNESCO 1987: 2). Reframing the issue in terms of 'reverse transfer of technology' served two purposes.

First, it picked up on and amplified a framing of highly skilled international labour migration as an issue of international trade and its labour content. In particular, it emphasised uneven development and inequality as drivers of international migration, such that both resided at least as much in the working conditions and opportunities available to highly skilled workers in source countries as in the 'superior' conditions and opportunities available to potential emigrants in recruiting countries.[31] As had been pointed out a decade previously (UNESCO 1968a), highly skilled labour migration was a 'sign of internal difficulties and disproportions due to legacies from the past'. These included the legacy of colonial histories, and how developing countries' work to build up institutional capacity and increase national highly skilled workforces was being thwarted by weaknesses in their economies generally and by scientific and technological dependence on developed countries. This dependence was sustained by weakness in scientific infrastructure, research centres, leadership, and lack of professional and wider social status of highly skilled workers who emigrated to seek better opportunities, conditions of work and standards of living abroad. Advanced countries exploit this dependence by continuing to draw on developing countries' pool of highly skilled labour to meet the insatiable needs for trained personnel generated by advances in science and technology. Such resource transfers are underpinned by favourable immigration policy of advanced countries and facilitated by private firms tasked to recruit 'talent' from overseas (UNESCO 1968a).

Second, it placed a spotlight on the significant resource transfer involved in highly skilled migration from developing to developed countries, and the corresponding loss of investment by developing countries resulting from permanent migration. The new terminology added a conceptual dimension by shifting emphasis from loss of 'brains' to the resource content of skills flows. As UNESCO put it:

> knowledge and skills are acquired as the combined result of investment in education, training and nurture and maintenance of the persons concerned, they could be considered as a form of productive resource embodied in human beings (human capital).
>
> (UNESCO 1987: 2)

'Human capital' implies that skilled migrants embody capital and knowledge, and effect a reverse transfer of resources and technology, from countries that are usually technology recipients to those that are predominantly technology suppliers (Papademetriou 1984, cited in D'Oliveira e Sousa 1989: 197). Framing the phenomenon as an issue of loss of resources resonated with many governments. This was reflected in the work of UNESCO and the World Health Assembly (Chapter 3) where developing countries pushed the reframing of 'brain drain' in terms of lost resources inhibiting development capabilities, rather than in terms of individual decisions responding atomistically to 'push and pull' factors.

More striking still was the way in which UNCTAD's ideas about reverse transfer were accompanied almost from the outset by consideration of the need for stronger international action and global agreement. Following its 1968 Conference UNCTAD began a global campaign. Over six years from 1972, it led an intense programme of research into the issues faced by developing countries in the transfer of technologies that included those of human capital. The immediate outcomes of this campaign were policy proposals to undertake action instituting responses to the identified issues on a global scale. By 1978 UNCTAD had set up intergovernmental machinery to negotiate an international code of conduct to address reverse transfers of technology (UNCTAD 1978d, 1985c). By the first meeting of intergovernmental experts UNCTAD had produced or was producing studies on reverse transfers (UNCTAD 1975, 1978a, 1978b, 1978c, 1978d, 1978e, 1979a, 1979b, 1979c, 1979d, 1979e), and had passed two resolutions. The 1977 UNGA Resolution (32/192) stated that the development process of developing countries, particularly their capacity to strengthen their domestic technological potential, is crucially dependent on the supply of highly trained personnel, and that the outflow of such personnel represents a significant loss of to these countries.

The group of governmental experts also moved quickly to a Resolution (UNCTAD 1978d) which was endorsed subsequently at the ILO General Conference in 1977 (ILO 1977a; UNESCO 1987: 19).

### 4.2 Elaborating global policy ideas: financial recompense and international resource flow accounting

These two Resolutions mandated continuing emphasis on global policy work. Two significant policy initiatives emerged, broadly directed at elaborating principles and methods of redistributing gains and benefits accrued by the countries of immigration and losses incurred by countries of emigration. One concerned a proposal to establish an international facility to compensate developing countries experiencing significant losses of skilled personnel (UNCTAD 1979e). A second concerned a proposal to measure international human resource flows (UNESCO 1987: 20).

Proposals to mitigate the losses incurred by developing source countries and to temper the gains accrued by developed countries included: revenue-sharing proposals that entail sharing a portion of income taxes paid by skilled migrants by destination countries with home countries; taxation proposals (levy of a surtax on incomes of 'brain drain' immigrants by the developed country of residence, and transfer of receipts to developing countries (Bhagwati 1976a, 1976b), or levied by the developing country of origin (Guhman 1978 cited in d'Oliveira e Sousa 1989); and a system of voluntary contributions to international human resource funds to channel resources to general development, or link to specific development programmes designed to mitigate international migration of skilled personnel (d'Oliveira e Sousa 1989: 205). These proposals were based on a compensation approach, involving payment for another country's loss of human capital. By far the most important proposal (in terms of attention within the UN system and durability) concerns the establishment of a global labour migration compensation mechanism for channelling resources back to source countries.

As noted earlier, the question of compensation to mitigate the loss of source countries' investment in human capital and its economic impacts arose as early as 1966 in UNESCO's work. It reported that:

A number of writers have made suggestions for working out an international system to offset the economic losses incurred by individual countries through the brain drain, these losses being reckoned as expenditure by the State on the education and professional training of the emigrants. For example, Professor Brinley Thomas defined the problem on the lines that if the import of physical assets had to be paid for why should human assets financed by society be imported free from abroad, while Professor G. Falchi suggested that the losses of the loser countries should be compensated by the winner countries.

(Thomas 1966 and Falchi 1966, cited in UNESCO 1968a: 40)

Although UNESCO did not take these ideas forward, others did. From the early 1970s, the issue of international compensation was worked on extensively, and various were iterated. Their elaboration took place during the UN's New International Economic Order (NIEO) initiative.[32] The proposals themselves were discussed in UN bodies – in UNCTAD in the context of its transfer of technology initiative, and in ILO (UN 1979).

ILO was at this time entering a period of activism regarding its standard-setting work on international migration as well as on matters of employment and working conditions. A proposal to establish a compensatory facility was made to ILO (ILO 1976b) conference on World Employment by HRH Crown Prince Hassan bin Talal (Jordan), on behalf of the G77 group of developing countries. It was supported by several developing country delegates who proposed that explicit measures of financial compensation for emigration by means of an international fund be included in the ILO Programme. The proposal of an International Labour Compensatory Facility followed the IMF's Trust Fund for Compensatory Facilities (d'Oliveira e Sousa 1989), the idea being that the Facility would be financed from contributions made by labour-importing countries, supplemented by other ILO members on a voluntary basis, and administered by the UN. The resources of that fund would be allocated to sending countries suffering from the effects of the 'brain drain', and disbursed either as direct aid or as soft loans in proportions relative to the estimated cost incurred by the loss of labour (International Labour Conference 1977, in d'Oliveira e Sousa 1989: 203). Such financial support would be earmarked for training projects or the purchase of capital equipment (UN 1979: 8). The proposed facility was designed to cover migration in general and was especially applicable to highly skilled migration (d'Oliveira e Sousa 1989: 203).

Although this proposal was not included in the ILO Programme of Action, the statement that multilateral and bilateral agreements should 'provide ways of limiting losses in source countries of origin, particularly developing countries, which may result from departure of skilled personnel whose education and training they have provided' was incorporated (UN 1979: 4–5). This was an open door for further work, and greater traction. It was supported by UNCTAD, ILO, the United Nations Conference on Science and Technology for Development (UNCSTD), G77 and UNGA (e.g. UNCTAD 1977, 1978a, 1978b, 1978c, 1978d, 1978e, 1979a, 1979b, 1979c, 1979d, 1982, 1983a, 1983b, 1983c, 1984a, 1984b; 1985a, 1985b, 1985c; Böhning 1977, 1978; UNCSTD 1979; UN 1979; UNSG 1980). The work that ensued linked the financing of technological development of developing countries and the channelling of resources via a dedicated global mechanism.

The 1979 UNCSTD conference and the ensuing Vienna Programme of Action on Science and Technology (UNCSTD 1979) were important sources of support for the compensatory approach. UNCSTD went beyond recommending assessment of the 'brain drain' problem by developing countries at the national level to urge accelerated *international* discussions about ways and means to 'curb and reverse' the brain drain, encourage absorption of highly skilled and trained personnel within developing countries, and mobilise support for UN agencies seeking urgent solutions to the problem. Such solutions included provision of technical assistance to developing countries to identify measures to tackle and reverse 'the exodus' of highly skilled personnel (UN 1979: 4). The Vienna Programme also supported the idea that additional resources could be channelled to developing countries for scientific and technological activities, and that the financing system 'may use other resources, such as ... resources that may accrue from the proposed international labour compensatory facility' related to the reverse transfer of technology (para. 115) (UNCSTD 1979, in d'Oliveira e Sousa 1989: 204). The G77 similarly urged action to rebalance the distribution of losses and gains from the international migration of highly skilled labour:

> the emigration of skilled manpower represents a transfer of productive resources and there is evident need to take systematic account of this in international resource flow accounting. The gains associated with skills flows between the recipient and source countries should therefore be shared on the basis of reciprocity.
>
> (UN 1979: 7)

A UN Secretary-General report dedicated to an international labour compensatory facility was commissioned following a request from the UNGA in 1979 to carry out a feasibility study of HRH Crown Prince Hassan bin Talal's proposal (UNSG 1980). The report noted the different positions of developed and developing countries on this matter. Developed countries contested the assumption that developing countries experienced net losses, arguing that emigration relieved local unemployment problems of developing countries and benefited those countries in other ways such as through emigrants' international remittances and acquisition of skills abroad (transferable to 'source' countries) (UNSG 1980: 7). Nevertheless, the UNSG argued the need to move beyond ad hoc remedial and unilateral measures by individual countries to reduce the scale and impact of outflows of highly skilled workers. It stated that 'there is general consensus that individual national policies in themselves could not lead to the desired levels or improvements and that *collective international policy measures would be required to strengthen the national efforts*' (UNSG 1980: 3, our emphasis). Perhaps anticipating objections from labour-importing states to such a global facility, UNSG strongly emphasised its broader purposes and the initiatives that could potentially be engendered:

> principally, the facility is expected to undertake efforts to continuously assess the dynamics of migration of trained and skilled personnel, collect and evaluate data on a uniform and consistent basis, evolve policy measures

for consideration at national and international levels, assist in the implementation of steps to reduce the adverse effects of migration.

(UNSG 1980: 11)

The report outlined two broad approaches that compensation schemes could
take. 'Rigorous schemes' included options to levy a direct assessment on
developed countries that 'import' migrant labour according to specific criteria,
tax-sharing arrangements, voluntary (tax-exempt) contributions, ear-marked
taxes for donation to development financing, and levying supplementary tax on
incomes of skilled migrants from developing countries for development spending within developing countries. 'Generalised schemes' entailed all (not just
highly skilled) economically active migrants who continue to maintain their
nationality from the source country being included in a system of accounting of
human resource flows. General liability to pay compensation would occur when
a certain percentage of workforce in any given occupational category is derived
through migrant workers – developing countries with per capita GNP below a
certain level being exempted from liability. Entitlement to compensatory payments would be on the basis of resources incorporated in the budgetary processes of recipient countries, and the amount paid to them would bear some
relationship to the size of the migrant population without necessarily requiring
detailed and cumbersome accounting procedures.

'Generalised' compensation schemes should be negotiated in the spirit of
solidarity, good will and mutual advantage rather than as a charity or a penalty,
and the value of migrant labour accruing to recruiting countries should be recognised. Such arrangements could be agreed on a multilateral or bilateral basis, but
the advantage of the global labour compensation fund that Crown Prince Hassan
proposed was that it was a global (multilateral) arrangement and therefore free
from the boundary and consistency problems inherent in bilateral agreements.
The UNSG also argued that this approach would meet some of the demands
raised in the context of financing systems for international development strategies and that it would constitute a transfer of real resource (UN 1979: 8–9).
Objections to 'rigorous schemes' came from advanced industrialised countries at
the fifth session of UNCTAD: 'they did not believe that this highly complex
phenomenon – the full dimensions of which had not yet been determined – could
be remedied by compensatory means' (UN 1979: 8). Suggestions in support of
compensatory schemes were made by Italy, Finland, Yugoslavia and Germany
(ibid.: 10).

The final report of the study, presented at UNGA's thirty-sixth session, in
1981–1982 (preparation of which was carried out with UNCTAD, ILO and other
UN organisations (UNSG 1982: A/36/483)) concluded that, in the light of the
contestability of the principles and operation of such a facility, the complexity of
the issues, the extent of resources and the scope of ultimate benefits that could
be derived from such as facility, a group of experts would be needed to consider
the issues further. In effect, the proposal was kicked into the long grass. Thus, no
consensus on a multilateral basis emerged, but the proposal nevertheless

remained a focus of UNCTAD's attention within its transfer of technology initiatives (UNCTAD TD/B/AC.35/6; d'Oliveira e Sousa 1989: 204). Supporting the UNSG study and UNCTAD work on this issue was ILO. A study it commissioned (Böhning 1982) lent important support to the moral case for the concept of recompense to inform the development of global policy in this area. It drew up an outline model agreement, on the basis that international labour migration gives rise to significant economic and legal inequities between countries in ways that compound extant inequalities, and that the principle of international distributive justice warrants a compensatory approach.

If the establishment of a facility raised complex questions and could not sustain the support of governments on a multilateral basis at the time, the idea of a global mechanism of some kind which would redistribute financial benefits resulting from emigration from developing to developed countries was far from defeated. A number of subsequent proposals were made in UN forums to establish international funds to 'backfill' the losses experienced by countries experiencing significant emigration of highly skilled workers. These include a proposal by the President of Egypt at the International Labour Conference (1983) to set up an International Fund for Vocational Training 'to enable those countries which suffer manpower outflows to implement programmes for training substitute elements, thus filling the gap left behind by migration' (ILO 1983). An address to the UNDP Governing Council the following year by the Prime Minister of Jamaica proposed the creation of an International Fund for Manpower Resources. Like Jordan, in Jamaica's case, the Prime Minister pointed out that his country had lost $194 million in trained skilled migrants between 1977 and 1980. The Fund, he indicated, would be used 'to finance the recruitment of skilled manpower on a medium-term basis with whatever concessions may be affordable from the use of grants, operational projects or any other concessional resources available to the Fund' (d'Oliveira e Sousa 1989: 203). The idea of a global policy based on recompense to source countries continues to have appeal among developing countries, and sustains intellectual interest to the present day. It forms the basis for policy recommendations advocated, for example, by Mensah *et al.* (2005), the West Asia–North Africa Institute (2015) and Van de Pas *et al.* (2016). Notably, the concept of compensation is inscribed in the WHO 2010 Global Code, albeit in a quite different form from proposals based on financial recompense (Chapter 4).

The idea of a global policy founded on the concept of recompense and justified by a global approach to distributive justice required, amongst other things, a method of calculation of differential gains and losses from labour migration incurred by each country. In 1982 UNCTAD's Intergovernmental Group of Experts on the Feasibility of Measuring Human Resource Flows met to consider and progress work to this end. This work intertwined issues of a technical and political nature. The technical problem revolved around the absence of data on highly skilled labour migration and how to place an economic value on it. The UNCTAD group considered only the measurement relating to the value of human capital embodied in the migrants. In focusing on the value of the skills that are transferred, and considering different approaches to assigning values to skill flows, it excluded considerations of wider economic and non-economic effects that the movement of (human) capital produces in the countries of immigration and emigration (d'Oliveira e Sousa 1989: 206). As the political implications of these 'technical' issues became apparent, the Group was unable to agree conclusions and a remit for follow-on work acceptable to all governments. The two main 'regional' blocs, G77 and Group B (advanced industrialised) countries, presented separate conclusions and recommendations, differences which the Chair nevertheless managed to reconcile. However, the Group failed to agree the terms of reference for the following meeting. G77 concluded that the measurement of international human resource flows is feasible, with difficulties, and urged that rapid progress on policy-oriented action be pursued. The advanced industrialised countries emphasised the uncertainty and contestability of the methods to measure such flows, concluding that 'further detailed study of the problem and of the requirements for realistic measurement of human resource flows is therefore required before any definitive decision on the issue could be taken' (UNCTAD 1982, Annex II).

### *4.3 Global policy legacies*

Although none of the proposals to regulate international highly skilled labour migration or establish a compensatory system that were mooted came into existence, the idea that there should be a global policy response could not be shelved. UNCTAD's work on the reverse transfer of technology directly informed the Third UN International Development Strategy (Resolution 35/36, Annex, 1980). Following recommendations by UNCTAD at its fifth session in Manila 1979, the Third UN International Development Strategy (Resolution 35/36, Annex, 1980) committed the UN and member states to taking 'comprehensive action' on the international migration of skilled personnel and the 'brain drain'. This aimed to better protect the interests of all countries and minimise the economically-disruptive impacts on countries experiencing large-scale highly skilled labour outflows. Crucially, it included a commitment to elaborating 'arrangements whereby developing countries experiencing large-scale outflows of their skilled nationals which cause economic disruption could secure assistance in dealing with the adjustment problems arising therefrom' (d'Oliveira e Sousa 1989: 202).

This defined highly skilled migration as a priority area during the 1980s and kept the need for better global responses on the agenda. A 1981 UNGA Resolution (A/RES/36/141) took note of the international labour compensatory facility idea and mandated continued work on the reverse transfer of technology by UNCTAD and ILO. By the mid-1980s it was apparent that the prospect of concluding a multilateral Code of Conduct on the Transfer of Technology was highly unlikely, despite support by G77 and socialist countries, not least due to Group B boycotting negotiations (UNCTAD 1986, 2001). The UN had not however given up on reaching some kind of agreement. The Fortieth UNGA passed a Resolution (40/191) restating that outflows of highly skilled personnel damage development and that there is an 'urgent need to formulate national and international policies to avoid the brain drain and obviate its adverse effects' (d'Oliveira e Sousa 1989: 208).

Amongst the intangible outcomes of this process were the experiences gained and lessons learnt. First, regarding multilateral approaches, 'long-term solutions to the brain drain had to be sought in a blending of different proposals and implemented in a flexible way' (d'Oliveira e Sousa 1989: 207). Underpinning this was a recognition that the 'brain drain' was a complex, multi-faceted phenomenon which no single approach or mechanism could hope to address by itself. Second, progress was made on technical, conceptual and methodological aspects of the reverse transfer of technology (d'Oliveira e Sousa 1989). In this, 'policymakers in the developing countries have now at their command well-reasoned substantive arguments and precise enough tools to measure human capital embodied in skill flows' (UNCTAD 1985c: 169). Third, the detailed and systematic consideration given to international migration of highly skilled personnel enabled important linkages to be made between population, economic development, employment, human rights, health, and science and technology. In this, a better understanding, and a more balanced and integrated approach to development aspects of 'brain drain' emerged (d'Oliveira e Sousa 1989: 208–209).

Fourth, the relationship between uneven development and international migration was firmly established. It was now understood that highly skilled migration was a structural feature of the world economy which could not be seen simply in terms of decisions by individuals whether to migrate and whether to return. It needed to be understood within a wider structural framework of uneven development within and between countries. Fifth, recognition of the resource dimension of the catastrophe for source developing countries, including loss of investment entailed by mass transfer of (human) capital to developed countries, was firmly established. Finally, international migration of skilled labour was delineated as a prime matter of global strategic significance requiring international responses.

Yet translating abstract principles underpinning those responses into a concrete agreement posed considerable difficulties. This was *especially* the case for a multilateral agreement that instituted the principle of global redistribution – as the Code of Conduct and the Global Labour Compensatory Facility had aimed to do. The lessons from this period in the development of the global policy field are not reducible to a lack of political will: developing countries repeatedly supported institutionalised global (UN) mechanisms capable of realising a fairer distribution of benefits and costs. The advanced industrialised (health worker-recruiting) countries were responsible for opposing and blocking progress on this front.

## 5 Conclusion

This chapter has charted the range of initiating actions relating to highly skilled labour migration carried out by the UN system. The seeds of what rapidly became a substantial global policy field were sown in the early years of the UN system, starting with the establishment of UN norms and principles establishing the right to migrate, and with ILO's and WHO's implementation of their mandates in relation to conditions of work, social protection, migration, and the training of health professionals. Development of the scope of the field and clarification of the issues at stake gained momentum during the First UN Development Decade as a result of UNGA and ECOSOC activism in relation to the 'brain drain' of highly skilled labour, and established the development dimensions of the issue. Further momentum came from the development of global human rights and equality regimes, which were directly relevant to labour migration. The dynamics UNGA and ECOSOC spearheaded drew in progressively more UN bodies and specialised agencies. WHO was among the first to take up the issue of shortages of highly skilled personnel, but it was largely absent from broader discussions taking place in UNESCO, ILO and UNCTAD, as supported by UNSG and UNCSTD. WHO's interest in health worker-migration, such as it was, was confined to physicians, whereas ILO's expanded to include nurses and midwives in a context of its actions on gender equality and social protection.

This period was formative in the emergence and elaboration of foundational ideas about the principles underpinning the global governance of international highly skilled migration. A characteristic theme was the need to expand and strengthen global action to develop a global policy, as distinct from a plethora of domestic measures pursued unilaterally. Credit for this is largely due to UNESCO whose intervention in 1966 stands the test of time today. The strong intellectual and political lineages of its work are evident in the work of ILO and UNCTAD during the 1970s. UNCTAD's concept of 'reverse transfer of technology' connecting with the international trade agenda and emphasising the significant material resource transfers involved in highly skilled labour migration from developing countries to developed ones was especially innovative. Indeed, this catalysed the series of proposals revolving around global compensatory mechanisms and human resource flow accounting. The global policy field was teeming with proposals of all kinds, ranging from declarative statements to binding codes of conduct. They were radical, including as they did binding regulatory and redistributive measures, and these ideas were strengthened by the combined efforts of UN agencies more rooted in 'third-worldism' (UNCTAD), labourism (ILO) and anti-racism (UNESCO). Global 'social' (compensatory) facilities attracted significant and serious attention. Crucially, such actions and proposals were propelled by UN initiatives on human rights and equality, as well as efforts to improve the overall terms of developing countries' participation in the global economy, not least by directing a greater share of resources to developing countries to support 'accelerated industrialisation'. The UN's NIEO initiative reflected and sustained the radicalism of this period.

The period covered by this chapter can be read as one of intensive efforts to initiate a global policy field. It was one of significant activism by multiple UN agencies and bodies elaborating their mandates. Through these wider processes they grappled with wide-ranging questions relating to international highly skilled migration and recruitment. It was one of the most exciting periods in global social policy. Key ideas were proposed, developed and tested. At the same time, the limits to a global regulatory policy aimed at redressing uneven development and realising international redistribution were encountered. The blocking actions of advanced industrialised countries against the many initiatives proposed was a tangible manifestation of these limits. The legacies of this time can be seen in the later stages of the development of the global policy field. In the next chapter we continue our historical discussion of this first phase of the global policy field by focusing on key WHO and ILO initiatives specifically in respect of the international recruitment and migration of health workers.

## Notes

1  Although the Executive Board is elected by the WHA, members are supposed to serve in an individual capacity as technically qualified in the field of health, rather than as representatives of governments. This could conceivably mean that WHO is able to act as more of a technical bureaucracy than some other IGOs, although this is undermined by its lack of resourcing from high-income country governments. We thank Chris Holden for this point.

2  However, WHO is increasingly involved in global PPPs with businesses and is also open to civil society input (mainly health experts) through its technical work.

3  The focus was on 'constant activity to promote the exchange of knowledge available within Europe and elsewhere', providing direct assistance to individuals rather than countries (WHO 1958: 344). WHO reported that '[i]n nearly all the less advanced countries a serious obstacle to the flow of graduates from the medical schools is the lack of teachers' (ibid.: 374).

4  'It has found countries everywhere eager to offer services and institutions for the instruction of WHO fellows, and to supply teachers ...' (WHO 1958: 154). During this period, most fellowships were awarded to physicians (56 per cent), nurses (16 per cent) and sanitary engineers (5 per cent). The remaining 23 per cent covered other types of health worker or were students (WHO 1968: 87).

5  Between 1947 and 1966 WHO awarded almost 24,000 fellowships, latterly to newly independent countries for basic medical studies, comprising 10 per cent of all studies by 1966 (WHO 1968: 86–88).

6  ECOSOC Resolution 797 (XXX) 1960 advocated 'more concerted efforts to assist the under-developed countries in the improvement of education and in the rapid formation of adequately trained cadres, particularly in the administrative and technical fields'. UNGA resolution 1515 (XV) 1960 mandated 'concerted action for economic development of economically less developed countries' (para. e) through technical training, education, technical assistance and the supply of development capital tailored to the needs of recipients.

7  For example, in 1961 ECOSOC requested that the UN Secretary General act to address labour shortages and their adverse impacts upon industrial development (Resolution 817 (XXXI)). UNGA Resolution 838 (XXXIII) (1961) recognised 'the need for a systematic assessment of human resources and the need for trained personnel ...'.

8  In 1962 ECOSOC Resolution 906 (XXXIV) on education and training called for 'manpower' surveys to 'safeguard against the waste of scarce resources'. UNGA resolutions 1824 (XVII) and 1515 (XV) and ECOSOC Resolution 898 (XXXIV) highlighted the importance of training national technical personnel in the developing countries themselves, and of the training of technical personnel in fostering economic development.

9 ECOSOC Resolution 1090 (XXXIX) (1965) commended the Recommendations of ILO and UNESCO (1962) concerning vocational training and technical education.

10 For example, resolutions on vocational training were adopted by ILO regional conferences in Africa, America and Asia; UNESCO held yearly conferences of Ministers of Education (UNSG 1964).

11 See ECOSOC Resolution 1029 (XXXVII) (1954): 'the main scientific and technological resources of a country lie in its trained people'; and 'the provision of trained personnel … is an essential element in the achievement of the rapid and self-sustained economic growth of developing countries' (ECOSOC, 37th Session, Annexes, agenda item 12, documents E/3901 and Add.1 and 2).

12 UNSG's (1964) conference on education and economic and social development and its report on *Training of National Technical Personnel for Accelerated Industrialisation of Developing Countries* was based on research involving ILO, FAO, UNESCO, WHO, ITU and WMO.

13 UNSG (1964) estimated that an additional 1,400,000 engineers, scientists and technicians would need to be trained by 1975 to meet developing countries' industrialisation requirements; that 'the training given [to teaching staff] is not always sufficiently comprehensive' (UNSG 1964 E/3901: 10); that large numbers of personnel go to developed countries to avail of their training facilities; that programmes in developing countries are frequently 'inspired by those in use in industrialised countries' and that

> standards and programmes will not be sound unless they are based on the analysis of occupations as practised in the country in which the standards and programmes will be used … action is being taken by some [developing countries] to establish standards and programmes consistent with their own circumstances and requirements.
>
> (UNSG 1964 E/3901/Add.1: 66–67)

14 This would build on the UNESCO and ILO Recommendations (1962), producing technical standards in the form of guides or manuals (UNSG 1964 E/3901: 21).

15 ECOSOC Resolution 1090 (XXXIX) (1965) requested that competent organisations prepare programmes of action for promoting training and utilisation of human resources in developing countries; and that ILO, UNESCO and other agencies increase their activities to develop and utilise human resources.

16 UNGA Resolutions 2083 (XX) and 2090 (XX) (1965) asked these agencies to 'intensify concerted action … with regard to the training of national personnel for the economic and social development of the developing countries'.

17 This focused on social and economic statistical data and scientific information on the brain drain and its economic, social and cultural causes and consequences at country level.

18 The report adds that 'migration to the United States also appears to occur among workers of a lower level: thus, more than 6,000 Philippine nurses are reported as working in that country and 300 Iranian nurses in New York alone" (ILO 1967: 30).

19 See UNGA Resolution 2259 (XXII), 1967. Also UNGA Resolutions 2320 (XXII) (1967) and 2350 (XXII) (1968).

20 T. J. Mills, "Scientific personnel and the professions", Annals of the American Academy of Political and Social Sciences, September 1966. Cited in footnote 91 page 54 of UNSG 1967 report.

21 It recommended further study by the UN Statistical Commission, ILO and WHO regarding the collection of statistical data, encouragement to governments to improve their data on migration, and a study 'in the form of concerted international action' on 'the extent to which the multilateral exchange of skills … is in fact a two-way transfer of identical skills which could be avoided' (UNSG 1967: 55).

22 The report refers to recommendations

> intended to provide the necessary basis for the consideration, in due course, of possible measures of international action without which it currently appears unlikely that the emigration of technical and especially scientific talent from developing countries can be slowed down, let alone halted.
>
> (UNSG 1967: 55)

23 ECOSOC Resolution 1274 (XLIII) Development and utilisation of human resources (1967).

24 UNGA Resolution 2417 (XXIII) (1968).

25 The Resolution also requested that the UN Secretary-General undertake studies of developing countries most concerned with the 'brain drain', 'to assess its consequences for their economic development and to make appropriate recommendations for practical action at the national and international level in tackling this problem'.

26 'The international organisations, and first and foremost the Specialised Agencies of the United Nations, must assist in solving this problem [of keeping trained nationally highly-trained personnel in the services of their country] which is exercising developing countries' in order to 'halt the brain drain' (UNESCO 1968a: 36).

27 A major UNESCO (1971) study of the movement of scientists was published out of this programme. UNITAR also supported diagnostic studies on the migration of highly skilled personnel (Henderson 1970, Glaser 1978), including the motives of individuals in leaving and returning.

28 UNESCO Recommendation adopted on the report of the Commission for Science at the 38th plenary meeting, 20 November 1974.

29 See also Ramaswamy, N. S. and Shah, R. (1973), United Nations Publication ESA/ SAT/AC.3/4, October 24, 1973.

30 UNCTAD secretariat is held to be a key driver of this campaign (UNCTAD (1985c). The studies and the policy departures it proposed were picked up by interested governments, particularly G77 (UNCTAD 1985c), and amplified back into the global debate.

31 For a refinement of this argument see UNCTAD 2014: 19.

32 The NIEO aimed to institute measures capable of evening out unequal development by enhancing the bargaining positions of developing countries in UN and other fora.

# 3 Elaborating the global policy field

## The 1977 Nursing Personnel Recommendation

## 1 Introduction

This chapter continues tracing the historical antecedents to the contemporary global policy field on health-worker migration and recruitment. Whereas Chapter 2 discussed the broad institutional structures propelling UN initiatives on highly skilled labour migration, this chapter focuses on the UN's elaboration of global initiatives specifically relating to highly skilled health-worker migration. The emerging implantation of a *global* policy had taken root during the UN's First Development Decade, and this was institutionally embedded and further elaborated during the mid-1970s by WHO and ILO.

Discussion centres on the institutional conditions and dynamics leading to the first global agreement on health-worker migration in 1977 – the ILO Recommendation on Nursing Personnel – and its immediate outturn. This period precedes the restructuring of architectures of global health and migration governance of the 1980s and 1990s (see Chapter 4) but it was one in which global neo-liberal political and economic priorities were nevertheless starting to emerge. WHO and ILO were both at the 'centre of gravity' within the UN system on health-worker migration at this time, as they have been ever since. The main institutional policy dynamics during the period from the late 1960s to 1979 were played out within and between WHO and ILO. WHO entered a field whose parameters were already framed by ILO and other UN agencies (see Chapter 2). It was tardy in proposing concrete actions to address health workforce shortages, migration and recruitment. Indeed, as we discuss, WHO was primarily oriented towards the responsibilities of developing country governments that were experiencing chronic shortages of health and medical personnel whereas ILO's sights were set on the necessity of global policy instruments. In this, the main propelling force behind the elaboration of this global policy field was not WHO but ILO. Thus, the proposal and conclusion of the first global agreement in this policy field emanated from ILO activism on global migration governance, and its labour migration initiatives conditioned the pace and nature of the global agreement on nurse migration. WHO had struggled to make headway on its own, and its collaboration with ILO helped produce the ILO Recommendation on Nursing Personnel in a matter of months. Despite the limitations of the Recommendation, it is a remarkable agreement in that it defined a high threshold for subsequent global initiatives and in many ways exceeded the provisions of the 2010 WHO Code of Practice on the International Recruitment of Health Personnel.

This chapter is organised around four principal sections. We first trace the entry of WHO into the global policy field on health-worker migration and discuss the principal WHO initiatives in this area during the 1970s. Section 3 discusses the ILO Recommendation on Nursing Personnel (1977), the dynamics leading up to it and debates during its passage into the ILO labour standards canon. Section 4 attends to the aftermath of the ILO Recommendation in terms of WHO's engagement with this policy issue. We argue that WHO fundamentally disengaged from it and failed to capitalise on the advances gained by the ILO Recommendation. This disengagement occurred despite the repeated protests of member state governments at WHA about the adverse development impacts of recruitment by developed countries. The concluding section considers the main findings in the light of the key developments and themes during the first phase of development of this global policy field.

## 2  WHO joins the debate on highly skilled labour shortages and outflows

### 2.1  WHO enters the global policy field

1967 was the first year that WHO made any real impression upon the global health-worker migration policy landscape. Six years had elapsed since its first and (until this point) only WHA Resolution (1961) on the training of national health and medical personnel, and the field had since developed substantially and rapidly (see Chapter 2). The migration of highly skilled health workers, its development consequences and international policy responses to it were widely studied, discussed and initiated across multiple UN fora. Outside the UN system, research evidence about the extent and nature of medical labour migration, alongside other highly skilled personnel (scientists, engineers, professors) was mounting and gained considerable traction. In health worker-migration alone, our re-analysis for this study of a bibliography compiled by the US Department of Health Education and Welfare shows that by 1967 some 70 studies had been published. Most were academic publications and publications in 'popular' political periodicals; state departments, medical colleges, medical and hospital associations were actively commissioning research into this issue (US DHEW 1975).

WHO not only arrived into the global policy field late: it was 'behind the curve'. Its work programme during the 1960s had failed to reflect the growing concerns. Whereas references to serious health workforce shortages as issues for health services provision had featured relatively prominently in WHO's first report on the World Health Situation (WHO 1959), they were accorded little attention in the second (WHO 1962) – despite WHO's 1961 Resolution on health workforce training. However, by the Third report (WHO 1967) it gave the matter greater prominence, warning that worsening staffing deficiencies impeded the extension of health services, the elimination of disease and improvement of public health:

> Altogether 21 countries spread over all the regions regarded these defi-ciencies as detrimental to the efficient working of their health services, and three felt they were their most urgent problem. [Doctors and nurses] are still the two categories in which the shortages are greatest, but the demand for midwives is larger than before. There is also a definite lack of the specialized skills of X-ray and laboratory technicians ... the statement of these deficiencies is usually accompanied by a request for improved training facilities.
>
> (WHO 1967: 34)

> [I]n four major areas at least where governments are seeking to discharge their health responsibilities to their citizens, there are serious deficiencies. These deficiencies ... include shortages in health service manpower, and the dearth of training facilities ... and inadequacy of available financial resources.... There is, however, at least one point of encouragement. It is the expressed desire of so many countries to organize their health planning in association with the systematic planning for economic and social devel-opment. These then are amongst the basic requirements and needs under-lying all else. When they have been even partially satisfied, other important objectives such as malaria eradication, rural development, perhaps also some elements of environmental improvement, will be more readily achieved.
>
> (WHO 1967: 61)

However, none of the three WHO World Health Situation reports linked these shortages to international migration. This is puzzling given that health workforce shortages were already the focus of considerable attention by the Pan-American Health Organization (PAHO), the WHO regional office for the Americas. Indeed, since the early 1960s PAHO had paid considerable attention to the education and training of professional and auxiliary health personnel in its ten-year plan, adopted in 1963 (WHO 1968: 10), and in 1966 it published a compre-hensive study of the migration of highly skilled personnel from Latin America (PAHO 1966). The study, commissioned by PAHO's Advisory Committee on Medical Research, contained invaluable insights into the scale and significance of medical migration. It showed, for example, that in 1956–1965

> a total of 4,265 physicians was admitted to the United States from Latin America ... equal to the total production of four United States medical schools over the decade.
>
> (WHO 1967: 35)

Yet PAHO study's findings and conclusions barely registered in WHO's decennial review of its own programme (WHO 1968).[1] WHO's main priority seemed to be to strengthen its authority as the expert agency regarding the extension of health services to wider population groups. At the same time, its advocacy of the need for governments to adopt a systematic approach to health workforce planning and management encouraged a focus on migration. In 1967 the UN Commission for Social Development (one of ten commissions set up by ECOSOC since 1946) invited WHO to report on extending health services (UN CfSD 1967: 23). The WHO submission duly highlighted shortages of health workers as a factor affecting the availability and use of health services, though this was in the context of a wider discussion focused principally on the potential for planning, education and training to harness health labour more effectively in the interests of public health (WHO 1967). From this study's perspective, the real significance of the report lies in its attention to medical migration. This was the first time a WHO-authored report had ventured into this realm. A two-page subsection in the chapter on training and education of health personnel covered the 'brain-drain of medical personnel to high-income countries' (WHO 1967: 34–36) which outlined the impact of emigration of health and medical personnel on the quality and development of health services, principally in relation to developing countries:

> These migratory movements have recently attained considerable dimensions and have obtained no or little publicity…. The importance of the popularly designated 'brain-drain' of university-trained and qualified people lies not only in the loss of the money invested in their education but also in the fact that the place they should have taken in national development has to be filled from another source or not filled at all.
>
> (WHO 1967: 34–35)

The report emphasised the uneven development impacts of medical migration, and noted that although 'the quantitative loss can be largely absorbed by an annual increase in the production of doctors' (WHO 1967: 35) this was far from true for developing countries which 'cannot as yet afford to train medical personnel for export' (ibid.). It was attuned to the global dynamics of medical migration in its case study of the UK and Ireland,[2] showing that developing country graduates were filling posts in these countries' health systems vacated by the emigration of British and Irish doctors to other advanced industrialised countries.[3]

The WHO report was disappointingly unspecific about policy responses, confining itself to rejecting restrictions on medical migration while highlighting the need for the medical curriculum to be fully adapted to the needs of source countries, improved professional facilities, working conditions, and a stable, organised health service (WHO 1967: 36). The Commission 'noted with concern the serious drain of trained medical manpower from the less developed countries to the more developed countries' (UN CfSD 1967: 25) and pointed to the need for research into 'the motivation of those physicians and other health personnel practising their profession outside their own countries and the measures and incentives used to keep such personnel in developing countries' which 'might offer the basis for international recommendations on this subject' (ibid.: 25 para. 1). WHO was invited to prepare a further study for the following year's session of the Commission on the availability of basic health and medical services, but there was no suggestion that this would or should incorporate medical labour migration.

WHO continued to pursue its mandate to provide technical assistance in training and education systems to developing countries. Its objectives were to increase numbers of qualified workers and improve curricula to serve identified national needs (WHO 1968). Regarding the latter, WHO passed two resolutions (1968, 1969) aiming to enhance the comparability (equivalence) of medical curricula and qualifications internationally. This work was WHO's most substantial engagement to date with international medical migration issues. The Resolutions implicitly addressed the issue that the qualifications and experience of those participating in overseas education and training schemes were either not recognised by the source country or that the education, training and other experience they received while abroad was ill-matched to its circumstances and needs. In a context where professional development and advancement often depended upon some overseas training, barriers to returning also meant loss of potential health dividends for source countries.

It helps to understand that the WHO initiative on equivalence of medical degrees had been promoted by the UN Regional Committee for Africa (AFR/RC17/R4) which was primarily concerned with inadequate health provision in Africa:

> The countries of the Region were poorly equipped in trained manpower to face this situation. In a large measure this was due to mediocre levels of general education, lack or inadequacy of national (or even regional) training facilities, poor terms and conditions of service, and less availability of expatriate personnel.
>
> (WHO 1968: 5)

The problem of skilled health worker shortage the Regional Committee identified was somewhat 'lost in translation' in WHA's 1968 Resolution WHA21.35 (WHA 1968). It stated that countries possessing medical or paramedical teaching institutions needed to understand 'the importance of ensuring that the level of recruitment and training of candidates always conforms to the standards required in their own countries'. Behind this seems to be a vague concern that the standards of recruitment and training for African medical students were lower than for 'home' nationals. In any case, a consultancy report commissioned following the Resolution (WHA 1968) was considered by WHA in 1969 (WHA 1969a). It noted the report's conclusions that an inter-country agreement on basic medical qualifications was needed, and recommended follow-up work 'to collect and make available to members information on medical education practices'. Thus began a strand of long-term activity within WHO and the UN leading to programmes of work to harmonise medical (and nursing) education and training internationally.

The issues that WHO chose to address first were not the loss of resources or the impacts of international migration on the capability of developing countries to extend their health services provision, but improving the 'dividends' to developing countries from international medical migration by 'smoothing over' anomalies and barriers in that dynamic. The principle that qualified doctors from developing countries who emigrate for professional development should be encouraged to return to their countries voluntarily following a period of international placement is foundational to the UN governance of health worker-migration (see Chapter 2). WHO's focus on medical education and training at this time is best understood in this context. The irony is that harmonisation of curricula and recognition of qualifications internationally have been significant factors enabling increased international migration in the health professions (as in others). This critical point was predicted by WHO years afterwards (as discussed later). Over time, a growing body of research evidence has corroborated the concerns of some in WHO. Health workers from countries that have aligned their curricula to international (usually US) standards are better placed to emigrate to high-value economies, while those from countries that align to regional standards often tend to be restricted to lower-value economies (Yeates 2009a, 2009b).

Despite its late entry into this global policy field, the late 1960s witnessed a flurry of WHO activity aimed at catching up. In addition to resolutions on medical curriculum equivalence, a further resolution directly addressing health worker-migration was passed in 1969. This called for initiatives to increase local medical training and education capacities in developing countries), and for developed countries to cooperate in this, and also take part in the training of physicians from developing countries to encourage graduates to return to work in their countries (WHA 1969b).[4] These were not the first UN Resolutions on medical migration, but they were the first passed by WHO. The crucial questions were what would its programme of action comprise, and how would it pursue it in the context of the evolving UN debate and institutional dynamics?

### *2.2 WHO's first landmark study of international health worker-migration*

Amongst the outcomes of Resolution WHA22.51 was a draft resolution on the training of national health personnel[5] which requested that WHO commission a major study of the outflow of highly skilled health personnel from developing to developed countries. WHA25.42, adopted in 1972, referred to the 'magnitude and complexities of the problem of international migration of national health personnel', and mandated WHO to conduct a study of health worker-migration 'to determine its causes and find appropriate solutions' (WHA 1972). It requested WHO 'seek[s], if necessary, additional resources outside the regular budget to finance such a study' (WHO 2008: 162). The US and Germany, both major recruiting countries, funded the study. A group of experts reviewed the study protocol. Collection of available information began in 1974, led by Alfonso Mejia, WHO's Chief Medical Officer in Health Manpower Development. The study was a decidedly multi-agency collaboration, involving many UN agencies, particularly UNESCO and UNITAR (WHA 1975: 348). It was descriptive and prescriptive in intent and scope (Mejia 1978). The original plans for a comprehensive study were reduced to a streamlined study, produced in 1977,[6] and published as Mejia (1978, 1981) and Mejia *et al.* (1979).

Whereas the focus of debate on medical 'brain drain' referred to doctors, the WHO study notably included nurses. This picked up an issue that ILO had previously highlighted (see Chapter 2), and helped to feminise a global policy field that was otherwise focused on health professions dominated by men. This inclusion of nurses was an important starting point for a strand of WHO activity that grew into more substantial programming over several decades. Nursing proved to be a common meeting ground for WHO and ILO, and one from which the first global policy agreement on health-worker migration was launched (see Section 3, below). Decades on, nursing and midwifery were also the 're-entry' point for the WHO campaign to institute a Global Code of Practice (see Chapter 4).

The pressure on WHO to address the growing problem of health worker-migration was increasing, and not only as a result of accumulating reports by ILO, UNESCO and UNSG referring to the scale of recruitment: developing country governments too were exerting considerable pressure through annual WHAs. Our detailed analysis of WHA proceedings at this time finds that governments were increasingly vocal about the financial and wider development costs they bore as a result of losing to developed countries significant numbers of the health and medical workers they had trained and educated. For example, at the 24th WHA in 1971, a government delegate from Ceylon (Sri Lanka) described the problem of the 'outflow of health personnel' in dramatic terms. Ceylon, he said, belonged to a group of countries that he described as 'over-exploited' rather than 'developing', the exploitation having lasted in Ceylon for 'nearly five centuries'. The country's two medical schools (built in 1870 and the 1960s) were producing some 200 physicians a year, 'which was just enough for a nation of 12 million people'. In the previous year (1970), however, '101 young doctors had resigned from the government health services to go abroad'. The delegate pointed out that 'all those doctors had been educated at the cost of the State, which should therefore receive compensation from the countries to which they had emigrated'. He added that Ceylon allocated about 30 per cent of its national budget to health and education, and it 'would not be happy to see other more prosperous countries benefit from that' (WHA 1971: 569–570; see also WHO 2008: 161). Four years later the Sri Lankan government delegation made this lucid and powerful intervention to the WHA:

> … between the years 1971 and 1974 something like over 575 doctors left
> my country for employment in two of the most developed countries of the

world. The loss in investment this involved was something like 12 million dollars. The gain to the developed countries where these doctors ultimately found employment was estimated at something like 325 million dollars. The loss to my country over this migration of doctors alone can best be judged when it is pointed out that the total amount of foreign aid received during this period from the countries to which these doctors migrated was not more than 60 million dollars for the whole period.

(WHA 1975: 264)

Sri Lanka was not alone in providing such evidence and pressing WHO into action. Throughout the 1970s many developing and socialist country government delegates at the WHA commented on how the emigration of health workers compromised their ability to meet strategic national and global goals, leaving WHO and developed country governments in no doubt about the scale and severity of the problem.

The findings of the WHO study confirmed what governments were saying in the WHA: the volume and scale of migration of physicians and nurses had increased. By 1972 6 per cent of the world's physicians (c.140,000) were practising in countries other than those in which they were either born and/or trained, and 'one-eighth of the world's production of physicians in 1970 migrated annually during the period under study' (Mejia *et al.* 1979: 399–400). Almost 0.5 per cent of nurses (c.14,000) were moving internationally each year (Mejia *et al.* 1979). The report also highlighted broad changes in the global dynamics of migration:

Prior to World War II the movement of physicians had generally been a bidirectional flow among developed countries and a unidirectional flow from the more developed countries to the less developed. During recent years, however, increasing numbers of physicians have been going not only from the less developed to the more developed countries, but also from the less to the more affluent developing countries.

(Mejia *et al.* 1979: 27)

The principal direction of flows remained from developing to developed countries (c.90 per cent of cases) – mostly physicians to the US, UK and Australia, and nurses to Europe, North America and developed Western Pacific countries (Mejia *et al.* 1979). The study predicted a continuation of these trends.

To its credit, the study, cognisant of the already-substantial evidence (collated in the US's DHEW project (1975)), and pointing to the serious adverse impacts on source countries' health systems and socio-economic development, found an inextricable link between such migration and the quality of national health workforce planning and wider development strategies:

The complex interrelationship between health and other socioeconomic factors makes it inappropriate to isolate health, and thus the phenomenon of health manpower migration, from the rest of the development process.

National administrations concerned about the outflow of health manpower will need to seek long-term solutions. Such solutions will, of necessity and at the minimum, involve a revision of policies concerning the supply, distribution, productivity, and utilization of health manpower.

(Mejia *et al.* 1979: 414)

The study highlighted that 'measures taken by certain countries to foster migration have been, on the whole, more effective than the measures to curb it' (Mejia 1978: 214) and that '[t]he record shows that migration policies and practices in highly developed countries have nearly always been more influential in determining the pattern of migration than have those in developing countries' (Mejia *et al.* 1979: 171). Its overall recommendations were poorly aligned to this finding, however. It recommended further country-level studies and actions on the part of developing ('donor') countries on the basis that 'the only measures that can have any hope of resolving the migration problem for donor countries are those that aim at eliminating or neutralizing the push factors in those countries' (Mejia *et al.* 1979: 415). None of the recommendations were addressed to the recruiting countries, notwithstanding general points about needing better health workforce planning and management. The closest the report comes to criticism of the major recruiting countries is acknowledgement that:

The general structure of international politics and economics will no longer make it practical for the developed countries to attempt unilaterally to arrange, on their own terms and in their interest solely, the major issues between them and the developing world. Thus, as regards the migration issue, it is not sufficient that the major recipient countries individually and unilaterally take measures – as they are doing – to curb the inflow of physicians. Such measures will not automatically and immediately solve, for the donor countries, the problems underlying the migration, one such problem being the overproduction of physicians to meet the export market – *a market which the major recipient countries either explicitly or implicitly have stimulated over the past decade.*

(Mejia *et al.* 1979: 423–424, our emphasis)

Given that the recruiting countries of US and Germany helped fund the study it is perhaps not surprising that their recruitment practices (and those of others) avoided critical scrutiny. It is also disappointing that the study shied away from advocating a robust global policy initiative, as proposed by UNESCO and others (see Chapter 2). Instead, the global policy component of the report stipulated greater emphasis on WHO-led bilateral negotiations through technical cooperation/assistance, through which 'perhaps a more mutually beneficial approach to regulating health manpower migration may be found' (Mejia *et al.* 1979: 424). In essence, WHO rejected the idea that it could or should do more than provide technical assistance to individual countries. The study gave no clues that it supported a robust global, collective response – *despite* its recognition that the upsurge in demand for medical and health workers cannot be managed by countries unilaterally. WHO's 'technocratic' and anti-globalist politics of global policy in this area is aptly encapsulated in the study's conclusions: 'No country can really rely on another country to solve its problems, including the migration problem, which is merely one of a number of undesirable symptoms of … managerial deficiencies' (Mejia *et al.* 1979: 420).

Despite these omissions, which seem especially pronounced given the pace at which UNCTAD was proceeding with establishing negotiating machinery to conclude a Code of Conduct (Chapter 2), it would be unfair to overlook the extent to which the study critically engaged with emergent global policy on health-worker migration. The report made the important critical point that 'International agreements such as those of the European Economic Community, of the Andean Pact countries and of the Mediterranean States … facilitate migration.' (Mejia *et al.* 1979: 400). This referred to the role of regional integration in generating labour market dynamics that draw health workers into international labour migration streams. The report also highlighted how 'International agreements promoting the international recognition of (medical and nursing qualifications facilitate and, possibly, encourage migration' (ibid.: 405). This can be interpreted as a thinly veiled critique of WHO's own initiatives to progress the 'equivalence' of medical qualifications. Thus, it seemed to point the finger at itself, highlighting WHO's own complicity in bringing about conditions facilitative of physician and nurse migration. The authors deserve full credit for identifying how international integration strategies pursued by the developed and developing countries alike (albeit under different conditions of power and agency) were as much a part of the 'story' of medical and nurse migration dynamics as were the unilateral health workforce management strategies of those countries.

## 3 The first global policy instrument: the ILO Nursing Personnel Recommendation

Given that the Mejia study was the first WHO (and UN) comprehensive multinational study examining the international migration of physicians and nurses, and taking into account the study's mild policy recommendations and the growing calls for international action, WHO might reasonably have expected to build on the momentum it started. It did not do so, at least within its own organisational framework. Instead, the initiative passed to ILO, where a Recommendation on nursing personnel, which included provisions on international migration and recruitment, was successfully concluded even as the Mejia study was underway.

### 3.1 *Resurgent ILO activism on global labour migration*

The mid to late 1970s were a period of intensifying ILO activism in standard-setting across social policy areas, including international migration and recruitment.[7] New instruments were concluded. The 1975 Migrant Workers Convention and Recommendation took a more robust line than its 1949 predecessor. The 1975 instruments affirmed that migration policy should be based on the social and economic needs of source countries *and* countries of employment, and should take account of short-term labour needs and resources and the long-term social and economic consequences of migration for migrants as well as for communities in source and recruiting countries. This constituted a very different approach from the 1949 Migration for Employment Convention which stated that countries should 'facilitate the international ... movement of manpower [*sic*] from countries which have a surplus of manpower [*sic*] to those countries that have a deficiency', having 'due regard to the manpower situation in the country' (ILO 1949)

The 1975 Convention was in fact an important milestone in ILO's campaign to 'socialise' the UN's NIEO initiative, and it was an important achievement in the run-up to ILO's Tripartite World Conference on Employment, Income Distribution and Social Progress, and the International Division of Labour (1976). The Programme of Action agreed at this conference pressed ahead in setting out the aims of national and international policies on labour migration:

> to provide more attractive alternatives to migration in the country of origin ... to protect migrants and their families from the difficulties and distress which sometimes follow migration ... [and] to take care that neither migration nor its alternatives are prejudicial to the rest of the population or harmful to economic and social development in either the country of origin or the country of employment.
>
> (ILO 1976b: 389, para. 35)

The Programme of Action (together with the 1975 Migrant Workers Convention) reiterated equality of opportunity and treatment as a guiding principle to be embedded in all key areas of national labour policy and in international action, in particular in multilateral and bilateral agreements governing labour migration. It emphasised that agreements should be based on mutually-accepted policies to 'even out fluctuations in migration movements, return migration flows and remittances, and make them as far as possible predictable, continuous and assured so as to facilitate the implementation of long-term programmes of economic and social development' (para. 42). The Programme also elaborated the aims of such agreements in relation to skilled migration as being to:

> provide that countries of origin should adopt appropriate measures so as to avoid the departure of skilled workers;
>
> provide that countries of employment should refrain from recruiting skilled and highly skilled works when there are recognised or potential shortages of such workers in the country of origin;
>
> provide that the countries of employment could take complementary measures to aid the developing countries to minimise their loss of qualified manpower;

provide ways of limiting losses in countries of origin, particularly developing countries, which may result from the departure of skilled personnel whose education and training they have provided.

(ILO 1976b, para. 43)

The Programme mandated ILO to provide support to countries and regional organisations to implement these measures. Although the call by Crown Prince Hassan of Jordan for an international compensatory facility could not be resolved (see Chapter 2), the Programme kept the issue alive within ILO by recommending that it should 'initiate studies on the economic and social effects of different kinds of migration for employment' (para. 46). This was a landmark intervention in the development of the global (UN) migration governance framework and provided an important 'vanguard' initiative for ILO work on nursing personnel (see Section 3.2).

This ILO migration initiative was long overdue. As pointed out by the Workers' delegate during the passage of the 1975 Migrant Workers Convention, and the proposed Resolution concerning the future ILO activities concerning professional and similar workers, ILO had 'not kept a constant watch' on the 'brain drain' issue since 1967 when it reported on the problems of highly skilled staff (engineers, managers, technical, medical and health staff) (ILO 1967) (see Chapter 2). Moreover, the delegate pointed out, ILO had failed to discuss the issues of professional staff, migrant or not, in ILO Conferences or in the Advisory Committee on Salaried Employees and Professional Workers (ILO 1976c: 14). He called upon ILO to thoroughly activate itself on 'the problems of the "brain drain" from developing countries and means of putting an end to it' (ibid.).

The ILO Programme of Action was highly significant in marking the beginning of UN action on global migration, the most recent manifestation of which is the UN Global Compact on migration (2018) (see Chapter 7). The Programme also, de facto, established ILO as *the* leading UN agency dealing with labour migration, skilled or otherwise. It provided for further ILO initiatives and ensured ILO's authority as lead UN agency dealing with global health worker-migration policy. More critically, although the Programme was by far the most radical and substantial initiative proposed, it fell short of what UNESCO had proposed a decade previously. The ILO Programme was confined to identifying policy objectives and principles rather than proposing any concrete regulatory initiatives. Prefiguring the role that WHO would three years later define for itself through the Mejia study, ILO defined its own role as principally providing technical assistance to countries to attain international labour (migration) standards.

## 3.2 The ILO Nursing Personnel instruments

Against the backdrop of ILO activism on labour migration ILO codified the first set of global policy principles explicitly concerned with nurse-migration and -recruitment. In 1977 it simultaneously adopted a Convention and a Recommendation on Nursing Personnel. The immediate contextual origins of these instruments lay in ILO's resurgent activism on labour migration and increasingly loud calls for international action on highly skilled labour migration. Such calls had been gathering pace over the decade, and were amplified by high-level interventions by Crown Prince Hassan of Jordan for a multilateral facility on migration (which remained unresolved during ILO's 1976 World Conference) and the Sri Lankan Prime Minister Bandaranaike at the 1975 Conference. The latter's plenary conference speech highlighted the 'situation' of highly trained personnel, 'trained at considerable expense to the nation being attracted to affluent countries of the developed world' (ILO 1976c: 190) and, in the words of the ILO Secretary General, urged ILO to take action to address this (ILO 1978: 735).

Drawn up in collaboration with WHO through ILO's tripartite policy formation mechanisms, ILO formally 'owned' the global initiative on nursing personnel. In many ways, though, the instruments can be regarded as a successful outcome of a genuinely multi-stakeholder initiative, involving joint collaboration by the two UN agencies, in full consultation with and agreed by ILO's tripartite constituents (employers, workers, governments). Informed by WHO's work on health personnel shortages and developing of nursing and midwifery personnel and ILO's own expertise and competence in respect of labour migration, supported by its institutional relations with governments and employers' and workers' groups, ILO propelled the process to a successful conclusion within 12 months, translating the need for such instruments into the elaboration of key principles, agreement on instruments to be used, and the means of implementing them.

Both ILO and WHO had good reasons to support ILO's instruments to a successful conclusion. For ILO, they were key developments in its standard-setting on international labour migration, and an opportunity to demonstrate tangibly its engagement with highly skilled labour migration. They also furthered ILO's work to promote gender equality in relation to a highly feminised profession in the health workforce. Indeed, ILO regarded the nursing personnel instruments as integral to the 'second' phase of its action programme to promote women's working conditions and prospects at work through equal pay and equality of opportunity and treatment in employment (ILO 1978). For WHO, the instruments were a chance to demonstrate Mejia's point about the 'policy applications' of its work, as well as to shore up its other on-going work in the nursing and midwifery workforce and the training of health and medical personnel.[8] For both ILO and WHO, then, the Nursing Personnel instruments were an opportunity to pursue action jointly relating to their own institutional mandates as well as to collectively pursue action relating to a key global development issue. Above all, the instruments would help realise multiple goals in a single health profession: strengthen international standards on gender equality and labour migration; address health-worker shortages and the development of health professions; promote wider UN principles on migration as a human right; and promote international development cooperation through provision of technical assistance and international agreements to realise a range of social, health and economic goals.

The Convention (ILO 1977b) and Recommendation (1977c) covered the occupational category of nursing personnel only, defined as 'all categories of persons providing nursing care and nursing services', and apply 'all nursing personnel, wherever they work' (Article 1). WHO would have preferred that midwives be included within these discussions, as their conditions of work were similar to nurses' (ILO 1978). The instruments did not do so, but were the first to address an identified occupation in the health field and they remain the only ones to do so to date. This focus on nurses was not without controversy (see Section 3.3). The instruments were mainly concerned with nurses' working conditions: they set out a range of provisions concerning working hours, rest periods, paid annual holidays, educational leave, maternity leave, sick leave and social security, and the settlement of disputes relating to terms and conditions of employment. They also incorporated the principle that nursing personnel should be enabled to participate in the planning of nursing services, and provided that 'nursing personnel shall enjoy [working] conditions at least equivalent to those of other workers in the country' (Convention 149, article 6).

The Convention did not incorporate any principles on international migration, referring only to shortages of health personnel in its preamble and the fact that nursing personnel were not always utilised to best effect. However, the Recommendation did. It brought together various UN principles developed over the decades into a single framework and confirmed the longest-held UN principle that international migration should be voluntary and freely chosen. It acknowledged WHO's recognition of positive development impacts of organised exchanges of personnel, and exchanges of ideas and knowledge, as part of efforts to improve nursing care and professional development (Articles 62, 63.2), and the promotion of international mobility through harmonisation and mutual recognition of qualifications initiatives. It affirmed ILO international labour standards in emphasising that participation in such exchanges, and/or to study, train or gain experience abroad, should be under good, non-discriminatory working conditions that maintain participants' social security rights (Articles 64.1, 65, 66.3, 68, 69).

The ILO migration framework that set out the need to avoid adverse human and wider social consequences of excessive or uncontrolled increases in international migration (ILO 1976b) was interpreted and applied in the statement that countries *should not rely on overseas nursing personnel to staff their health services*. Thus, Article 67 set out two conditions under which international recruitment would be permissible: if there is a lack of qualified personnel for the posts to be filled in the country of employment, and/or if there is no shortage of nursing personnel with the qualifications sought in the source country. These conditions were more stringent than the WHO 2010 Code, which only referred to the avoidance of recruitment from countries suffering from serious health personnel shortages (see Chapters 4 and 5).

The ILO Recommendation also notably inscribed a conditional element into the principle of international migration in the context of its support for international professional exchanges. Article 64.2 stipulates that financial aid provided to nursing personnel for education or training abroad 'may be made dependent on an undertaking to return to their country within a reasonable time and to work there for a specified minimum period'. This reflected and responded to the 'anxieties' of many that exchanges and periods of overseas professional development turned into permanent emigration. Otherwise, the Recommendation encouraged governments to enter into multilateral and bilateral arrangements to promote international nurse migration according to these (and other) principles.

In all of these respects, the Recommendation remains unrivalled as a UN statement on health worker-migration and -recruitment. Yet the Recommendation was ultimately no more legally binding or enforceable than a WHO resolution. However, there is a key difference: the Recommendation automatically benefits from ILO's institutional governance of labour standards, in the form of implementation and reporting mechanisms (including access to them by a range of constituencies) by virtue of the general institutional provisions of ILO binding governments, employers, workers. While the Committee of Experts on the application of Conventions and Recommendations monitors both types of instruments, there is no ratification process for Recommendations however and, consequently, the reporting process for them is less rigorous. Moreover, the Recommendation itself only contains 'suggestions' for its application.[9] The Annex's model policy specification concerning the migration/recruitment elements of the Recommendation (International Cooperation) (see Box 3.1) relates only to financial aid given to nursing personnel education or training abroad and how periods of leave or detachment for such purposes should be taken into consideration in the calculation of seniority, particularly as regards remuneration and pension rights.

---

**Box 3.1 ILO Principles on International Cooperation in Nursing Personnel**

*Article 62*

In order to promote exchanges of personnel, ideas and knowledge, and thereby improve nursing care, Members should endeavour, in particular by multilateral or bilateral arrangements, to:

a   harmonise education and training for the nursing profession without lowering standards;
b   lay down the conditions of mutual recognition of qualifications acquired abroad;
c   harmonise the requirements for authorisation to practise;
d   organise nursing personnel exchange programmes.

*Article 63*

1   Nursing personnel should be encouraged to use the possibilities of education and training available in their own country.

2    Where necessary or desirable, they should have the possibility of education and training abroad, as far as possible by way of organised exchange programmes.

*Article 64*

1    Nursing personnel undergoing education or training abroad should be able to obtain appropriate financial aid, on conditions to be determined by multilateral or bilateral agreements or national laws or regulations.
2    Such aid may be made dependent on an undertaking to return to their country within a reasonable time and to work there for a specified minimum period in a job corresponding to the newly acquired qualifications, on terms at least equal to those applicable to other nationals.

*Article 65*

Consideration should be given to the possibility of detaching personnel wishing to work or train abroad for a specified period, without a break in the employment relationship.

*Article 66*

1    Foreign nursing personnel should have qualifications recognised by the competent authority as appropriate for the posts to be filled and satisfy all other conditions for the practice of the profession in the country of employment; foreign personnel participating in organised exchange programmes may be exempted from the latter requirement.
2    The employer should satisfy himself that foreign nursing personnel have adequate language ability for the posts to be filled.
3    Foreign nursing personnel with equivalent qualifications should have conditions of employment which are as favourable as those of national personnel in posts involving the same duties and responsibilities.

*Article 67*

1    Recruitment of foreign nursing personnel for employment should be authorised only:
     a if there is a lack of qualified personnel for the posts to be filled in the country of employment;
     b if there is no shortage of nursing personnel with the qualifications sought in the country of origin.
2    Recruitment of foreign nursing personnel should be undertaken in conformity with the relevant provisions of the Migration for Employment Convention and Recommendation (Revised), 1949.

*Article 68*

Nursing personnel employed or in training abroad should be given all necessary facilities when they wish to be repatriated.

*Article 69*

As regards social security, Members should, in accordance with national practice:
a    assure to foreign nursing personnel training or working in the country equality of treatment with national personnel;
b    participate in bilateral or multilateral arrangements designed to ensure the maintenance of the acquired rights or rights in course of acquisition of migrant nursing personnel, as well as the provision of benefits abroad.

Source: ILO Nursing Personnel Recommendation (R157) (ILO 1977c)

Despite the obvious limitations of the policy instrument, the robustness of the Recommendation is supported by having a 'natural' constituency – notably as represented by trade unions, as well as employers and governments, supported by ILO. However, the extent to which these constituencies make the Recommendation a 'living document' is dependent upon their activism after the instrument is concluded. In this respect, the results are extremely disappointing. Our archival research at ILO carried out for this study found that historically none of the General Reports by the Committee of Experts on the Application of ILO Conventions and Standards (including the only three dedicated to migrant workers (ILO 1980, 1999, 2016d)) cover nursing personnel, whether migrant or not. Nor do they follow up any issues to do with the implementation of the Recommendation (or the Nursing Personnel Convention). Consequently, the question of the extent of implementation of the Recommendation has never arisen in the Conference Committee on the Application of Standards (a standing tripartite body of the International Labour Conference and an essential component of ILO's supervisory system). If this follow-up work had been undertaken it would have come up in the Conference Committee, since each year it examines the report published by the Committee of Experts on the Application of Conventions and Recommendations. The Conference Committee may, under article 19 of the ILO Constitution, request a report on a specific Convention or a General Survey (on a theme or collection of Conventions), but it has never requested a report on the Nursing Personnel Instruments. Indeed, the Nursing Recommendation does not even seem to be considered as a migration instrument: of the two instances when the Conference Committee has requested a report on ILO labour migration instruments (1999 and 2016) it did not include the Nursing Personnel Recommendation. This collective failure by ILO constituencies means that the normative power of the Recommendation to effect potentially transformative change remains unexploited.

Prior to considering the political negotiation of the Recommendation, we conclude this discussion by highlighting that WHO deserves credit for forming this first comprehensive statement of global health worker-migration policy. The contributions of ILO and WHO are both reflected in the Recommendation's international cooperation principles. We can therefore conclude that the outcome of WHO's work on health worker-migration did not so much evaporate as shift over to ILO where it was worked into an historic milestone in this global policy field. If the locus of global policy-making was shifted to another UN agency (ILO) this reflected the more propitious conditions there: ILO's tripartite governance structure was more conducive than WHO's, which interfaces only with governments, while ILO interfaces with employers and workers' groups and governments. Even if governments can never be out-numbered by Employers' and Workers' groups at ILO, it nevertheless produces a quite different political and policy-making dynamic. It is one that is favourable towards collectively negotiated global policy instruments elaborating the principles underpinning health worker-migration and -recruitment.

### 3.3 The institutional passage of the Recommendation: a case of non-contestation?

Although WHO would have preferred that the ILO nursing personnel instruments had included midwives, its concerns did not derail the successful conclusion of the instruments. More pressing issues were raised during the passage of the Recommendation's international migration provisions which needed to be dealt with. Of particular interest for the purpose of this discussion are the occupation-specific focus of the instruments and provisions concerning emigrant nurses' employment relationship with their source country, and the conditions under which countries recruit nursing personnel from overseas.

A first set of concerns revolved around Article 65, regarding the maintenance of nurses' employment rights in the source country when working abroad, whether under the auspices of organised exchange programmes or not. The concern was that maintaining these rights would further encourage emigration of qualified nursing personnel and disrupt the proper functioning of the health service in the source country. Thus, an amendment, tabled by the government of Belgium, and supported by government members of seven African countries, requested that provision to maintain employment rights should only pertain to nurses participating in organised international exchange schemes, and that it should exclude anyone wishing to work abroad outside of these schemes. The amendment was opposed by both workers' and employers' groups, and the governments of Australia and Italy, on the basis that the text of Article 65 was already flexible enough. The amendment was an indication of the anxieties of many governments that the coordination of employment rights among source and destination countries would greatly facilitate highly skilled labour migration, to the detriment of developing countries. This concern had already arisen in the context of the Migrant Workers Convention (1975), in relation to a proposal by the Employers group that references the UN human rights recommendations that the right to migrate be included in the Convention's preamble to strengthen its governing principles. The amendment to the draft Recommendation was not accepted, following discussion in which the Government members of Algeria, Colombia, France, Mexico, Spain and the USSR, the Employers' members of Mexico and Sweden, and the Workers' members of France, Germany, Mali and the USSR took part, and during which it was emphasised that the adoption of this amendment might be interpreted as encouraging 'brain drain' (ILO 1978).

A second set of concerns revolved around what was to become Article 67.1, concerning the conditions under which recruitment of overseas nursing personnel for employment should take place. Such conditions were broadly scoped, applying to all operations designed to seek out nurses with a view to employing them in another country, whether such activities were organised under bilateral or multilateral technical cooperation or otherwise, and irrespective of the status of the nurses recruited. One aspect of the concerns about this article was that it was up to the source countries to take the necessary steps to prevent the exodus of qualified workers. Accordingly, the government members of France and the UK sought to delete this article, but this was opposed by government, employers' and workers' members of India and Uganda, on the grounds that the article effectively protected the interests of the country of employment as well as those of source countries by laying down conditions governing the recruitment of nurses. The article was however modified to reflect the opposition of governments (Fiji, Ghana, Kenya, Nigeria, USA) and workers to the requirement that there did not exist, in the country of employment, personnel 'ready to accept the conditions offered' (ILO 1978).

The third issue raised concerned the scope of the Recommendation (and the Convention). WHO had previously highlighted its preference that midwives be covered as well as nurses. But the fear was that introducing instruments for specific occupational groups (nurses) would gradually weaken attempts to have general standards for *all* workers, and lead to a proliferation of instruments. These would, in turn, undermine the effectiveness of ILO standard-setting activities. Indeed, the Nursing Personnel instruments are exceptions in the history of ILO's approach to labour standards: then, there were only two other specific categories of worker to have been the subject of such instruments, both in the agricultural sector.[10] All parties let such a concession pass on that occasion, given the level of support for the instruments, although one government member warned ILO that he expected not to see any further occupation-specific instruments being proposed or discussed in future (ILO 1978).

## 4 Developments at WHO

### 4.1 After the Mejia study: WHO disengagement

Given the success of WHO in contributing to making the first global policy instrument in this field (albeit institutionally located at ILO), it is surprising that the proposals made by its own study failed to make much headway within WHO structures. We reach this conclusion because the issue is absent from ensuing WHO resolutions and documents in the late 1970s. Furthermore, even before the study was concluded and the ILO Recommendation had passed a period of institutional disengagement from the issue within WHO more widely was already in train.

There were several signs of this disengagement. One was that the WHA passed just two Resolutions, in 1976 and 1978. In 1976 the Director-General was asked 'to collaborate with Member States in ... *the development of measures to control undesirable migration of health manpower*' (WHA 1976b, our emphasis). It requested 'a long-term programme of health manpower development ... in all regions' that would incorporate a study of 'the extent of actions taken by governments in modifying their health manpower training programmes'. Although this seemed to represent an advance in that the matter was not defined *principally* as pertaining to developing countries' lack of capacity, the programme did not include any specific element on international migration or recruitment. In 1978 the matter arose tangentially in the context of a highly specific discussion of the effects of the Israeli occupation of West Bank and members' concern about 'forcing the migration of Arab medical and health personnel, and imposing restrictive conditions on the inhabitants as regards the practice of the medical and health professions' (WHA 1978b).

A second sign was the omission of health worker-migration and -recruitment from WHO's medium-term programme for health staffing development 1978–1983 as well as from its long-term programme for maternal and child health. Even though child health otherwise highlighted needs for better socio-economic planning, and to 'review when appropriate present utilization of all health personnel including traditional health workers in order to ensure a better use of existing resources for maternal and child health' (WHA Resolution 32.42) (WHO 1979), WHO made no reference to health worker-migration as a factor of the sub-optimal utilisation of the health workforce.

International migration was similarly excluded from the WHO Declaration of Alma-Ata (WHO 1978) which identified primary health care and adequately staffed health services as the principal means for achieving public health goals (Article VII). Preparations for the international conference on primary health care which culminated in the Declaration were already underway during the period of the Mejia study, and the conference took place a year after the study was completed. 'The Declaration's demand for social justice in health matters and plea for urgent national and international action for health' may well have been 'at the heart of all of WHO's work during the period' (WHO 2011d: vii) but it failed to consider how the geographical maldistribution of health workers globally transferred capital resources to advanced industrialised countries or the significant subsidies those countries enjoyed as a result. These were clearly not regarded by WHO as a matter of health-related social justice.

To be fair, the WHO global strategic initiative, 'Health for All' (WHO 1981), did incorporate a commitment to addressing health worker-migration as part of its focus on health 'manpower' training as a vital factor of public health, and of its main target that 'all citizens of the world [should] attain by the year 2000 a level of health to enable them to lead socially and economically productive lives' (WHO 2011d: vii).[11] The strategy document states that amongst the actions to be taken 'at the international level' are that '[t]he developing and developed countries concerned will be brought together to agree on practical measures for preventing the brain-drain of health personnel' (ibid.: 67). Although WHO may have committed to promoting 'dialogues' between countries (WHO 1981: 84), in practice it went no further than the most tentative parts of the Mejia study. The focus of the strategy was the responsibilities of developing countries and the actions they would be encouraged to take with the support of WHO technical assistance and developed countries. In this, it was at least consistent with WHO Assistant Director-General, D. Tejada de Rivero, whose preface to the Mejia *et al.* (1979) study forewarned that:

> If 'Health for all by the year 2000' is to be more than an empty slogan, it is vitally important that the developing countries should turn away from the piecemeal solutions of the past and attempt not only to integrate all aspects of health care, including personnel, but to integrate the development of that health care with overall national development.
>
> (Mejia *et al.* 1979: xi)

WHO's lack of progress on this front may be explained by reference to the insufficient 'political will' available to translate the high levels of 'anxiety' and moral concern surrounding health worker-migration into a global agreement that would reduce, prevent or offset the impacts upon those countries unable to afford the losses. The presenting reasons for stalling WHO initiatives following the Mejia study were attributed to governments deciding they did not want to pursue the more detailed case-study analyses that were originally envisaged. These studies were intended to focus on contextualised patterns of migration in recipient and source countries and the domestic workforce planning measures needed to address these. Mejia's optimistic slant on this – that the original research programme was modified 'in the hope that its findings would be used in decision-making' (Mejia 1978: 208) and Mejia's appeal for a 'mutually beneficial approach to health migration in which developed countries would no longer unilaterally set the terms of health migration' (Bach 2004: 625) – may have been conditioned by wider institutional shifts in train.

The first aspect of this shift lay in apparent changes in the domestic governance of health worker-migration and -recruitment on the part of advanced industrialised recruiting countries. The WHO response may have been conditioned by evidence that some of these countries were tightening immigration and medical sector controls in ways that were impacting upon the international-national composition of health and medical workforces. Mejia *et al.* (1979: 28–31) showed a relative decline was taking place in the rate of growth of foreign physicians practising in the US and Canada. Immigration restrictions introduced by the US in 1977 were expected to restrict inflows of foreign physicians, while similar effects were foreseen as a result of other major recruiting countries (Australia, Canada, UK) also introducing registration restrictions.

A second aspect of the shifts was the changing balance of economic and political power within the UN. The rising power of developing countries was, by some accounts, expected to 'force recipient countries to pay more attention to the needs of donor countries' (Bach 2004: 625). It may have seemed that the tide was turning in favour of those who supported strengthening the UN's hand on the matter of brain drain of medical and other workers in support of developing countries. One aspect of this was the UN's New International Economic Order (NIEO) initiative (UNGA 1974a, 1974b) which set out a more influential role for the developing countries in all fields of international activity (UNGA 1974a) (see Chapter 2). This was to be implemented, inter alia, through a stronger role for the UN (via ECOSOC) to 'define the policy framework and coordinate the activities of all organisations, institutions and subsidiary bodies' within the UN system in relation to international economic cooperation (UNGA 1974b, article IX). It would build on the 'irreversible changes in the relationship of forces in the world', resulting not only from the liberation of countries from colonialism but also from the 'grave crises' which the world economy had undergone since 1970. These global crises disproportionately adversely impacted on developing countries not only in terms of economic downturn but also declining levels of financial and other assistance. They necessitated, in turn, 'the active, full and equal participation of the developing countries in the formulation and application of all decisions that concern the international community' (UNGA 1974a).

Coming at mid-point during the UN's Second Development Decade, the NIEO initiative represented a mid-term galvanising call for developed countries to support UN emergency measures and programmes for the most hard-hit developing countries. Yet its ambitions were clearly greater than this. The NIEO Programme of Action (UNGA 1974b) set out a range of measures to step up UN action with a view to realising a mode of economic development on more favourable terms to developing countries. These included promoting collective self-reliance and cooperation of developing countries to achieve an increased share of industrial production and world trade, better terms for access to development finance, and debt relief. It proposed codes of conduct in relation to transport and insurance, transnational corporations, and the transfer of technology as part of this programme. The UN did not shy away from proposing global regulatory initiatives in these areas to increase resources available to developing countries.

WHO may have lacked financial and political resources to assert a stronger discipline on governments, or to persuade them to change national policies, but activism elsewhere in the UN and wider movements in support of the NIEO could change the balance of power and force concessions from major recipient countries – even if largely symbolically. These wider shifts within the UN and ILO might, we contend, help explain why WHO did not advocate global initiatives to help curb the losses sustained by developing countries as a result of substantial emigration. WHO's was by any measure a timid response when the tide seemed to favour robust global policy approaches, backed up by international law, to regulate highly skilled (health) labour migration and recruitment.

## 4.2 Developing countries respond: activism at WHA

WHO's failure to build on its 'landmark study' in no way signalled the defeat of those calling for the global regulation of health worker-migration. Rather than conceding, developing country governments were increasingly direct in expressing frustration at WHO's failure. The Committees of the WHA were a crucial forum in which government delegates could freely express their 'anxiety' over the unfolding catastrophe, air their views about the unfavourable distribution of losses and gains of international medical and health worker-migration, and more generally keep up the pressure on WHO and developed recruiting countries to respond.

They made full use of their right to protest. At each WHA between 1973[12] and 1978[13] government delegates commented on the significance of health worker emigration for their countries' development prospects. Delegates were often excoriating in their criticisms. One from the government of Uganda, which otherwise expressed general appreciation of WHO's efforts to develop the medium-term programme for health manpower (1978–1983), offered damning criticism of it: 'His delegation deplored the absence from the medium-term programme of any mention of ways of reducing the undesirable migration of health manpower' (WHA 1978a: 408). There was no lack of appetite for assertive responses or calls for WHO to embark on more robust forms of international action to address the issues. Referring to an interim report to the 1976 WHA by Mejia on the study's progress, a government delegate from Gabon suggested that:

> The remuneration of health personnel was also an important question on which the Organization might make recommendations to Member States so that national health personnel would be suitably paid. That might contribute to preventing the migration or emigration of key personnel.
>
> (WHA 1976a: 438)

At the 1977 WHA, the delegate from the Syrian government said:

> It seems that, unless the countries receiving the migrants co-operate with the countries losing them in putting an end to such migration, any future effort in this direction will be fruitless. When newly graduated physicians and health technicians went to study abroad, this was presented as humanitarian assistance from the developed nations to the developing nations ... however, their assimilation and incorporation in the developed countries changed their training from a humanitarian service into egotism and selfishness; the impression is that it was never humanitarian, but just a means to overcome manpower shortages and to give our oppressed personnel the hard and exacting jobs that the citizens of the host country do not want. Once again we raise our voices and reiterate our demand to the beneficiaries from the 'brain drain' of physicians and technicians that they should limit residence permits to the period of specialization and training.... The trainees' country

of origin needs them more than a country that has hundreds or even thousands of such personnel.

(WHA 1977a: 182 part II)

In 1978 a government delegate from the German Democratic Republic commented that:

In view of the important effect of the 'brain drain' on training and research within the developing countries ... the multinational study being carried out by WHO on the migration of physicians and nurses might provide a basis for a convention on the prevention of the brain drain of medical manpower.

(WHA 1975: 343)

Other governments were more direct in urging WHO to continue its work beyond the Mejia study (and by implication the 1977 ILO Recommendation). From the government of Poland:

Migration takes away from the developing countries the most educated and most dynamic people, who could be useful not only for their health services but for the training of new personnel. I think that to have a full appraisal of the situation it would be necessary to estimate the financial consequences of migration and the resources invested by the World Health Organization and the developing countries in the training of doctors and nurses from the developing countries who now work in the developed countries. We are of the opinion that the Organization should study more thoroughly the problem of undesired migration....

(WHA 1978a: 156, part II)

And from the government of Bulgaria:

The [WHO] had now completed the first stage of the study on the causes and extent of the problem, and the various factors involved. The results should be published as soon as possible, so that WHO might proceed to the second stage: to find ways of stopping the 'brain drain'.

(WHA 1978a: 405 part II)

Over the decade, many developing country governments gave evidence of the nature and scale of the problem of emigration of medical personnel. In 1978, the government of India delegate, for example, testified that:

The number of physicians produced yearly in India was 12,500, and a total of approximately 190,000 physicians were registered at present. The loss of personnel, through emigration and through contractual service obligations to many developing countries, amounted to about 25,000 doctors, or approximately 12% of the national register.

(WHA 1978a: 392)

Of note is that developed recruiting countries were absent from those urging further work by WHO in the form of specific concrete follow-up to elaborate policy responses to curb the medical brain drain. One exception was the Canadian government, a major recruiting country of health personnel, whose delegate set out how his government was trying to help developing countries address their health workforce issues and suggested how WHO could assist:

> To diminish the migration of qualified health personnel, who were more useful in their countries of origin ... Canada would wish to have close cooperation with other Member States. Resolution WHA 29.72 (WHA 1976b) requested the Director-General 'to collaborate with Member States ... in the development of measures to control undesirable migration of health manpower.' It was up to WHO to find ways and means of doing more in that line. Such possibilities should be explored as contracts with individuals requiring them to return, or the award of qualifications not carrying with them or opening up the right to practise in the host country.
>
> (WHA 1978a: 410)

This otherwise reasoned exposition of the Canadian government's position probably did little to assuage the concerns of developing countries, highlighting as it did the depth of the gulf separating the delegate's proposals and those advocated by developing country governments.

Despite these protestations and helpful suggestions from governments, WHO did not pursue its work on the international migration of health workers. During the 1980s and most of the 1990s the issue of health worker-migration and -recruitment remained largely invisible in, if not absent from, WHO's agenda. References in WHO documentation to 'outflows', 'brain drain', and migration all but vanished. With the exception of a 'one-off' 1987 resolution primarily dedicated to 'balanced' health workforce development, no other resolutions, discussion papers or strategy papers were scheduled at the WHA. Seventeen years elapsed after the 1987 Resolution before WHO re-commenced work in this field. That work, which was understood to lead to a multilateral agreement, took a decade to culminate in the WHO Global Code of Practice (2010). Overall, 30 years elapsed since WHO's 1970s initiative before it was able to 'make good' on (some of) the demands from developing country governments (see Chapters 4 and 5).

In many ways, this silence was mirrored in the UN more widely. To the extent that the UNGA considered matters of staff development, training and workforce availability, the focus was purely on asserting the importance of 'developing human resources for development' with the framework of UN principles and did not include mention of international migration (1989 Resolution). References to 'brain drain' and migration of highly skilled workers were noticeably absent. The traction gained was brought to an abrupt halt. By the time it re-started, the economic, political and institutional landscape of global health-worker migration governance had altered radically. The intervening years brought significant changes to the institutional architecture and policy dynamics of global governance of health and migration. Neo-liberal globalisation brought a new focus on temporary and circular migration, systematic economic liberalisation, the creation of new institutional regimes governing trade, health, labour and development in which WHO and ILO were marginalised. These changes fundamentally altered the global policy 'space' which strongly conditioned prospects for any global action to curtail or mitigate health-worker migration. These developments are the subject of Chapter 4.

## 5 Conclusion

The events covered by this chapter are remarkable. The principal 'milestone' at this time was the first-ever multilateral agreement setting out the principles for international nurse recruitment and migration. ILO's 1977 Nursing Personnel Recommendation was exceptional by any standards. It was the first global policy instrument on any specific occupation of highly skilled workers or migrant care workers more generally (the only other to date being ILO's 2010 Recommendation on Domestic Workers). Despite reservations that its focus on one occupational category risked splintering ILO's international labour standards regime, it commanded universal support. It was a vital instrument in the elaboration of ILO's gender equality, labour migration and social protection regimes, WHO's right-to-health regime, and the UN's human rights and development regimes. It was a practical and feasible multi-stakeholder response to the growing 'moral concern' and 'anxieties' of the international community, most notably developing source countries, that were mounting in the wake of repeated warnings that unhindered health worker-migration and -recruitment would seriously compromise universal health care and global public health. Being occupation-specific and not principally about stemming health-worker migration no doubt rendered the proposal and conclusion of the Recommendation more palatable than a wide-ranging multilateral agreement dedicated to addressing the migration and recruitment of multiple categories of health workers.

At the same time, the status of the Recommendation as a non-binding instrument (and much weaker than ILO Conventions) probably contributed to its speedy successful passage. The political method met the conditions for a successful global agreement. It was issue-specific and containable: the constellation of pressure, interests and political will aligned (Sauvant 2015). Its passage was indirectly facilitated by the UN's NIEO initiative and directly by ILO's labour migration activism, as well as ILO's tripartite governance structure: all proved conducive institutional conditions for universal agreement. WHO was instrumental in raising health-worker-migration and -recruitment as a factor compromising the realisability of the global right to health and universal health care objectives, and in this respect it was a vital element of the pressure on governments and others to act. Its focus on health workers brought sector-specific knowledge to the UN debate that otherwise focused on highly skilled labour in general. Yet WHO was not a conducive organisation for concluding a global agreement. The problem was that it 'looked south', and was preoccupied with the responsibilities of developing countries to improve their production and retention of health workers, while neglecting the responsibilities of developed countries to desist from recruiting those workers. It failed to take forward the modest work undertaken by the Mejia study into its strategic priorities on universal health and health care, and confined its role in global policy development to those governments that specifically requested help.

Despite repeated, increasingly vocal, frustrated calls by developing country governments in successive WHAs that it should take action to address the international causes of health-worker shortages, WHO proved spectacularly incapable of responding within the confines of a governance and policy-formation structure constituted exclusively by national ministries of health. The challenges faced by WHO in consolidating its (modest) landmark study on physician and nurse migration provide an important insight into the constraints which it, like other UN agencies, faced in building on the momentum in global policy development gained at the time.

For all its strengths, the efficacy of the Nursing Personnel Recommendation was severely limited by its lack of implementation. In principle, it had great strengths: mobilised, active constituencies (governmental and non-governmental advocacy actors) with access to the implementation mechanism. That it is not legally binding is secondary to the fact that it remained so poorly implemented. The silence of the very constituencies on which the Recommendation was reliant to become a 'living policy' is remarkable. Especially noteworthy is the absence of the labour unions that had helped bring it into existence. This was a policy space vacated by employers and governments: while ILO and WHO successfully articulated a normative-based global policy framework it was undermined in terms of influence and effectiveness by the failure of ILO and its constituents to devise and embed a programme capable of sustaining pressure on governments to implement its principles. ILO's framework to regulate nurse migration and recruitment remains as valid today as it did in 1977. Indeed, as Chapters 4 and 5 show, many of the issues contained in this instrument later resurfaced in WHO instruments three decades later, notably in Resolution WHA54.12 on Strengthening Nursing and Midwifery (WHA 2001) and WHO's 2010 Global Code of Practice on the International Recruitment of Health Personnel.

Looking over the first phase in the development of this global policy field, following the initial mandate for UN action in the early 1960s, we can appreciate that it developed rapidly, moving from awareness-raising to scientific diagnosis to policy proposals. As the principal institutional locus of global policy-making at the time, the UN's authority was unquestioned. This was an expansionist period at the UN, which was building its institutional capacity, extending its competence, and building a cosmopolitan liberal ethical development framework. The global policy field was constructed by multiple social actors from the outset: UN bodies and agencies, governments, employers and workers organisations. The role played in global policy formation by non-state advocacy actors (scientific experts, NGOs) interacting with state actors was crucial.

WHO was a laggard in this nascent policy field. Its involvement was spurred by wide-ranging UN activism but its ambitions were decidedly limited in comparison with the radicalism of other UN agencies. The field was from the outset led by agencies other than WHO, notably ILO, UNESCO and UNCTAD. Latin American and African offices of WHO were also at the forefront of the multicontinental campaigns to elicit WHO action. Yet WHO seemed a reluctant participant. It was the sustained efforts of the combined forces of other social actors – governments, international civil servants, labour groups – that elicited an eventual response to their persistent calls for concerted attention to (and action on) the intertwined human health resource and public health crises enveloping many developing countries. Diverse initiatives across multiple forums and organisations outside of WHO were significant in keeping these issues 'alive', especially in the face of the challenges WHO faced in sustaining, let alone propelling, its modest study on international physician and nurse migration.

From its earliest days, the global policy field developed within a space carved out at the intersection of several UN normative and legal regimes: labour, international migration, health services, international development, equality and human rights. Our in-depth tracing of developments within them and the interactions between them has aimed to help improve understanding of the complex institutional conditions of global policy formation. Our close reading has elucidated how these multiple global regimes have together shaped the on-going institutionalisation of the global policy field. In doing so, we have aspired to situate global health worker-migration policy within the context of the broader global institutional order, not only as manifested in the 'internal' dynamics of the UN but also in the wider global political economy of inequality and uneven development.

This first phase in global health worker-migration policy – the 1960s to the early 1980s – reveals that the ethical and institutional contours of the field were permissive of a broad spectrum of global policy approaches. The liberal global development regime inculcated global policies that fostered international migration of health workers (through Fellowships, harmonisation of medical curricula, establishment of right to migrate and migrant rights). It also enabled more radical global policy approaches to be worked up (compensatory facilities, labour rights, new international economic order) that aimed to improve development dividends for developing countries and their populations. Progress on both fronts was made, but the more radical (redistributive) approaches failed to make as much headway in becoming enacted and institutionally embedded. In this regard, this period provides in many ways an important benchmark against which to compare the ideas circulated and initiatives promulgated in later phases. It is to this contemporary period that we turn next. Chapters 4 and 5 cover the second principal phase in the development of this global policy field when, after a lapse of two decades, a resurgence of global activism led to a second global agreement – the 2010 WHO Global Code of Practice on the International Recruitment of Health Personnel.

# Notes

1 Apart from a brief reference to the study there is just one further reference to difficulties in the Western Pacific region. The report did not elaborate further on this though US DHEW (1975: 6) cites a study and conference in the WHO Western Pacific region.

2 'Medical immigration from Great Britain and Ireland' J.R. Seale (cited by WHO 1967: 36)

3 See also WHO 1967: 36.

4 A WHO Resolution setting out WHO's global priority objectives for the Second UN Development Decade (1970–1979) focused on health workforce planning as part of health systems planning, organisation and operation (WHA 1969c).

5 The Resolution produced a range of substantial outcomes relating to existing themes and issues: expanding training programmes, medical curriculum equivalence, training of teachers/tutors, improved teaching methods, country-specific mechanisms for health planning (WHO 2008, passim: 162–172). It recommended a WHO study of physician and nurse migration.

6 Modified 'in the hope that its findings would be used in decision-making' (Mejia 1978: 208), it reviewed literatures, stocks and flows of migrant physicians and nurses for 137 countries, migration determinants and trends, countries' actions and policy options.

7 Once ratified by governments, ILO Conventions are legally binding. Recommendations complement Conventions, providing additional guidance and practical advice.

8 Resolution WHA30.48 (WHA 1977b) concerned the role of nursing and midwives in primary care teams. It did not directly refer to international migration as a factor in the availability of sufficient numbers of nurses and midwives in the health workforce.

9 Section XIV of the Recommendation concerning methods of application refers only to 'national laws or regulations, collective agreements, works rules, arbitration awards or judicial decisions, or in any other manner consistent with national practice which may be appropriate, account being taken of conditions in each country' (Article 70).

10 Plantations Convention, 1958 (No. 110); Protocol of 1982 to the Plantations Convention, 1958; Plantations Recommendation, 1958 (No. 110) and Tenants and Share-croppers Recommendation, 1968 (No. 132). ILO instruments have been adopted only for hotel and restaurant workers, home workers and domestic workers.

11 Cognisant that human resources are a vital part of the resourcing mix for health services necessary to attain universal health it stated that 'most governments will no doubt wish to take vigorous action to ensure the availability of adequate numbers of the appropriate types of health personnel required to devise and implement the plan of action.' (WHO 1979: 26).

12 1972 Progress update report from Secretary-General (WHO 1972).

13 WHAs in 1979 and 1980 were devoid of any attention to health worker-migration or -recruitment.

# 4 The rise of 'ethical recruitment'

## Momentum without enforcement

## 1 Introduction

The 1980s ushered in a global political climate that was hostile to building on the achievements of the previous two decades. The momentum gained during the 1960s and 1970s which could have been built on to strengthen and broaden existing initiatives, notably the ILO Nursing Personnel Recommendation, gave way in the face of radically altered economic and social policy priorities. As a result, the prospects for further gaining ground substantially receded. The new political priorities crashed through the UN's Third Development Decade, along with the main concerns embodied in WHO's Alma-Ata Declaration (WHO 1978) and ILO's World Employment Programme (ILO 1976b). The UN's authority as the prime institutional actor was diminished in a global policy field that more and more took its inspiration from Washington. The neo-liberal ideology that took hold emphasised modes of development founded on 'free' markets, export-oriented production and industrialisation, privatisation of industry and services, deregulation of wage and price controls, reduced public expenditure, cuts in progressive taxation and a depreciation in organisations representing workers (Yeates 2001). Even if this project was unevenly realised in practice, it nevertheless reframed global policy making. Policy space to extend regulatory initiatives significantly decreased while those that promised 'light touch' regulatory modes and methods increased. Globally, non-binding agreements and self-regulation prevailed, except aspects that related directly to the 'free trade adventure' (Dunkley 1997) which ushered in legally binding trade agreements assigning corporate enterprises unprecedented rights.

The period that is the subject of this chapter and Chapter 5 – the late 1980s to 2010 – constitutes the second phase in the history of this global policy field. It represents a qualitatively different political economy of global policy making and global development. The present chapter discusses how these large-scale shifts conditioned the global governance of health, labour, social protection, migration and development and their impacts on global policy on health worker-migration. It argues that neo-liberal globalising forces stalled on-going efforts to address health worker shortages while facilitating health worker-migration not least through a renewed emphasis on international recruitment borne from alliances forged between state and capital. In parallel, social forces of dissent and contestation regenerated social movements that spurred non-state global advocacy actors and the creation of new alliances. These worked alongside developing countries and some developed countries to establish and define 'ethical' recruitment principles which proved critical in garnering support and exerting leverage to bring into effect a raft of initiatives in this area.

This chapter discusses why and how 'ethical' Codes of Conduct and/or Practice became the prevailing global policy approach to address the deepening global health workforce and public crises. We show that ethical codes of conduct and practice became multilateral over the course of the decade, echoing the multilateralisation of health worker-migration itself (Yeates 2009a, 2009b, 2012; Connell 2010), culminating in a second global agreement in this area – the WHO Global Code of Practice on the International Recruitment of Health Personnel (WHO 2010a) which was universally accepted by all WHO member states. We trace the negotiation of the Global Code through the institutional process, showing the social actors involved and the ideational forces and global politics of policy making that propelled and channelled their efforts. Overall, this second phase elaborated international standards governing the international recruitment of health workers but this was at a cost of reinforcing the use of 'soft' law and the principles of voluntarism and self-regulation. Chapter 5 continues our coverage of this period, focusing on the implementation of the Global Code.

## 2 Changing institutional architectures and dynamics of global governance

The negotiating context for global policy on health worker-migration in the 2000s was markedly different from the 1970s. Globalising forces that had taken hold during the intervening period fundamentally altered the global institutional architecture, the range of policy actors, and the ideas and discourses across many policy domains to re-shape the governance of international trade, the economy, health, labour and social provision. Non-UN IGOs supportive of neo-liberal global restructuring – notably WB, IMF and WTO – increased their influence over the parameters of global policy formation, while the influence of WHO, ILO, UNCTAD and UNESCO was drastically curtailed. Having sought to regulate highly skilled international migration and outflows of capital investment in the interests of developing countries, the latter group of IOs felt these 'cold winds' most keenly. This section summarily outlines key contours of this changing global governance showing its pertinence for global policy on health worker-migration and -recruitment.

### 2.1 Global trade and business governance

The global trade in services agenda became increasingly relevant to global policy on health worker migration during the 1990s. The same countries that had pursued an 'empty seat' policy at UNCTAD negotiations on technology transfer were arranging to establish a new global institution, WTO (1995), with a mandate to promote and secure legally binding multilateral free trade agreements. Its General Agreement on Trade in Services (GATS) is the most relevant such agreement in our context because it bears on the cross-border supply and provision of services by firms and 'natural persons' in the health sector and others. As such, it potentially impacts on the recruitment of highly skilled health workers (South Centre 2004). We emphasis *potentially* because although WTO has argued that GATS is tangential to health workers and does not prohibit governments from regulating the 'brain drain'[1] there is uncertainty about the agreement's future significance.[2]

In this respect, it is important to note that GATS is regularly invoked as a model multilateral agreement in discussions about the value of temporary and circular migration and of strengthening trade in health services more generally. WB has invoked the value of international services trade agreements, including GATS, to manage health worker-migration in the Caribbean (Yeates 2005a, 2010). Francois and Hoekman (2010) from the WB and the Centre for Economic Policy Research have argued that GATS' rules on temporary and circular migration could mitigate the effects of 'brain drain' on source countries.[3] IOM's World Migration Report (IOM 2006) supported the position that GATS could 'enhance the positive contribution of migration by offering more predictability and market access for temporary labour migrants' (WHO 2006b: 15). The potential of GATS has also arisen in the GFMD process, not least because of the perceived value of a multilateral agreement available on a non-discriminatory basis to all WTO Member States over bilateral agreements:

> While limited in application, Mode 4[4] has the comparative advantage of eliminating the need for countries to negotiate a myriad of separate bilateral agreements. Efforts should continue to expand the application of Mode 4 to achieve the developmental impacts aimed for through bilateral channels.
>
> (GFMD 2008: 62)

This appetite for harnessing the potential of international trade agreements in support of temporary migration to enhance development dividends to source countries was not universally accepted. The concern was that multilateral trade instruments would promote greater reliance on trade-based temporary (and circular) forms of migration in the health workforce sector and that without checks on recruitment and compensatory measures trade agreements would become little more than agreements to provide quotas of temporary health workers with inferior working conditions and rights and without any of the corresponding development gains to source countries.

WHO has been surprisingly guarded about the significance of trade liberalisation for health worker-migration and health systems. Highlighting that GATS 'may be seen as having the potential to liberalize the temporary movement of people between countries, raising the earnings of skilled people, and enhancing their knowledge and competence' and that it is 'geared to a "brain circulation",

not a "brain drain", process' (WHA 2006b), it noted the 'opportunities and challenges' (WHO 2005: 4) of global trade and their increasing relevance to health
(WHO/WTO 2002). It requested that international trade agreements and remittances be the subject of research 'in order to determine any adverse effects and
possible options to address them' in Resolution WHA57.19 (WHA 2004) and
pledged to provide 'support and assistance to Member States in the development
of policies to address the relationship between trade and health' (WHA 2006c).

WHA, as always, reflected more diverse views, including outright opposition
to trade in health services. The EU representative urged WHO to 'provide
support to Member States for building a knowledge base and better understanding the public health implications of bilateral and multilateral trade agreements' (WHA 2006d: 136), but developing countries were far more forceful in
voicing their concerns. Summarising the views of the Eastern Mediterranean
governments, the Tunisian representative argued that free trade agreements
could exacerbate the depletion of qualified professionals from the region and
'create shortages that threatened the sustainability of essential health services'
(WHA 2006d: 134). The Venezuelan government argued that 'national public
health must come before the rights deriving from free trade', emphasised that it
rejected free trade agreements that created inequalities and worsened poverty,
and urged WHO member states to 'adopt energetic measures' to counter the
international migration of health workers in order to stem international trade that
impaired health care programmes in poor countries (WHA 2006d: 137). The representative speaking on behalf of African governments pointed to institutional
fragmentation threatening public health and health system capacities to deal with
the impacts of international trade on health. In particular, he identified the
'[limited] capability of national authorities to negotiate effectively at WTO
meetings in order to maximize health-related benefits, particularly since such
negotiations were usually led by trade ministries, which often collaborated insufficiently with the health sector in developing country positions' (WHA 2006d:
138). Several representatives expressed their disappointment that WHO's request
for observer status at WTO General Council had not been considered.

Even in the absence of tangible evidence about the direct impact of GATS on
migration policies in the health sector, the self-evident 'trade creep' (Koivusalo
2014) in health was a growing concern. This is because while WTO was instituting legally binding rules permissive of greater international trade, global initiatives that instituted human rights and social responsibility 'safeguards' on the
conduct of transnational corporations such as those operating in the health sector
and in workforce recruitment and staffing and to hold governments accountable
for monitoring such corporations' business practices were founded on non-
binding rules and voluntary agreements. Global initiatives such as OECD Guidelines for Multinational Enterprises (OECD 1976),[5] UN Global Compact[6]
(established 1999), and ILO Tripartite Declaration of Principles concerning
Multinational Enterprises and Social Policy (agreed in 1997[7]) – and much later
UN Guiding Principles for Business and Human Rights (UNGP 2011) (see
Chapter 7) – grew from concern about human rights abuses by corporations

across their supply chain operations and laid down minimum standards for businesses to adhere to and human rights monitoring mechanisms. However, they share a voluntary approach to compliance and are the subject of much criticism.[8] Although the updating of the UNGP in 2011 strengthened monitoring and implementation mechanisms, at the time the supervisory machinery of these initiatives was not at all robust. There was no mandatory monitoring or reporting requirement placed upon business or governments and those gaps were filled by NGOs and trade unions.

### 2.2 Global health governance

The global health landscape had changed considerably, becoming more crowded and more complex. Neo-liberal health reforms, a growing range of policy actors in global health and a declining budget combined to diminish the authority, leadership capacity and resources of WHO and, in turn, its ability to convene and lead global health initiatives. The entry of other IGOs, notably WB, IMF and OECD, together with non-state private corporate and philanthropic actors, some of which had explicit and central commitments to health and their own programmes (Youde 2012), altered the institutional, ideational and funding sources underpinning health sector reforms which momentous implications for health systems and population health especially in the global South (Martens and Seitz 2015; Adams and Martens 2015; Martens 2014; Storeng 2014).

The growing dominance of WB in global health during the 1990s was a significant development, especially for developing countries which formed the lion's share of WB lending recipients. WB did not have an overt policy on health worker-migration or -recruitment, but its effects on health workforces were felt through its health sector and social protection reforms.[9] Its population, health, nutrition and social protection agendas, bolstered by its lending on health and health-related projects and its generation of neo-liberal bodies of knowledge generation through research and policy analysis programmes, surfaced in its guidance that limited the options for governments wishing to extend socially equitable health services coverage, including more robust health workforce strategies. IMF loan conditions echoed those of WB (O'Brien 2014), further constraining the policy space available to expand health workforces and improve working conditions. OECD's work on health sector reforms was influential in OECD Member States, developing countries through the OECD Development Advisory Committee (an important influence on international development policies and aid agencies). WHO increasingly aligned itself with WB health care policies and OECD concerns about controlling rising health care costs (Koivusalo and Ollila 2014).

The proliferating structures and actors in global health governance, notably the growth of global health partnerships, reflected growing political support for global health (Lidén 2014) but also detracted from reforms that would strengthen existing organisations with explicit health mandates and made the work of coordinating global and national responses much more difficult (Youde 2012).

Funding for global health had increased but it was mostly channelled outside WHO. During the period 1990–1997 ODA and non-governmental funding for health increased by 49 per cent, most of which came in the form of bilateral funding and from a significant increase in WB health spending (Lidén 2014). That funding was, moreover, increasingly disease-led and donor-led at the expense of health sector strengthening as a whole.[10] WHO faced declining funding for its core activities (and had been forced to make prospective cuts to its programme budget on health personnel) (WHO 1993). The decline in its core funding in real terms was amplified by an apparent disconnect between the priorities of health ministries (which govern WHO) and ministries of foreign affairs and development assistance (which provide the bulk of financing for global health through ODA) (Lidén 2014). In addition, an increasing number of WHO activities were financed from extra-budgetary sources that nevertheless relied heavily on the regular budget for administrative and technical support, further aggravating the strain on WHO funding and its activities. This inevitably impacted on what WHO was capable of achieving, including in relation to technical assistance for health workforce strengthening (see Chapter 3). Its 'voice became less one of unquestioned authority but increasingly only one of several opinions' (Lidén 2014:145). Worse still, it was increasingly enlisted as a technical partner to other global health funds (e.g. Global Fund) and its normative work was reined in (Lidén 2014; Koivusalo and Ollila 2014). A further issue was WHO's apparent acquiescence to a trade-led global health policy. Global health policy increasingly came to be inflected by trade priorities and business interests and this was a contested interface around which national and international NGOs campaigned hard (Koivusalo and Mackintosh 2011).

Four consequences of these developments are worth highlighting. First, WHO's greater reliance on ad hoc sources of funding was increasingly tied to selective programmes based on donors' priorities rather than global health priorities (Lidén 2014), reducing that part of WHO's work which was less obviously outcome-oriented, such as its normative, research or monitoring activities. Second, although voting rights remained vested with ministries of health, they had less control over WHO activities that were (increasingly) financed from external funds (Koivusalo and Ollila 2014). Third, the increased tendency to define global health policy issues as development issues, and to realise them through international development policy, brought with it a move to target provision on the poorest populations and countries. This was at the expense of the Declaration of Alma-Ata which favoured universal primary health care for all in all countries on the basis of equality and justice. Fourth, the increasingly trade-inflected global health agenda reduced WHO capability to pursue policies that would constrain global business interests and activities. The effects of the diminution of its institutional capacity, power and resources have been critically commented on in relation to its interfaces with corporate and business interests across a range of health issues, and is reflected, as discussed later in this chapter and in Chapter 5, in the weakness of its regulatory approach to health worker-recruitment.

## *2.3 Global labour governance*

The globalisation of trade, de-regulation of labour markets and the rise of precarious and informal forms of work worldwide severely tested global labour standards. Government measures stripped labour of social protection and livelihood support and helped channel it into expanding export streams structured by global supply chains and 'fed' by export-oriented modes of domestic production. These, together with regulatory frameworks promoting 'free' trade, were behind increases in high-skilled migration in particular, including in the health sector (Yeates 2009b). These developments challenged ILO because they required it to address 'non-standard' forms of employment and a wider range of employment relationships. Marginalised as an advocate of high international labour standards, ILO's 'natural constituencies' – trade unions and social democratic political parties and labour movements – were discouraged about its capability to effect significant improvements in working conditions and they re-focused their attention on inscribing labour rights into 'free trade' treaties and agreements that were proliferating under the auspices of the newly-created WTO (1995) and backed by the World Bank (O'Brien 2014). Global labour struggles were increasingly fought over in the sphere of international trade to insert social clauses into trade agreements.

The challenge for ILO was how to counter its marginalisation in global policy and governance, while defending its relevance as an advocate of social equity and fundamental labour rights in a world economy markedly different from that in which it came into existence and enjoyed hegemonic authority for much of the twentieth century. Turning a defensive position into an offensive one, its Declaration on Fundamental Principles and Rights at Work (ILO 1998) pledged all ILO states to uphold four 'core' labour standards (collective bargaining, the elimination of forced or compulsory labour, the abolition of child labour and the elimination of discrimination in respect of employment and occupation) and recognised that economic growth alone is insufficient to ensure socially equitable progress. This message was reiterated six years later through the World Commission on the Social Dimension of Globalisation in 2002 (ILO 2004b).

As responses to a generalised onslaught against labour regulation and binding initiatives of all kinds, these ILO initiatives, along with its actions to strengthen business governance (see Section 2.2, pp. 88–89 above), reasserted ILO's standing as a norm-generating body and helped it regain a new edge. However, they did not extend the range of rights or strengthen enforcement of extant standards and instead focused on a circumscribed set of 'core' labour standards and so are seen by some as a retreat (O'Brien 2014). This was not helped by ILO's de-emphasis on strengthening labour rights through statutory instruments in favour of implementing existing rights and the use of recommendations, codes of practice and the provision of technical assistance, or by its acceptance of a greater role for non-state provision in social protection (Deacon 2007, 2013). These responses did however win some concessions, however limited. WB and IMF took steps to regularise (but not formalise) their relationship with trade unions and the WB integrated core labour standards into its contracts for major construction projects and recommended that other multilateral development banks do the same. At the same time, WB and IMF continued to support modes of economic development 'free' from labour regulation.[11] In this context the ILO Declaration was important for reaffirming adherence to 'core' labour rights at the heart of a socially just globalisation and providing a discursive and institutional counter-balance to neo-liberal social and economic reform programmes.

### 2.4 Global migration governance

Compared with global health and trade, there had been fewer developments in global migration governance. States remained reluctant to cede sovereignty and 'thin' multilateralism (Betts 2011) prevailed. Nevertheless, the profile of international migration as a global policy issue had been raised by a number of initiatives. These included the UN International Convention on All Migrant Workers and their Families (1990) which set out an approach based on human rights and equality to how states can treat 'regular' migrant workers and their families.[12] In the mid-1990s, states' calls for greater debate on the issue of international migration helped trigger further UN initiatives on labour migration and establish new institutional machinery.

A renewed focus on high-skilled migration from developing countries came about through ILO's World Commission on the Social Dimensions of Globalisation (ILO 2004a, 2004b). This specifically considered how the absence of a multilateral accord on migration led to 'the exodus from developing countries of highly qualified people' (ILO 2004a: 19) and proposed 'Policy Coherence Initiatives' to develop a common, integrated approach to global migration. The lead up to this was an ad hoc Commission on Human Security (CHS) (CHS 2003) which set an agenda for strengthening global migration governance based on 'managed and predictable migration policies'.[13] It underscored the need to ensure that countries could benefit more from the 'brain gain' rather than on stopping the 'brain drain', and in doing so emphasised national policies to facilitate migrants maintaining their links with source countries (through, for example, rights to own property, vote, hold dual citizenship) so as to attract the return of skilled migrants, either permanently or temporarily (CHS 2003). However, it failed to endorse the need to regulate highly skilled health (and other) worker recruitment as a global policy issue. Such was the pace of developments in this area that a new forum, the UN High-Level Dialogue on Migration and Development (2006), was established for states to openly reflect on the appropriate location for a multilateral debate on migration. It set in train a new inter-state, multilateral process for considering how more coherent international migration cooperation might be developed and led to the GFMD being established in 2007 that raised the migration-development nexus as a core concern of multilateralism in this area (Betts 2011; Yeates and Pillinger 2013). Finally, IOM, which works principally on forced/conflict-based migration and refugee programmes, including return programmes, and at the time was outside of the UN system, helped shape the turn towards circular migration as a core theme in these debates. Despite not having a regulatory or standard-setting role to rival ILO, or command over resources to rival WB, its promotion of diaspora exchanges and knowledge transfer through 'brain circulation' has influenced the rise of diasporic migration approaches, including in the health sector (see also Chapter 6).

### 2.5 Global advocacy actors and networks

By the early 2000s, two decades of neo-liberalist global disinvestment strategies had 'hollowed out' state powers, weakened national health systems worldwide and worsened health inequity. Little had been achieved in addressing the underlying causes of high indebtedness, social inequality and poverty, poor quality health services or health sector under-funding and under-performance. These injustices were, however, also sources of renewal. Civil society coalition campaigns involving 'new' and traditional social movements, NGOs and the labour movement were increasingly cooperating, most often in the sharing of information and debate, but increasingly also in their actions. Essentially oppositional in challenging growing corporate power and the global institutionalisation of 'free trade' norms, laws and modes of regulation, they provided an important countervailing force contesting the centralisation of power, especially bureaucratic and economic power, and increased the political and economic costs of pursuing 'free trade' agreements and neoliberal-inspired health and welfare retrenchment (Keck and Sikkink 1998, 1999; Tarrow 1995; Yeates 2001). By 'troubling' the smooth progression of such agreements and initiatives, they disrupted the ineluctability of neo-liberal globalisation and opened up political space for alternative initiatives to emerge.

Alliances of state and non-state social democratic forces campaigned globally during the 1990s for alternative modes of global development, and in 2000 the UN Millennium Development Goals (MDGs) were launched (Cheru and Bradford 2005). As a statement of global social policy goals, the MDGs were significant. Although they did not include any specific initiatives on health workforces or international migration and recruitment, they did contain health goals and spurred international organisations, notably ILO and WHO, to re-engage with these issues. Importantly, they stimulated global estimates of health worker densities needed to attain the MDG health goals. The 'return' of health workforce issues onto the global policy agenda was facilitated by a markedly changed advocacy environment in which key non-state actors such as GHWA, trade unions and other civil society organisations (CSOs) were extensively and effectively networked, organised and vocal in connecting advanced countries' recruitment strategies, the globalisation of labour markets for highly skilled workers, the dilapidation of national health systems, and the unfolding global public health crisis (see Section 4 below).

In an institutional landscape scarred by nearly three decades of neo-liberal globalism, these developments combined in different ways to focus attention on the ethics of international recruitment. They changed the balance of political power sufficiently so that by the early 2000s the momentum to institute a more socially responsible approach to the recruitment of overseas-trained health workers had taken hold. This impetus proved sufficiently dynamic, and was supported by a powerful array of state and non-state coalitions that enabled a second multilateral agreement to be secured within a decade.

## 3  The rise of ethical recruitment codes and frameworks

The opening years of the twenty-first century witnessed the introduction of a raft of ethical recruitment codes and frameworks broadly regulating the conditions under which overseas-trained health workers could be recruited. These initiatives were instituted by major recruiting countries in higher-income countries and negotiated outside of the UN system. Voluntary 'ethical' codes of practice developed through multi-stakeholder negotiations have been one route where 'the voices of employers, recruiters, unions, and migrants themselves' are involved (PSI 2012a: 2). During the course of the decade, what started off as unilateral initiatives increasingly became multilateral ones involving an ever-greater number of signatory governments.

The earliest of these was a unilateral initiative, spearheaded by the UK government. Its Code of Practice for NHS Employers (2001) is a binding instrument that specifies principles and standards for the recruitment and employment of overseas health workers, with a particular emphasis on prohibiting recruitment of health workers in developing countries experiencing severe shortages of health care workers.[14] Its original restricted scope to public sector employers (in the NHS) was a significant loophole because private companies are major recruiters of staff that often end up working in the NHS. The UK Code was subsequently strengthened in 2004 to require all public, private and independent health care organisations and recruitment agencies to align their practises with the Code's principles. It is unclear how effective the subsequent strengthening of the Code has been.

This Code was instrumental in revitalising a long-standing UN principle regarding the implementation of normative standards and goals through inter-state cooperation in the form of bilateral agreements (see Chapters 2 and Chapter 6). This is because under the Code recruitment is only permitted from countries that have consented to do so through bilateral agreements or Memoranda of Understanding (MoUs). The UK signed a series of bilateral agreements with the Philippines, South Africa, China, Pakistan and India on this basis (see Chapter 6). The UK–Philippines MoU (2002) enabled the UK to recruit registered nurses and other health care professionals, while the agreement with India stipulated that agencies can recruit health workers from India except the four states that receive DfID aid (Andhra Pradesh, Madhya Pradesh, Orissa, West Bengal). The UK Code marked a shift in its policy on international recruitment with greater emphasis on recruitment from EU countries. Nevertheless, its focus on limiting migration from poor countries to the UK without addressing the underlying inequalities that propel this migration in the first place has been judged as 'ethically unsatisfactory' for '[failing] to provide an effective response to the detrimental impact of staff loss on low-income, staff-short health systems' (Mensah *et al.* 2005: 11).

The Commonwealth Code of Practice for the International Recruitment of Health Workers (2003) is non-binding on the 53 member states of the Commonwealth. Like the UK Code of Practice, it discourages recruitment from countries that experience shortages, promotes ethical recruitment practices and emphasises the role of bilateral agreements in implementing the provisions of the Code. However, unlike the UK Code, the Commonwealth Code suggests that compensation should be made by the governments of recruiting countries to mitigate the impact of the loss of health workers in developing countries, particularly the loss of investment in training. However, only a small number of developing countries actually signed up to the Commonwealth Code and uncertainty remains over the its status. For this reason, other measures have taken precedence, notably the WHO Global Code (Labonté *et al.* 2007; Pagett and Padarath 2007).

The best example of multi-stakeholder initiatives that emerged during this time is the Alliance for Ethical International Recruitment Practices, which later formed into a division of the USA's CGFNS Alliance, the Commission on Graduates of Foreign Nursing Schools. This is the only international initiative on health worker-recruitment entered into or negotiated by the US government. Its Voluntary Code of Ethical Conduct for the Recruitment of Foreign-Educated Health Professionals to the United States (Alliance Code) was launched in 2008 when negotiations on the eventual WHO 2010 Code were already underway. The Alliance Code covers nursing only, and brings together in dialogue and cooperation the recruitment industry, regulators, professional organisations, trade unions, employers and recruiters, providing detailed guidance to individuals and organisations working in the USA's nurse recruitment industry. Adherence to the Alliance Code is voluntary and relies on self-monitoring by members and a system for certifying recruiters. The Code sets out minimum standards for employers and recruiters, including possibilities for applicants to review contracts and support for workers to adjust to living and working in the USA, and identifies best practices protecting the rights of foreign-educated nurses. It refers to mitigating the harms to source countries health care systems but does not refer to offering compensation to those countries (Shaffer *et al.* 2016).

The EPSU-HOSPEEM Code of Conduct on Ethical Cross-Border Recruitment and Retention in the Hospital Sector (EPSU/HOSPEEM 2008) stands out for being the first European social partner agreement to cover the hospital sector in Europe. An agreement between the European Hospital and Health care Employers' Association (HOSPEEM) and the European Federation of Public Service Unions (EPSU), it asserts the central role of employers and unions, along with governments and other stakeholders, in ensuring accessible, high-quality and sustainable public health services, including labour protection and effective management of health workforces. EPSU found that the Code had been used in varying and effective ways in Bulgaria, Denmark, Finland, Germany, The Netherlands, Norway, Slovakia and Sweden (EPSU/HOSPEEM 2012). The Code has promoted good cooperation amongst trade unions in Europe and helped inform health workers about ethical recruitment processes beyond Europe (ibid.).

Other non-binding instruments have been agreed by professional bodies such as the World Health Association and the International Council of Nurses. The Melbourne Manifesto (WONCA 2002) functioned as a 'call to action'[15] and is most notable for its focus on social justice and equity in health care and its elaboration of various measures to realise a 'just' global distribution of health workers. This includes the need for source and destination countries to improve workforce planning and retention, and measures to address rural and urban areas that face shortages of health care professionals. It emphasises providing education and training, improving working conditions, implementing ethical recruitment, exchanges and partnerships with training institutions between source and destination countries, making better use of skills in the workforce and only promoting outward migration in those countries that have an oversupply of health workers (WONCA 2002).

Despite the limitations of these ethical initiatives (Willets and Martineau 2004; Yeates and Pillinger 2013; Bourgeault *et al.* 2016) they paved the way for a multilateral agreement that all countries could support. They helped kickstart a 'new' global policy dynamic and trajectory by forging a pathway for voluntary initiatives to take hold as the 'default' mode of global regulation in this policy field. They also 'tested' the willingness of major recruiting countries to support a framework specifying the conditions under which they could embark on international recruitment. In addition, they generated new coalitions of state and non-state advocacy actors revolving around health worker-migration and -recruitment in ways that forged connections with the issue of equitable health care. Finally, they shifted the focus from migration to recruitment, and specifically 'ethical' recruitment practices (Dhillon, Clark and Kapp 2010). In this, they helped reframe the debate such that the responsibilities to manage migration were not only source countries (emphasised by WHO during the 1970s – Chapter 3) but also those of countries of destination, especially the higher-income ones (emphasised by the ILO Nursing Personnel Recommendation – Chapter 3). Next, we turn to the negotiating context and outcomes in relation to the second multilateral agreement in this global policy field – the WHO Code of Practice.

## 4  WHO Global Code of Practice on the International Recruitment of Health Personnel

### 4.1  Background to the negotiation for the Global Code

The WHO Global Code resulted from multiple institutional and political pressures for a global policy solution to the global maldistribution of health workers. The significant increase in health worker-migration since the Mejia study (see

Chapter 3) highlighted the misalignment of global development objectives, global policy instruments and national practices. The complexity of health work-force challenges, rising demand for health services, and the adverse impacts of inequitably distributed health workers globally strengthened and added urgency to renewed calls for global responses. These calls were borne of frustration with a global policy landscape comprising an ILO Recommendation on international nurse recruitment that had never been fully implemented let alone monitored (see Chapter 3), the liberalisation of highly skilled labour migration, and the new exigencies demanded by the MDGs' global health goals (Taylor and Dhillon 2011).

Civil society was highly influential in this process. The international multi-stakeholder Health Worker Migration Initiative (HWMI), established as a part-nership between the NGO Realizing Rights: the Ethical Global Initiative and the Global Health Workforce Alliance (GHWA) in 2006 in response to the height-ened concerns about the need for global responses to health worker-migration and -recruitment was a crucial actor during the negotiations. GHWA's advocacy role was also instrumental in the establishment of the high-level Global Policy Advisory Council to support the development of the Global Code. The secretar-iat for the Global Code comprised Realizing Rights and a WHO-led Technical Working Group formed by the WHO Department of Human Resources for Health. The Global Migration Policy Advisory Council brought together Minis-ters of Health, Labour and International Development from source and destina-tion countries, leading health, labour and migration experts, and ILO and IOM. Co-chaired by the Hon. Mary Robinson, former President of Ireland and UN High Commissioner for Human Rights and Dr. Francis Omaswa, Executive Dir-ector of GHWA, the Advisory Council played a significant role in international diplomacy through research and consultations and by engaging political support from amongst Ministers and governments and high-level representatives of IOs.

WHO's constitutional mandate on health personnel training plus its long-standing focus on nursing and midwifery workforces and strengthening health systems (see Chapter 3) proved to be its entry point into this renewed global policy landscape.[16] Resolution WHA54.12 (WHA 2001) formally initiated its work on nursing and midwifery migration and recruitment as a matter for global health policy.[17] Whereas WHO had previously defined this as an issue for, and the responsibility of, developing countries (see Chapter 3), it now defined it as a 'global' issue (i.e. for all countries). WHO was mandated to support Member States 'in setting up mechanisms for inquiry into the global shortage of nursing and midwifery personnel, including the impact of migration, and in developing human resources plans and programmes, including ethical international recruit-ment' (WHA 2001: para. 2.1). Three years lapsed before the matter came before the WHA (Resolution WHA57.19, WHA 2004). Curiously, this made no refer-ence to the 2001 resolution, but instead to two from three decades earlier (WHA 1969b, 1972). This broadened the focus on all health workers rather than just nurses and midwives. The 2004 Resolution formally requested that WHO initiate a programme of research on the international migration of health personnel including in relation to trade agreements and remittances, and to develop a Code of Practice.

As during the 1970s in the lead up the ILO Nursing Personnel Recommendation (see Chapter 3) WHA continued to be a key forum in which developing country governments testified to the extent, causes and impacts of health workforce shortages and voiced their demands that WHO act to address national health workforce shortages caused by the overseas recruitment of their 'capital assets'. Throughout the 1980s and 1990s they did so regularly, with an increased intensity during the 1990s. Most active and vocal were African and Caribbean governments, with India and Turkey also following suit (WHA 1983a, 1988, 1989, 1991, 1992, 1993, 1996). However, WHO showed itself to be lamentably disengaged and unresponsive to the demands of the governments raising them.[18]

By the end of the 1990s WHO had finally woken up to the issue, passing three resolutions on health system strengthening in as many years which also called for adequate funding for its work.[19] The 1997 Resolution was reminiscent of more radical times (see Chapter 2) in calling upon developed countries 'to facilitate the transfer of materials, equipment, technology and resources to developing countries for health development programmes that correspond to the priority needs of those countries'. Indeed, this request was a scarcely-veiled reference for developed countries to halt the 'reverse transfers' involved in the global dynamics of health care which included the medical brain drain. This approach was reiterated in the 1999 Resolution, and together the three Resolutions marked the return of WHO to health worker-migration and -recruitment as a global health policy issue. It was the first mention WHO had made of either its previous work in the 1970s – now some two decades ago – or that of UNCTAD, ILO and UNESCO on reverse transfers of technology and the brain drain (see Chapters 2 and 3).

Calls for WHO action arose through its own organisational structures. Amplifying African governments' calls in the WHA for over three decades, the 52nd session of the WHO Regional Office for Africa stated that Member States should prioritise health workforce issues and measures to address the moral and ethical implications of health worker-recruitment from developing countries (WHO-AFRO 2002). The previous year Health Ministers from the Southern African Development Community (SADC) had criticised poor health workforce planning by recruiting countries in a stinging attack. Countries that actively recruited health workers from Africa were vociferously declared 'immoral', whose actions were likened to 'looting' on a scale 'similar to that experienced during periods of colonisation when all resources, including minerals, were looted to industrialised countries' (SADC 2001: 33, cited by Pagett and Padarath 2007). Just as developing countries were active within WHO so were developed ones. The only developed country to make any significant intervention at WHA during this time was New Zealand, which managed to make an ill-judged intervention at the 1986 WHA.[20] Instead, they pressed the case elsewhere within WHO. The UK DfID, for example, pushed for an ethical code of practice within WHO, reflecting the greater role that government aid agencies, as opposed to ministries of health, played in priority-setting of WHO (see Section 2.2 above). Thus, developing countries, represented by health ministries, used WHA to raise their priorities, while developed countries impressed theirs via health ministries in WHA *and* by international development ministries outside of it.

As in the first phase of the global policy field (see Chapter 2 and 3), wider UN initiatives on global migration governance were significant drivers. By 2004, when WHO was asked to start work on global shortages of health workers and develop a new global instrument, UN initiatives on labour migration were already advanced (see Section 2.3 above). ILO was already preparing its own multilateral initiative on a rights-based global labour migration policy (ILO 2004a)[21] which paved the way for the 2005 ILO Multilateral Framework on Labour Migration, a non-binding framework on migrants' access to rights. UN institutional machinery was being established to take discussions forward on global migration governance (see Section 2.3).[22] In short, WHO was able to draw energy and support from major UN-wide initiatives on global migration in relation to global development goals.

### 4.2 The negotiations leading up to the Global Code

The context in which WHO found itself leading the negotiations on a global ethical code of practice was in many ways not especially conducive (see Section 2.2 above). Yet the prospect of the MDGs and a new global development agenda on health plus the increased political and economic resources available in support of global health were clear opportunities for WHO to assert its authority as *the* prime *global* health agency. WHO had already been forced to cede to ILO the first multilateral agreement on health worker-migration and -recruitment (see Chapter 3) in the 1970s, so for the new Director-General, Gro Harlem Brundt-land, who was seeking to lead WHO into a stronger position following two decades of decline, getting behind the prospective Global Code would be an important platform to develop and showcase a new global health agenda, a potential means for supporting WHO's primary health care goals, while also demonstrating WHO's continued convening power and authority in global health.

The decision by WHA in 2004 to draw up a non-binding Code (Resolution WHA57.19, WHA 2004)[23] reflected the unanimous agreement of Member States to work with WHO through non-binding measures.[24] The decision to have a non-binding Code along the lines of the only other international Code (on the Marketing of Breast Milk Substitutes agreed in 1981) was agreed from the outset. That it was already decided that the WHO Code would be non-binding is a reflection of the wider currents in the global political economy of global social policy making. A non-binding Code of Practice fell well within the realms of WHO's Constitution and the limits of what governments would all agree to. WHO also argued at the time that a Global Code would help to achieve its other goals around primary health care (WHO 2009a). According to Taylor and Dhillon (2011) the choice of a non-binding Code also 'reflects more nuanced understanding by Member States of the nature and utility of binding and non-binding international legal instruments to further global health'. Pre-agreed as it was that anything 'stronger' (i.e. with 'legal bite' or force) was out of the scope of any eventual agreement, the actual content of the Code was left open for negotiation.

The potential for global action to mitigate the adverse effects of international recruitment was reflected in Resolution WHA57.19 (WHA 2004) calling for a Code of Practice on international recruitment on health personnel which made explicit proposals for measures to:

> develop strategies to mitigate the adverse effects of migration of health personnel and minimize its negative impact on health systems (para. 1);

> frame and implement policies and strategies that could enhance effective retention of health personnel including, but not limited to, strengthening of human resources for health planning and management, and review of salaries and implementation of incentive schemes(para. 2);

> use government-to-government agreements to set up health-personnel exchange programmes as a mechanism for managing their migration (para. 3);

> establish mechanisms to mitigate the adverse impact on developing countries of the loss of health personnel through migration, including means for the receiving countries to support the strengthening of health systems, in particular human resources development, in the countries of origin (para. 4).

WHO was also requested to:

> support efforts of countries by facilitating dialogue and raising awareness at the highest national and international levels and between stakeholders about migration of health personnel and its effects, including examination of modalities for receiving countries to offset the loss of health workers, such as investing in training of health professionals (para. 6);

> mobilize all relevant programme areas within WHO, in collaboration with Member States, in order to develop human-resources capability and to improve health support to developing countries by setting up appropriate mechanisms (para. 7).

Despite the UNGA mandate, the initial development of the Code 'lacked political support, resources and policy direction' (Taylor and Dhillon 2012). However, this shifted from 2006 when the World Health Report *Working Together for Health* (WHO 2006a) set out the global nature of the challenge of health workforce shortages. It estimated a shortage of more than 4.3 million health personnel across the world and highlighted that of the 57 countries with a critical shortage, 36 were in sub-Saharan Africa, and underlined growing awareness of the costs, often in human lives, of shortages of health workers. Following this, momentum for a Global Code increasingly came from developing countries which become more vociferous in their arguments for global action, particularly action that would compensate for the unfair effects of international recruitment on their capacities to realise core health goals.

Discussions at the World Health Assembly deliberating the draft text of Resolution WHA59.23 (WHA 2006a) indicated the negotiating challenges that lay ahead (WHA 2006d). One issue was the incorporation of compensatory mechanisms. A draft resolution proposed by the delegation of the government of Thailand suggested radical new measures were needed to tackle the chronic shortage of health workers through health system strengthening measures, including:

> encouraging direct financial support by global health partners, meaning bilateral donors, priority disease and intervention partnerships and global funds for health training institutions according to the prescription in *The World Health Report 2006* that of all new donor contributions for health, 50% should be dedicated to strengthening health systems, and 50% should be dedicated to the health workforce.
>
> (Ibid.: 141)

However, a weaker amended version stated that:

> establishing mechanisms to mitigate the adverse impact on developing countries of the loss of health personnel through migration, including means for the receiving countries to support the strengthening of health systems, in particular human resources development, in the countries of origin.
>
> (Ibid.: 148)

Also central to these discussions was the importance of the principle of the rights of health workers and the applicability of national and international human rights law, as embedded in existing voluntary Codes. As a result, the draft Article 4 referred to the human rights of health workers, and stated that their rights were to be treated in a manner consistent with the principles of fairness and equality. High-income countries rejected the relevance of this to the matter at hand. A further issue centred on the role that the Global Code should play in shaping bilateral cooperation. The language in the draft Code referred to the principle that 'states should refrain from active international recruitment unless there exist equitable arrangements to support recruitment activities'. This was deleted from the final text of the Global Code (Taylor and Dhillon 2012:10). There was also significant global pressure for governments to address ethical recruitment in the widest sense by taking into account the impact of health worker migration on the health systems of developing countries. Despite the efforts of high-income countries in shifting the focus of the Code towards recruitment in a more restricted sense, skilful negotiations and constant pressure from developing countries, whose presence in the negotiations involved senior diplomats and international lawyers, ensured that the final text kept some focus on health system sustainability (Article 5) and the collection and exchange of information on health worker migration (Articles 6 and 7) (Taylor and Dhillon 2012).

In terms of sources of political support, Norway was a leading country arguing that 'all countries abstain from targeted and active recruitment of health personnel from developing countries with critical shortages of health workers' (WHO 2010b: 5).[25] Its political leadership in advocating for the Global Code and supporting the engagement by developing countries during the negotiations helped secure its subsequent unanimous passage. As importantly, the issue galvanised WHO and was backed by political leadership at the 2006 UNGA Special Session on Migration and Development. It was also supported by the activism of HWMI (Taylor and Dhillon 2012).

Clearly, with a range of national and international ethical recruitment initiatives already, it would be hard for reluctant governments to ignore all of this. And this meant not just developing source countries, but developed recruiting countries too. It was vital that the agreement would have genuinely global applicability. The Global Policy Advisory Council, in particular, along with other leading advocates and several developing country and European governments, including Norway, argued strongly for an approach based on global solidarity and shared responsibility. WHO regional meetings also helped to raise the voice of governments in developing countries and bring the issue of global social justice and global responsibility into the centre of discussions.[26] This call was reflected in the discussions held during WHO regional meetings and consultations on the second draft code.

### 4.3  Gaining agreement for the Global Code

Negotiating the Code involved WHO in securing agreement from governments with a wide range of health systems and political interests. The agreement was particularly difficult to achieve in two key areas – provisions on the mutuality of benefits and the monitoring of health worker mobility – because of the resource implications of these provisions for countries (Buchan 2010). Despite this, the first draft of the Code drew on, but went further than, the texts of existing national and regional codes of practice on health worker-recruitment. It also drew on the detailed research and advocacy carried out by HWMI. On the basis of the first draft further consultations took place, including a global web-based public hearing held between September and October 2008. National and regional consultations were also carried out through WHO Committees of the European Region, South-East Asia Region and Western Pacific Region. Questions were raised at an early stage about how the Global Code would be implemented, with several destination country governments opposing a monitoring system. This issue was addressed in the first draft of the Code, with a mechanism for a 'robust and transparent framework for global governance, including voluntary mechanisms for effective and periodic information sharing, reporting and supervision of implementation' (Taylor and Dhillon 2012: 4).

A revised text was produced in January 2009 and presented to the 124th WHO Executive Board. This prompted a call for further consultations and parti-cipation with governments to gain support for the final text and its adoption. All six regional committees held further consultations on the Code during 2009, expressing support for a non-binding Code, but with some suggested revisions to the draft. The Africa, Europe and the Eastern Mediterranean committees sup-ported the draft Code. During the 144th session of PAHO's Executive Com-mittee (Washington DC, 22–26 June 2009), PAHO Member States raised the challenge of addressing the responsibilities of both source and destination coun-tries (WHO 2009b). Following the consultations through the regional commit-tees a number of new issues were addressed in the Code. During discussions on the second draft of the Code, at WHO Executive Board in 2009, several govern-ments (Mauritania on behalf of WHO Africa office, South Africa and Malawi) stressed the importance of enforcing the Code; other governments stressed the importance of the rights of health workers (Taylor and Dhillon 2012).

Two main thematic issues were addressed in the revised draft Code. The first concerned Member States' roles in achieving a balance between the rights, obligations and expectations of source countries, destination countries and migrant health workers. The second concerned the view that health worker-migration should have a net positive impact on the health system of developing countries and countries with economies in transition. This led to strengthening Article 5 on the mutuality of benefits, with a revised text stating that inter-national health personnel 'should be recruited in a way that seeks to prevent a drain on valuable human resources for health' (WHO 2009b: 3). Some regional committees went as far as suggesting that countries should not engage in active international recruitment of health personnel unless there were equitable bilat-eral, regional, or multilateral agreement(s) in place for this. Changes to Article 11 were also proposed relating to voluntary technical and financial mechanisms to strengthen the development of health systems in developing countries and countries with economies in transition. The revised draft Code also recom-mended that Member States seek

> to strengthen the balance between the rights of health personnel to leave their countries and the right of everybody to the enjoyment of the highest attainable standard of health in order to mitigate the negative effects of migration on health systems.
>
> (WHO 2009b: 3)

Further revisions included strengthening the text on national health workforce sustainability, with new provisions recommending that Member States consider a variety of measures to retain health workers.

A further contentious issue during the discussions on the draft Code (WHO 2010b) was the inclusion of strong procedural mechanisms in the Code, covering data collection, monitoring and implementation. These were opposed by many of the high-income countries, including the USA, Canada and the European Union, with some arguing that these provisions could only be fully implemented if the Code was binding and that they had no place in a voluntary code (WHO 2010b). In fact, the introduction of these procedural mechanisms helped to appease the concerns of some developing countries that a non-binding code would lack strong incentives and mechanisms for implementation. Several African states (South Africa, Zimbabwe, Kenya and Botswana) took a firm stance on the maintenance of strong legal and institutional provisions in the draft text (Taylor and Dhillon 2012). The final text of the Code retained this approach by including detailed legal, institutional and data sharing mechanisms (Articles 7 and 8) and implementation (Article 9). This was a significant breakthrough, ensuring a mechanism for monitoring the implementation of the Code every three years with first reporting starting in 2012 (Article 10).

One of the strengths of the draft Code was that it brought mutuality of benefits to the centre of international health worker recruitment discussions (Buchan 2010). During discussions in 2009 on the second draft of the Code, several governments from developing countries, amongst them governments from the WHO-AFRO region and Sri Lanka, argued strongly for the WHO Code to include compensatory mechanisms for developing countries negatively affected by the outward migration of health workers to developed countries (Taylor and Dhillon 2012). This focus on compensatory mechanisms was closely tied to ethical recruitment practices which needed to take into account the impact of migration on developing countries' health systems, shortages of health workers and the loss of resources and investments in education training health personnel (Pillinger 2013; Agwu and Llewelyn 2009; Mensah *et al.* 2005). In terms of mechanisms for compensation, the likelihood was that these would be excluded from the Global Code, although they remained on the table during the final stages of negotiation for the Code (WHO 2009b). This proved one of the main difficulties for the negotiations. African countries, which lose a large proportion of their trained doctors to Europe and America, sought stronger measures to mitigating the negative impact of outward migration. The issue of compensation was dropped as developing countries represented in the final negotiations for the Global Code in the UNGA were aware that funding for developing countries was an issue that high-income countries would not budge on. As the delegate of Brazil noted, 'the Code effort should not be held back by lack of agreement on compensation that maybe, in the future, there could be meaningful discourse on compensation' (Taylor and Dhillon 2012:10). Destination countries were opposed to incurring any direct financial costs or establishing systems for compensating source countries for their loss of health workers. These consultations led to a revised wording based in paragraphs 3.3 and 11.3 and formed the basis for heated debate in WHA.

The final Code reflected these concerns of destination countries and included weakened provisions relating to mutuality. The language of mitigation was framed in terms of 'should be considered' and 'to the extent possible', rather than in terms of stronger provisions that require governments in developed countries to act to mitigate the loss of health workers:

> The specific needs and special circumstances of countries, especially those developing countries and countries with economies in transition that are particularly vulnerable to health workforce shortages and/or have limited capacity to implement the recommendations of this Code, should be considered. Developed countries should, to the extent possible, provide technical and financial assistance to developing countries and countries with economies in transition aimed at strengthening health systems, including health personnel development.
>
> (WHO Code, para. 3.3)

### *4.4 Adoption of the Global Code*

The WHO Global Code of Practice on the International Recruitment of Health Personnel was agreed at the 63rd World Health Assembly in May 2010 (WHA 2010; WHO 2010a), led by the governments of Norway and Thailand (GHWA 2012). Margaret Chan, the-then WHO Secretary General heralded the passage of the Global Code as a 'real gift to public health everywhere' (Taylor and Dhillon 2012: 11). Its unanimous adoption was the outcome of skilful negotiations, health diplomacy, effective multi-stakeholder advocacy networks in a context of political recognition of the 'magnitude and urgency of the challenge of health worker migration' (Taylor and Dhillon 2012: 11).

Even though the ILO 1977 Nursing Personnel Recommendation had already laid the groundwork (see Chapter 3), the Global Code is seen to reflect the long-established need for a global instrument to regulate and assure ethical international recruitment covering all health workers. Nevertheless, the Code recognises that ethical recruitment is an issue that goes beyond national workforce planning and recruitment and that it is an issue of a truly global dimension. It fills an important global policy gap in recognising the need for global action to address the transnational nature of migration and public health. Although it is voluntary and therefore non-binding, it brought the debate about ethical recruitment firmly back in to the global arena after three decades of global policy obscurity. It recognises, at least to some extent, the need for measures to mitigate the effect of outward migration and to ensure there is a more even distribution of social and economic costs and benefits associated with health worker-migration and -recruitment.

The Code's principles aim to promote dialogue on, and good practice in, international recruitment of health workers, encouraging countries to achieve greater sustainability, while recognising the importance of ethical recruitment and the basic human right of every person to migrate. It goes beyond recruitment in other respects, as a multilateral framework for tackling shortages in the global health workforce and addressing challenges associated with the international mobility of health workers. It aims to 'establish and promote voluntary principles and practices for the ethical international recruitment of health personnel' (Article 1.1) and 'discourages the active recruitment of health personnel from developing countries facing critical shortages of health workers (Article 5.1). It calls for multilateral dialogue and cooperation:

> The Director-General shall: (c) maintain liaison with the United Nations, the International Labour Organization, the International Organization for Migration, and other competent regional and international organizations as well as concerned nongovernmental organizations to support implementation of the Code.
>
> (Article 9.3)

The Code contains a preamble and ten articles that provide guidance for source and destination countries. The Code's guiding principles are wide-ranging, setting out ethical norms and legal and institutional arrangements for national and multilateral cooperation, alongside a strong focus on developing sustainable health systems, protecting migrant health workers' human rights and the need to support through technical and financial assistance health systems in low- and middle-income countries. Principles of ethical international recruitment and norms for recruitment practices include: recognition of the right to migrate; the responsibility of recruiting countries to adequately inform migrant health workers of their rights and provide the same working conditions enjoyed by nationals; and the avoidance of recruiting from countries facing a health workforce crisis. The Code also addresses the need for stronger, sustainable and self-reliant health systems, the need for the planning of the education and training of health workers to meet future service needs and the associated development of working environments to retain health workers. Specific reference is made to the need for countries of destination to support the sustainability of health care systems in source countries.

Other measures referred to in the Code include financial reimbursement for source countries for the loss of investment and human capital or investment in education and training in the source countries. It offers support to countries like the Philippines and others producing health workers 'for export' to benefit from the Code's provisions on reciprocal compensation arrangements between source and destination countries in the future. The multi-stakeholder mechanisms for information-sharing and monitoring of the implementation of the Code (Article 2.2) allow for transparency. These mechanisms have been important in mobilising a wide range of professional groups, CSOs, trade unions and others to engage in dialogue around the Code and its monitoring. We discuss this point further in Chapter 5.

## 5 Conclusion

Reviewing the changed ethical and political environment conditioning the second principal phase of global health worker-migration policy, this chapter has focused on how a series of voluntary 'ethical' recruitment initiatives emerged to define this global policy field during the first decade of the twenty-first century. This was a 'cold' political climate, hostile to global initiatives aspiring to strengthen public institutions and statutory regulation or institute programmes of redistribution. The 1980s and 1990s were marked by the roll-out of neo-liberal globalisations, the reconstruction of global governance regimes relating to health, trade and labour, and the instituting of new multilateral institutional machinery on international migration. These were all significant in shaping this second phase, but it was the growing calls for a common international framework on migration negotiated through multilateral spheres of governance that were especially significant for the successful conclusion of the WHO Global Code.

The materialities of political economy the issues with which negotiators were dealing entailed the globalisation of social reproduction (Yeates 2009a, 2009b) which widened existing social inequalities and created new ones coupled with accelerated trends in the 'reverse transfer of technology' between countries, regionally and beyond. As the apparent contradictions wrought by neo-liberal globalisation became seen increasingly as incompatible with the need to upgrade institutions capable of providing key public goods, such as health and human resources, a new dynamic took hold. By the late 1990s, WHO and ILO regained assertiveness in promulgating the values and, crucially, the realisability of a socially just globalisation. Their 're-awakening' was spurred on and enabled by new UN initiatives on global migration governance and the MDGs. Throughout this time many developing countries of origin continued to protest at the conditions under which they were urged to strengthen their health sectors and the massive resource transfers entailed by recruitment of health workers to advanced industrialised countries, while non-state advocacy groups from within the health professions and labour movement elaborated health workforce strategies and the idea of 'ethical' international recruitment. Collectively, these developments combined to propel a series of initiatives on 'ethical recruitment' of overseas health workers that began in advanced industrialised countries, drew in developing countries, and became multilateral over the course of the 2000s, culminating in the WHO Global Code.

The political and institutional environment in which these initiatives and agreements unfolded was significantly different in many ways from the 1960s and 1970s. It was overtly hostile to legally binding global agreements and measures especially those promoting the progressive redistribution of resources. It was also far more complex in terms of there being a wider range of global actors, structures and sources of funding for global-level activities. The positive benefits of international migration for individual migrants and their families, countries of origin and destination/employment were increasingly emphasised at the same time as a discursive and institutional shift in favour of temporary and 'circular' migration emerged. Time-limited international exchanges of health workers had always been emphasised by the UN as desirable and legitimate (see Chapter 2), but because such little progress had been made in instituting a global labour and social protection regime in health or any other sector, and because the new discourse engendered erosions of permanent rights of settlement for labour migrants at the same time as it facilitated the liberalisation and integration of international (health) labour markets, the emphasis on temporary and circular migration amounted to a substantial change in the material conditions governing health worker-migration.

On the recruitment side, the neo-liberal erosion of a swathe of labour and social protection rights and de-commitment from progressive domestic taxation structures built up over the course of more than a century, combined with rising demand for health care and new treatment technologies and public expenditure constraints on public social provision, produced a widespread demand for 'new' international solutions to health workforce issues. The circumstances that created these adverse outcomes were state-sponsored: advanced industrialised states raided the health workforces of developing countries, which, in turn, received economic benefits from the repatriation of a share of their overseas nationals' earnings. These kinds of inter-state 'solutions' that operated in practice were of a very different kind to the bilateral and multilateral agreements into which they formally entered to manage migration. It was also clear that what was required was a wider picture: 'solutions' to structural issues that went way beyond the domain of health workforce planning were needed.

Given this challenging set of circumstances, the Global Code was a significant initiative and a real achievement. It represents an attempt to address important challenges in global health and was among the most noteworthy of WHO initiatives at this time (Lidén 2014). One the one hand, the agreement for a Global Code reinforces the importance of a common framework that is applicable to all countries – irrespective of whether they are a source or destination country – and reflects the global nature of health worker-migration as well as its negative impacts on source countries, especially low(er) income countries which account for the overwhelming majority of those with health worker shortages and are most affected by outward migration. It is clear that developed countries bear particular responsibility for desisting from recruiting the health workers and resources of most vulnerable countries. The symbolic power of the Code is therefore significant given that several high-income countries are set to remain dependent on foreign health workers. As a tool for awareness-raising and dialogue, the Code is an important tool for promoting ethical international recruitment practices, stimulating international debate about the effects of health worker-migration, keeping these issues on the global agenda and, prospectively, 'may lead to a deepening of commitment over time' (Taylor and Dhillon 2012: 12).

Taylor and Dhillon (2011) argue that political leadership and civil society engagement in global negotiations at WHO were highly important and marked a new development in the global health agenda. They are right in pointing to the importance of advocacy actors pushing for the Code and supporting its institutional passage to final agreement, and a multi-stakeholder approach to the negotiations was a vital part of that. However, regarding their point that the Code marks a new development in the global health agenda we are more equivocal. Certainly, it is an important, and in many ways innovative, multilateral policy instrument. Yet it is not the first such instrument. It was the culmination within one phase rooted in a much longer trajectory within the global policy field that had been established and active since the 1960s and to which WHO was marginal for the most part (see Chapters 2 and 3). The Global Code may have been a new development for WHO, but it was not unprecedented for the global policy field at large.

We concur with Taylor and Dhillon that the Code marked a new development in the global health agenda – but not for the reasons they give. As this chapter has argued, it copper-fastened an approach to global policy that accepted minimal concessions within a global governance framework structurally predisposed towards and dependent on international migration and recruitment of health workers. In this, the Code reflects states' reluctance to engage in global institution-building and regulation that surpasses what is minimally necessary to address some of the direst social consequences of labour market and services trade liberalisation. It is voluntary in nature, relies largely on self-regulation, and is devoid of an enforcement mechanism. The absence of a binding Code makes it difficult to realise a global system of health worker-migration governance consistent with the global challenges presented by the globalisation of health labour markets and financial investment to support the objectives set out in the Code. It is ill-equipped to address global inequalities in health workforces that undermine achieving universal health care for all.

While we accept that the Code *potentially* has wider leverage and is important in the context of the global commitment towards universal health coverage, there is no getting away from the fact that it secures wealthy countries' continuing access to the health resources of less wealthy ones, and that neither WHO or any other multilateral or national organisation has the power to enforce its 'restraining' conditions beyond the exertion of moral leverage. It is predicated on the fact that governments, along with other stakeholders, will voluntarily conduct international recruitment in ethical ways and work towards sustainable human resources for health institutional mechanisms in their own countries without binding regulation that would hold them to account if they breached international standards. These weaknesses ultimately reflect the unwillingness of governments, particularly in richer parts of the world, to accept binding global regulatory measures that have a redistributive element. They embody the continuing hold of state sovereignty in matters of international labour migration governance and the weakness of multilateral migration governance on this matter. In this sense, it is arguably little more than a set of global aspirations and a 'call for action' for governments, other national stakeholders and multilateral organisations to collaborate around good practice approaches to health workforce issues.

The final content of the Code not only reveals a lack of progress in global institutional strengthening but points to the toll of decades of its weakening. As the organisation designated to lead negotiations, WHO was spectacularly constrained in its ability to do so. Years of resource austerity linked to loss of authority in a highly complex and crowded global health and migration policy field compounded already-existing constraints engendered by its governance structure and other internal (leadership) issues significantly compromised its capacity to negotiate and conclude a new global policy initiative in this area in a way that was forceful enough to deal with the scale and nature of the problems. Just as multiple constraints shaped the negotiation of the Code, and conditioned what it could ultimately achieve, so they also impacted upon the implementation of it. It is to this latter issue that we turn in the next chapter.

## Notes

1  WTO self-consciously absented itself from UN HLD-MD, GFMD and GHWA on the grounds that the GATS is not a migration agreement even though health worker-migration is included in a review of GATS Mode 4 (WTO 2009) and medical technology (WHO/WIPO/WTO 2012). The latter concluded that:

> Governments wishing to contain brain drain remain free to do so, as such measures are not subject to GATS disciplines which relate – particularly for Mode 4 – only to the temporary inward migration of foreign health workers. The limited scope of Mode 4, both its definition and specific commitments, means that GATS *probably* plays an insignificant role in the international migration of health personnel.
>
> (WHO/WIPO/WTO 2012: 80, our emphasis added)

2  Also, so much of GATS' significance for health services generally is dependent on its potential implications should more progress be made in WTO negotiations on extending countries' commitments. Part of the issue is that there aren't currently many commitments for health services, so debate is speculative until and unless WTO talks on services progress which they look unlikely to. Further negotiations are with the Trade in Services Agreement (TiSA) (see Chapter 8) and bilateral agreements (see Chapter 6). Much depends on whether these cover the health services sector. The main issue is about the contracting of workers for temporary needs rather than employment. However, this has not significantly moved for health workers, and most trade agreements now seek something on mutual recognition of qualifications in order to provide a service within a country. There is also an issue about intra-corporate transfers: if a (health) corporation provides a service in another country it can bring its staff over. We thank Chris Holden and Meri Koivusalo for these points. See also Holden (2014) and Yeates (2005b).

3  They argue that

> [t]emporary movement of service suppliers through [GATS] mode 4 offers arguably a partial solution to the dilemma of how international migration is best managed given the substantial political resistance that exists against it in many high-income countries. It could allow the realization of gains from trade while addressing some of the concerns of opponents to migration in host countries, while also attenuating the brain drain costs for poor source countries that can be associated with permanent migration.
>
> (Francois and Hoekman 2010: 671)

4  'Mode 4' concerns 'movement of natural persons' – individuals travelling from their own country to supply services in another. Government commitments tend to be restricted to higher-level personnel, notably professionals and specialists, whose mobility is related to foreign direct investment.

5 These OECD Guidelines (OECD 1976) were most recently updated in 2011 following the adoption of the UNGPs. Adopted by 42 governments to date, the 2011 revisions strengthen risk-based due diligence and responsible supply chain management principles. Implementation procedures specify that governments should establish National Contact Points to provide mediation and conciliation services. Responsibility for enforcement rests with governments. A built-in grievance mechanism can be used by CSOs.

6 Signing up to the UN Global Compact enables businesses to associate themselves with the UN in return for demonstrating their adherence to human rights, labour, environmental or anti-corruption standards (Deacon 2014). It has developed into a global network involving UN agencies, companies, governments, employers' organisations, trade unions and NGOs. Over 12,000 organisations, two thirds of which are businesses, from 170 countries presently participate in it.

7 The ILO MNE Declaration was adopted in 1977 and last revised in 2017. It promotes fundamental rights and a broad range of good industrial relations practices.

8 The UN Global Compact has been supported and criticised in equal measure. 'It has won support from companies precisely because it is voluntary and it provides good opportunities for corporations to associate themselves, or their products, with the UN's positive "brand"' (Farnsworth 2014: 95). It is also dismissed as 'blue-washing' and for over-reliance on NGOs and others to monitor on-going corporate abuses – including of those signed up under the initiative (ibid.).

9 WB promoted selectivist forms of health care targeted at the poorest sections of the population; user-fees; non-governmental (including commercial) provision of health services, and 'vertical' interventions over more 'horizontal'-type interventions directed at public health sector strengthening. In social protection its 'social risk management' approach supported commercial and family provision as social security systems of the 'first resort', bolstered by philanthropic and voluntary efforts to compensate for withdrawn or pared down 'last resort' public provision with weakened labour and welfare rights. Its social policy reflected neo-liberals' preference for individual responsibility, 'choice', self-interest and enforceable contractual rights over collective responsibility that enhances social cohesion, integration and equity (Dixon and Hyde 2001, cited in Yeates 2007).

10 The Roll Back Malaria and Stop TB Partnership provide advocacy and technical advice independently of WHO. The Global Fund engaged NGOs as grant recipients and as formal stakeholders. The Gates Foundation is the single largest non-governmental funder of health research and exercises a 'strong –if informal – authority in setting global health priorities and influencing policies' (Lidén 2014).

11 'Doing Business' (World Bank 2004) was published with a mandate to identify regulation constraining business. Despite objections from the International Trade Union Confederation (ITUC) the publication continues to praise countries that have reduced social protection for workers (O'Brien 2014: 143). '[T]he IMF supports the policy of core labour standards, but continues to push labour market deregulation wherever it can' (ibid.: 143) – particularly in borrowing countries where organised labour is relatively weak (ibid.).

12 The effectiveness of this Convention is limited by low ratifications. As at September 2018 there were just 52 state party signatories, mainly in central and south America and north and west Africa. A total of 131 countries, many of which are migrant-receiving ones, were not signed up to it (OHCHR 2014)

13 The gathering momentum for a global migration policy was also reflected in two independent initiatives in 2003: the Hague Declaration on the Future of Refugee and Migration Policy of the Society for International Development (Netherlands Chapter) and the Berne Initiative. These urged for humanitarian principles to be incorporated in migration management (ILO 2004a).

14 The Departments of Health and Social Care (DoH) and International Development (DfID) produced a list of countries that the UK should not recruit from. The list of

countries is periodically updated. Recruitment companies are monitored for compliance with the Code. The Code was introduced under the NHS' comprehensive human resource management reforms that provide for overseas health care staff to be employed on the same pay and conditions as UK nationals and aimed to make health work more attractive and increase the flow of students into medical and nursing schools. DfID's support for ethical recruitment was a way to avoid a situation where aid programmes in health failed because of the outward migration of health workers to the UK, amongst others.

15 The Melbourne Manifesto (2002) was adopted by the World Organisation of National Colleges, Academies and Academic Associations of General Practitioners/Family Physicians representing 128 national professional associations and 37 academic institutions worldwide.

16 A WHO Resolution on health manpower (WHA 1983b) referenced an earlier (1977) WHO Resolution on Nursing and midwifery personnel, and re-emphasised nursing and midwifery personnel in realising Health for All.

17 Resolution WHA54.12 (WHA 2001) elaborated the issues thus: '[c]oncerned about global shortages of nurses and midwives' and '[r]ecognizing the importance of nursing services and midwifery services as the core of any health system and in national health', countries were urged 'to establish comprehensive programmes for the development of human resources which support the training, recruitment and retention of a skilled and motivated nursing and midwifery workforce within health services....'

18 Discussion of the implementation of the Alma Ata Declaration and HfA strategy at the 1988 WHA made no mention of international migration, brain drain or health workforce shortages (see Chapter 3). Its 1992 report on HfA implementation sidestepped the worsening health workforce crisis, while a WHO DG report to the 1994 WHA emphasised staff shortages as a factor in the struggling WHO drug strategy, but failed to elaborate. The disconnect between WHO Executive's priorities and the concerns raised by developing countries surfaces in WHA 49 (1996) which omitted any reference to labour shortages. The Jamaican and Botswanan delegates protested, emphasising these severely constrained the efficacy of their health care systems.

19 WHA50.27, WHA51.18 and WHA52.23 (WHA 1997, 1998, 1999). The first coincided with WHO's 50th anniversary, just three years prior to the MDG period. The 1997 and 1998 Resolutions were the most direct about sufficient health labour for effective health systems capable of preventing and controlling non-communicable diseases. The 1999 Resolution elaborated these same points when reaffirming WHO's commitment to the goals of equitable, affordable, accessible and sustainable health care systems based on primary health care in all countries.

20 The New Zealand delegate's report on its health sector reforms, which included increased spending and improved planning capacity, concluded with this: '[w]e expect these improvements, coupled with a vigorous immigration policy for health professionals, to put us in a position where we shall at least have enough people to provide basic services' (WHA 1986: 111–112). The bitter irony of this cannot have been lost on anyone.

21 ILC debated how it could 'further strengthen and expand assistance to governments and to employers' and workers' organizations in translating [rights-based] principles into policy and practice at national levels' (ILO 2004a: 140). A new plan of action, it mooted, could include ILO establishing an international forum on migration for work bringing together 'all the relevant actors on a regular, frequent and tripartite basis to consider appropriate responses to the issues raised by increasing migration' (ibid.).

22 This work started in 1994 at the International Conference on Population and Development, continued through a UNSG-commissioned study, 'The Doyle Report' (2002), an ad hoc Global Commission on International Migration (GCIM 2005), the appointment of a Special Representative on Migration and Development and a UN High-Level Dialogue on Migration and Development (2006) (Betts 2011).

23 WHA57.19 (WHA 2004) 'requests the Director-General to develop a code of practice on the international recruitment of health personnel, in consultation with Member States and all relevant partners.' A footnote in the Resolution stated that it was 'understood that this will be non-binding'.

24 The alternative would have been to negotiate it through ILO. However, ILO was at a low ebb with problems of low implementation of its labour standards instruments. For ministries of health the problems that the Code sought to address were very practical and immediate ones, and WHO was an easier forum in which they could discuss health-specific issues. We thank Meri Koivusalo for drawing this to our attention.

25 Reflecting the Norwegian framework for global solidarity (2007), Norway was an important advocate for the interests of low-income countries. It committed to refraining from recruiting health workers from developing countries and set out a policy approach linking national level health workforce planning, increased capacity in home-based training, international recruitment of health workers, and donor aid to developing countries.

26 For example, Dr Danzon, the Chair of the consultation held by WHO's Europe office concluded that 'global solidarity must become both our goal and one of our central planning principles.' He went on to say that 'new approaches to both national and international health development need to be identified, hopefully through multilateral mechanisms. Only through the principle of global solidarity will our goal of equity in health be attainable'.

# 5 Implementing the WHO Global Code of Practice

## Momentum sustained?

## 1 Introduction

Although governments and global organisations recognise the relevance and importance of the WHO Global Code there are significant challenges in terms of it being a transformational global instrument capable of contributing to the goal of universal health care to which it aspires. Where Chapter 4 discussed how the global political economy of global policy making conditioned the Global Code in respect of its mode (multilateral), basis of adherence (voluntary), aims ('ethical' recruitment), discursive orientation (mutuality of benefits) and procedural methods (periodic reporting and review), this chapter focuses on its implementation in practice. Implementation was a major weakness of the ILO Recommendation on Nursing Personnel (see Chapter 3), so scrutiny of the Global Code's implementation can help ascertain whether this is also an issue for this second agreement.

The discussion responds to two questions. The first question is whether the Global Code's provisions are being implemented and to what extent. The answer to this is a pre-condition for any broader conclusions about the efficacy of the Global Code. We review the evidence from studies by WHO, advocacy actors and academic researchers on the implementation of the Global Code. We supplement this existing base through secondary analysis of countries' returns in the reporting rounds (2013–2018) and of data from the stakeholder engagement mechanism. We identify areas which the evidence points to implementation being strongest and weakest. The second question is whether the provisions of the Global Code are adequately defined. This relates to the provisions (other than the implementation mechanism) inscribed into the Global Code. We identify several issues originating in the body of the Global Code itself and show how these give rise to a number of operational problems that are factors in the weaknesses of the Global Code in its implementation phase. These include the absence of a definition of ethical recruitment, weaknesses in the equality provisions, narrowness of the implementation mechanism, problems with the reporting framework, ambiguities regarding the workforce aspects of the means of realising the conditions necessary for universal health care, the limited accessibility of the implementation mechanisms, and the narrow range of entities to which the Global Code's provisions apply.

We thus distinguish between different sources of problems of implementation – the design features of the Global Code and its institutional mechanisms and the conditions under which it is being implemented. We scrutinise the decision to restrict the Global Code to governments in the light of the poor implementation track record by states and the growing significance of private recruitment agencies in health worker-recruitment. In this light, we ask whether existing global provisions and initiatives to regulate private enterprises that were developed outside of the Global Code might provide a potential basis for future policy development aiming to strengthen the global policy 'toolbox' to realise sustainable health workforces.

## 2 Implementation mechanisms established under the Code

The Global Code encourages information exchange on issues related to health personnel and health systems in the context of migration. Resolution WHA63.16 (WHA 2010) set out mechanisms reviewing and monitoring the Global Code through periodic reporting. Under Articles 9.2 and 7.2(c) of the Global Code, Member States are encouraged to submit national reports to WHO every three years on measures they have taken to implement the Global Code. Following the first review of the Code the WHO Director-General (WHO DG) is mandated to make proposals, if necessary, to revise the Code which may enhance its application (paragraph 3(4)), as well as to keep the implementation of the Code under review with periodic reports to the WHA. Article 9.4 encourages the WHO Secretariat to consider reports from all relevant stakeholders on activities related to implementation of the Code. The Global Code is directed to, and expected to be, implemented, disseminated and reviewed by governments and 'other stakeholders' which are defined in the Code as:

> health personnel, recruiters, employers, health-professional organizations, relevant subregional, regional and global organizations, whether public or private sector, including nongovernmental, and all persons concerned with the international recruitment of health personnel.
>
> (Article 2.2)

This is one of the strengths of the Code: its drafter wisely understood that a multi-stakeholder approach would help with transparency, accountability and future monitoring of the Code, and the wider stakeholder advocacy that could persuade governments to agree the Code and implement it.

From WHO's perspective, its monitoring activities will assist in assessing the implementation of the Code and keep track of trends in international recruitment. The quality of data available is central to this objective, and guiding principles for a minimum data set (MDS) were developed jointly by WHO and the OECD in time for the second round of reporting (WHO/OECD undated). Although the guidelines initially focused on doctors, nurses and midwives there is provision for these to be expanded to other health care professionals in the future. At this stage it is not known what type of permanent monitoring system will be put in place.

In order to promote country reporting, WHO requested Member States to designate a national authority (Designated National Authority – DNA) for reporting purposes. DNAs are responsible for providing WHO with information on the implementation of the Code (Campbell *et al.* 2016). The monitoring provisions have led to the development of a national self-assessment tool – the National Reporting Instrument (NRI) – containing qualitative and quantitative indicators covering the rights of migrants, international agreements, research on health personnel mobility, statistics, and regulation of authorisation to practice, amongst other areas. The NRI was also updated to enhance the reporting process and improve the Global Code's monitoring. Comprising 18 questions, the updated NRI 2018 enables WHO to collect and share current evidence and information on the international recruitment and migration of health personnel. Common use of the periodic NRI aims to promote comparability of data and regularity of information flows. An NRI reports database (WHO undated) provides a valuable source of evidence on the implementation of the Global Code. We draw on this database in this chapter and in Chapter 6 in relation to bilateral agreements.

To date, three sets of reporting on the Global Code have been carried out, in 2013, 2016 and 2018. The results of the second round helped to inform the WHO's Review of Code Relevance and Effectiveness (WHO 2016a). The main differences between the 2013 and 2016 reporting rounds are that the latter increased the number of self-assessment questions under the NRI relating to health workforce development and sustainability, legal rights of migrants, bilateral agreements, research on personnel mobility, statistics, regulation of authorisation to practice, partnerships and technical cooperation. In addition, the OECD and Eurostat, in cooperation with WHO, drew up a module on health workforce migration providing new disaggregated data on foreign-trained health personnel (OECD/WHO 2016), the results of which were incorporated in the second round of reporting. Furthermore, the second round of reporting introduced the possibility for stakeholders, including civil society, to provide information relevant to the implementation of the Global Code independently of governments through a specific reporting mechanism. The results from the first and second reporting rounds are presented and discussed in the following section.

## 3  Overview of results from the first two reporting rounds

As Table 5.1 illustrates, in the first round of reporting 85 countries had established DNAs for reporting on the Global Code, which increased in the second round by 37 per cent in 2016 to 117 countries. In some regions there was a significant increase in the number of DNAs. Notably, the Western Pacific saw a fourfold increase (WHO 2016a). In the first round 56 countries submitted a completed report to WHO and this rose to 74 countries in 2016, reflecting an increase of 32 per cent from 2013 (WHO 2016a). Overall, little progress on reporting was made in Africa, which has the highest number of countries with

*Table 5.1* Designated national authorities by WHO region and number of reports received

| WHO region | 1 Countries with critical HRH shortages 2013 | 2 Designated National Authority established 2013 | 2016 | 3 Completed reports received by the WHO secretariat 2013 | 2016 |
|---|---|---|---|---|---|
| Africa | 36 | 13 | 14 | 2 | 9 |
| Americas | 5 | 11 | 15 | 4 | 9 |
| South-East Asia | 6 | 4 | 7 | 3 | 6 |
| Europe | 0 | 43 | 43 | 40 | 31 |
| Eastern Mediterranean | 7 | 8 | 14 | 3 | 7 |
| Western Pacific | 3 | 6 | 24 | 4 | 12 |
| **Total** | **57** | **85** | **117** | **56** | **74** |

Source: WHO (2013a, 2016a).

critical shortages of health workers. Reporting on establishment of DNAs and completed reports were higher in other WHO regions, notably Europe, which represents the majority of the known source and destination countries for health worker-migration (WHO 2016a).

According to WHO's (2016a) analysis of the reports received, 49 (66 per cent) of the 74 countries with completed reports in 2016 had taken steps to implement the Code at national and subnational levels. WHO also reported that the geographical diversity and quality of reports had improved between 2013 and 2016 (ibid.). Despite increases in levels of reporting between 2013 and 2016 in all regions except for Europe, this is still a very low response rate overall. According to WHO's Expert Advisory Group on the Relevance and Effectiveness of the WHO Global Code of Practice (WHO-EAG)[1] this low response rate makes it difficult to make a full assessment of the effectiveness of the Code:

> Contributory factors to successful implementation in Member States include the level of awareness, political commitment, technical and financial resources to support systematic implementation and reporting on the Code, and whether there is engagement by all stakeholders to deliver the promise of the Code. The implementation gaps constrain a full assessment of the effectiveness of the Code's potential.
>
> (WHO 2015a, para. 16)

Although 38 per cent of all WHO member states sent completed reports in 2016 (having risen from 29 per cent in the 2013 round) such a low rate of reporting is unpromising given that the Global Code was the outcome of multilateral negotiations and that its agreement confers reporting obligations upon all of the 194 WHO Member States. This low response rate highlights the key problem of the voluntary, non-statutory nature of the Global Code: WHO has no means of enforcing adherence other than through moral leverage. Furthermore, as our own analysis of the WHO data shows, the proportion of countries with critical health shortages that reported having set up a DNA and/or reporting in the first and second rounds did not rise significantly. In 2015 only just over one-third (36.1 per cent) of the 36 countries with critical health shortages in Africa had established a DNA, rising by one country, to 38.8 per cent in 2016. Similarly, only two countries (5.5 per cent) in Africa submitted completed reports in 2013, rising to only nine (25.5 per cent) in 2016 (WHO 2016a).

Furthermore, despite the greater geographical diversity of countries having completed an NRI under the second round, it remained the case that most engagement was by European countries. Thus in 2013 and 2016, the majority of responding countries were from within the Europe region, covering 80 per cent of countries in the Europe region. These countries have received implementation support from the EU and the WHO Office for Europe, and have active civil society engagement around unethical recruitment practices. However, the numbers submitting completed reports in Europe dropped from 40 countries in 2013 to 31 in 2016. In the 2016 reporting, eight countries reporting were from the top ten countries of destination for international migrants (Australia, Canada, France, Germany, Ireland, Spain, UK and USA), which amongst them accounted for 75 per cent of foreign-trained doctors in OECD countries (WHO 2016a). Migration from countries with serious shortages accounted for 84 per cent of foreign-trained doctors (Scheil-Adlung 2016, cited in HEEG 2016).

Reporting on measures taken to implement the Code was highest in destination countries, particularly in Europe, although Australia, Canada and the US have larger absolute numbers of overseas-trained health workers in their domestic workforces (OECD 2015; see also Table 5.1). This suggests that these are the countries that have the most capacity and resources to undertake monitoring and reporting; they also have the most to gain as they know they will have to continue international recruitment in the future (Dhillon 2015). Lower levels of reporting by low- and middle- income countries are evident and these are countries which tend to lack the resources, institutional and data collection capacity. In the Eastern and Southern Africa (ESA) region, for example, the Code has a relatively low profile and there have been limited resources and policy support to implement the Code. A further issue is that the Code is largely written with destination countries in mind and reflects concerns about recruitment by higher-income countries. This issue was raised at the multi-stakeholder consultative forum held in Manila, Philippines in 2011, which recommended that changes be made to the national reporting instrument to make it more relevant to source countries (Yeates and Pillinger 2013).

Table 5.2 shows reporting on the Code for 2013 and 2016 on key elements of the Code. There was some progress in reporting on several of the monitoring indicators of the Code in core areas. For example, responses to the question 'Migrant health personnel enjoy the same legal rights and responsibilities as domestically-trained health personnel' (Article 4) rose from 46 (out of 56)

Table 5.2 WHO monitoring: country responses by Article in the Global Code (based on returns from 2013 and 2016 reporting rounds)

| Monitoring indicator | Number of countries reporting compliance, 2013 (out of 56) | Number of countries reporting compliance, 2016 (out of 74) |
|---|---|---|
| Migrant health personnel enjoy the same legal rights and responsibilities as domestically trained health personnel (Article 4) | 46 | 70 |
| Countries undertaking measures to educate, retain and sustain domestic health workforce (Article 4) | n/a | 67 |
| Migrant health personnel are hired, promoted and remunerated based on objective criteria as domestically trained health personnel (Article 4) | 34 | 58 |
| Countries adopting measures to address geographical maldistribution and improve retention in underserved areas (Article 5) | n/a | 58 |
| Mechanisms exist to regulate the authorization to practise by migrant health personnel and maintain statistical records (Article 7) | 32 | 50 |
| Statistical records of health personnel whose initial qualification was obtained in a foreign country (Article 7) | 31 | 44 |
| Actions have been taken to communicate and share information across sectors on recruitment and migration (Article 9) | 31 | 39 |
| Migrant health personnel enjoy the same education, qualifications and career progression opportunities as domestically-trained health personnel (Article 4) | 29 | 47 |
| Government and/or nongovernment programmes or institutions are undertaking research in migration (Article 6) | 23 | 29 |
| Recruitment mechanisms allow migrant health personnel to assess the benefits and risks associated with their employment (Article 4) | 17 | 36 |
| Measures have been taken to involve all stakeholders in decision-making processes involving migration and international recruitment (Article 8) | 15 | 27 |
| Actions are being considered to introduce changes to laws/policies to conform with the Code recommendations (Article 8) | n/a | 24 |
| Database of laws and regulations related to international recruitment in place (Article 7) | 11 | 14 |
| Records are maintained of all recruiters authorised to operate (Article 8) | 10 | 13 |
| Countries providing assistance to other countries or stakeholders to support the Code implementation (Article 10) | n/a | 10 |
| Countries receiving / requesting assistance from other countries or stakeholders in support of the Code implementation (Article 10) | n/a | 7 |

Source: WHO (2013a, 2016a).

Note
Additional items were added to the National Reporting Instrument in 2016, thereby extending the range of questions and issues to be covered in national reports in 2016. The absence of data in the 2013 reporting round reflects this.

countries in 2013 to 70 countries (out of 74) in 2016. However, a low level of reporting on some indicators is an issue. For example, only ten countries in 2013 and 13 countries in 2015 reported on the question 'Records are maintained of all recruiters authorised to operate' (Article 8). Only one country, Germany, reported that it had implemented the provisions of the Code into its national laws (WHO 2016a). In 2016, 70 countries (88 per cent) reported having implemented measures to meet health workforce needs within domestically trained personnel, with 58 countries (78 per cent) reporting that they had taken measures to address geographic imbalances in workforce distribution within their countries. On the issue of bilateral, regional and multilateral agreements, 36 countries in 2016 were engaged in implementing measures, with agreements reached at a regional level (ASEAN, Nordic countries and Middle Eastern countries) for dentists and pharmacists (WHO 2016a). However, many of these measures pre-date the Code. Chapter 6 further analyses NRI reports in relation to these international agreements.

The 2016 reporting round elicited data under the health workforce migration module, which reflects a set of voluntary indicators for monitoring stocks and flows of physicians to inform data on health worker-migration drawn up by the OECD. Of the 74 countries that completed the NRI, 37 provided information on the stock of foreign-trained physicians, 26 gave information on the annual inflow of foreign-trained physicians, 27 on the stock of foreign-trained nurses and 19 on the annual inflow of foreign trained nurses. No countries were able to provide data on outflows of their workforce at the aggregate level or which countries they departed for. This is because such data can only be gained from requests for verification of qualifications prior to migration, which is not always an indicator of actual migration. Otherwise, according to WHO (2016a), the reporting provides some extremely useful data on developments in health worker-migration, including data on intra-regional, South–South, and North–South health worker-migration patterns, as well as information about temporary migration and employment in multiple jurisdictions.

## 4 Assessing the implementation of the Code: achievements and challenges

### 4.1 Key achievements and strengths

According to the WHO-EAG the Global Code has helped raise awareness and inform policy dialogue, especially among health workforce planners and policy-makers, and this underpins better understanding of the relevance of the Code in the light of projected continued reliance on foreign-trained health workers (WHO 2015a). The Global Code, though largely focused on destination countries, has been used as a basis for governments and other stakeholders in source countries to argue for ethical recruitment standards. Indeed, the Code's periodic reporting and review provisions have led it to become an important global platform for dialogue and engagement with WHO Member States and other relevant stakeholders:

Long ignored, the issue of health worker migration is and, thanks to the Code's reporting requirements, will remain on the global health agenda for the foreseeable future. In particular, African governments, underrepresented in global negotiations, played a key role in addressing an issue of significant concern to African health systems.

(Taylor and Dhillon 2011: 22)

The WHO-EAG has highlighted the extent to which the Code's principles and provisions have been incorporated into national health systems plans. It reported that provisions of the Code have been incorporated into government policy in Ireland, Norway and the Philippines, implemented into national legislation in Germany, while Moldova had incorporated principles of the Code into the bilateral agreements it was in the process of negotiating (see Chapter 6). Other examples came from health ministries, which stated they were using the code to promote multi-sectoral dialogue on health system sustainability (the Maldives, the Philippines, Indonesia and El Salvador). Further achievements are the implementation of the Global Code into regional plans of action such as the WHO/SEARO Resolution and Decade for health workforce strengthening in South-East Asia and the European Commission Action Plan for the EU Health Workforce. Further measures to integrate or plans to integrate the principles into regional actions were reported from member states in the EMRO network (Arab League), the Andean network, the Ibero-American General Secretariat (SEGIB), and the Council of Health Ministers of Central America (COMISCA) (WHO 2015a).

A tangible example of where the Code has prompted changes in national health workforce policy is South Africa, where the negative impact of the migration of health workers has been addressed through multinational, bilateral, and domestic policies. Starting with the Commonwealth Code and later with the WHO Global Code, policies tended to focus on public recruitment and their voluntary nature had limited impact on South Africa along with other African countries (Labonté *et al.* 2015). While in South Africa the decline in outward migration of health workers since the early 2000s has been affected by a slowdown in recruitment of nurses particularly to the UK, tighter migration rules along with better retention of health workers following salary rises introduced under the Occupation Specific Dispensation (OSD) policy (2007) were also important factors (Pillinger 2013). Notably, the South African Department of Health developed a policy to promote high standards of practice in the recruitment and employment of health professionals in the health sector in South Africa. Its policy on the Recruitment and Employment of Health Professionals in the South African Health Sector (2010), which was approved by the National Council on Health in the South African Health Sector on 5 February 2010, drew on the principles and guidance set out in the WHO Global Code, as well as on the bilateral and multilateral agreements in the Southern African Development Community (SADC) and the African Union (AU). The policy discourages the active recruitment of health professionals from developing countries unless there are government-to-government (bilateral) agreements for this in place. The policy specifies that foreign health professionals 'shall enjoy the service benefits and comply with all the conditions of service' on the same basis as their South African counterparts, including 'support for their professional development to enhance their clinical skills'. The policy states that recruitment shall be limited to health facilities in designated underserved or rural areas.

A further positive outcome is multi-stakeholder participation in implementation and monitoring of the Code. This has been facilitated by later adjustments to the implementation mechanism, which improved its accessibility by introducing an Independent Stakeholders Reporting Instrument (ISRI) for the second (2016) and third (2018) reporting rounds.[2] The ISRI has helped monitor states' implementation of the Code by including a range of stakeholders in the implementation and monitoring process (see Section 2, this chapter). As with state reporting, multi-stakeholder involvement in monitoring has largely predominated in the WHO-Europe region, for which a roadmap for implementing the Code in the European Region was drawn up. There is also evidence of a participatory process involving stakeholder dialogues in a number of European countries supported by the European Parliament's Committee on Development. The NGO 'Health Workers for All' partnership submitted a report under the second round of reporting documenting initiatives and case studies from eight European countries illustrating the extent of engagement by NGO and trade unions with the implementation the Code (HealthWorkers4All 2014). They show the implementation of practical measures on the ground, alongside the campaigning call from NGOs to fully implement the Code in a more systematic and coordinated way. This partnership has created a civil society Call to Action 'A health worker for everyone, everywhere' (HealthWorkers4All 2014) with 179 signatories from European and global NGOs, including Equinet, GHWA and Health Workers for All and All for Health Workers (ibid.), to raise awareness amongst policymakers at EU and national level of the need to develop and maintain strong health systems and sustainable health workforces within Europe and elsewhere (ibid.).[3]

Not all success stories were confined to Europe. Several countries (El Salvador, Indonesia, Maldives and the Philippines) reported that the Code had led them to promote multi-sectoral dialogue on health system sustainability. In the Andean and ASEAN networks, the Code led to a framework for health worker mobility dialogue (WHO 2016a). A similar process to the one undertaken in Europe was carried out through the Asia-Pacific Action Alliance for Human Resources and through a meeting organised by the WHO-Europe in Amsterdam in May 2013. In the Philippines, the government has been advocating for improved practices and procedures on ethical recruitment through a multi-stakeholder approach (WHO 2014; DoH, Philippines/ILO 2012). The EU-funded ILO *Decent Work Across Borders* project supported innovative monitoring through multi-stakeholder partnerships and multi-stakeholder engagement (DoH, Philippines/ILO 2012). Led by the Philippine Department of Health, it involved the Department of Labor and Employment in the Philippines, ILO, WHO, trade unions, employers, recruitment agencies and professional associations. Two participatory workshops helped to raise awareness about the WHO Global Code and gain stakeholder feedback on its implementation. Workshops in advance of the formal engagement events were held to ensure that participants were fully informed about the Code and could play an active role in the implementation and monitoring of the Code (Pillinger 2013). The multi-stakeholder approach also led to discussion about adjusting the NRI to enhance its relevance to source countries. A key message from stakeholders was the need for WHO to develop an instrument to capture the perspectives of source countries (Pillinger 2013). The monitoring process also generated further evidence about the inherent constraints in a voluntary code and suggestions to strengthen implementation (e.g. better dissemination of the Code, high-level state dialogues and incorporation of the Code's provisions in higher education and government civil service policies) (WHO 2014).

This example from the Philippines shows that it is possible to promote multisectoral engagement with the Code and demonstrates what is possible if resources and effective leadership drive the process. The monitoring of the Code was particularly important in the Philippines, because as a major source country the Code has been used as a basis for embedding ethical recruitment into bilateral agreements. This work is notable for having gone beyond setting up a register of recruitment companies. However, this country example appears to be the only one of a comprehensive multi-stakeholder consultation in the first reporting round and it was not repeated during the second round of reporting in the Philippines. However, it established a model of a participatory approach used as a basis for consultations on the Global Code in the WHO Europe region.

Well-established civil society organisations, including trade unions, have played an important role in mobilisation around the Code. In Europe, civil society mobilisation has grown in recent years, culminating in a European civil society network on the issue. The Code has become a tool around which both CSOs and trade unions have mobilised to advocate for ethical recruitment to be formalised to play a role in the fair distribution of health workers, particularly in ensuring that health worker-migration does not lead to inequitable access to health services in the global South. In this respect, the annual 'Civil Society Days' run in parallel to the GFMD have been instrumental in helping civil society and workers' organisations to network and develop common strategies around the implementation of the Global Code. Such initiatives are significant because they have brought a wide range of stakeholders into a monitoring process. Outside of Europe, the PSI's training programmes with affiliates in East Africa, West Africa, Southern Africa and Asia have helped to build advocacy, skills and capabilities for trade unions to participate in discussions about the implementation of the Code at the national level, as well as to ensure that trade unions in those regions actively participated in the review process of the Code at the national level. Such initiatives are important in the ongoing development of multi-stakeholder approaches which, as we discuss in Chapter 7, often prioritise the corporate sector over CSO and trade union engagement.

## *4.2 Weaknesses and challenges*

Major challenges remain to be addressed, with large scope for significant progress to be made in implementing the Code. As Buchan (2010) argued at the time, '[a] global code on international recruitment will have sustained impact only if its signatories support monitoring and also tackle the related issues of workforce planning and retention' (Buchan 2010: 1). Clearly, a major early priority was to put in place systems at the country level capable of ensuring the ongoing implementation of the Code's various provisions on workforce issues and the monitoring of the 'roll out' phase internationally. This may have been a priority for WHO and advocacy networks around the Code but it does not seem to have been high on the priorities lists of most member states given the evidence we reviewed in Section 3. Our interviews with multilateral organisations in 2012–2013 raised the concern that although the Global Code led to much initial activity and engagement, particularly in Europe, some momentum had been subsequently lost (Yeates and Pillinger 2013).

WHO's understanding of the depth of the implementation gap has grown over time, such that by 2015 it was publicly appealing for support at all levels 'to expand its capacity to raise awareness, provide technical support and promote effective implementation and reporting of the Code' (WHO 2015a). One channel for gathering information and evidence underpinning this call for resources to step up implementation and reporting has been events run by WHO to engage with stakeholders. An example is the 2011 WHO public hearing (WHO 2011a) involving 38 organisations, associations, institutions and governments, during which they gave feedback on the Guidelines. This has been part of broader efforts WHO has made to address implementation challenges in its Europe region (WHO 2012) and provide a steer for other regions.

A second channel has been the WHO-EAG (WHO 2015a). This has drawn attention to the political and resource deficits undermining the Code's implementation, it has otherwise largely affirmed that the Global Code's value is in providing a set of guiding principles for policy makers and confirmed that its impact has largely been confined to raising awareness and promoting dialogues about ethical recruitment. In other words, despite some notable achievements, implementation of the Code has been uneven, fragmented and under-resourced, even though pressures on health workforces and health workforce planning remain as significant as ever. WHO's own reviews of the Global Code have also concluded similar points (WHO 2013b, 2015a).

In what follows, we identify specific weaknesses and challenges across the implementation process. We identify two 'classes' of issues affecting the Global Code's efficacy as a global policy instrument. The first concerns design features and content of the Code (section 4.2.1). The second concerns the resources available to implement the Code and to monitor its implementation (section 4.2.2). We discuss how implementation problems in part originate in the design of Global Code.

*4.2.1  Design features of the Code*

A ENFORCEABILITY OF THE CODE

The voluntarism underpinning the Global Code is a reflection of the unwilling-ness of destination country governments to engage in binding measures (see Chapter 4). This has created a fundamental major problem with the Code: legal unenforceability. Indeed, this problem is widely regarded as the Code's main weakness (Bourgeault *et al.* 2016). The Code's recommendation that it be incorporated into national policies and laws as a way to make it legally binding (Article 8.2) has been systematically ignored by most governments. The only major example to date of a government doing so, turning this voluntary code into binding national law, is South Africa (see Section 4.1, this chapter). There are no instances of the Code being invoked in national legal cases.[4]

With most member states not participating in implementing the Code (as judged by submission rates in the reporting rounds to date), or domesticating the Code's provisions into national law this raises the further issue that non-state actors involved in health workforce management, recruitment and migration are not direct subjects of the Code. The provisions of the Code do not apply directly to 'other stakeholders' such as private enterprises and private employers which are not obliged to comply with them, unless required by national law to do so (multiple stakeholders only participate in *monitoring* the implementation of the Code but no obligations are conferred upon them to implement the Code). To the extent that the Code has any leverage at all, it is only over WHO member states whose responsibility it is to ensure that their systems adhere to the standards set out in it. We return to this issue in Section 5 of this chapter in relation to private recruitment and staffing agencies.

B DEFINITION OF CORE CONCEPTS

The Global Code contains no precise operational definition of 'ethical recruit-ment' that would enable countries to be fully compliant with ethical recruitment principles and procedures as defined by the Code. In this respect, the Code falls short in defining a recognised global standard to attain. Failure to define such a global standard is a set-back in the quest to realise greater coherence across other policy instruments, such as bilateral or regional labour agreements, also aiming to achieve the same goals. There is a further lack of clarity in the Code in that it asks Member States to '… observe and assess the magnitude of active inter-national recruitment of health personnel from countries facing critical shortage of health personnel' (Article 8.7) without explicitly calling for active support for developing countries in doing so beyond the general level of support for health systems strengthening.[5]

C EQUALITY OF TREATMENT

The Global Code's provisions on the protection of workers give insufficient attention to equality of treatment of migrant health workers in accordance with ILO Conventions on fundamental rights at work and migration (see Appendix 3). One of the main difficulties is that there are different global governance regimes relating to rights to equality of treatment. Domestically-trained workers and their citizenship rights are the responsibility of Justice Ministries which impose restrictions on the length of stay and other rights of migrant workers, such as the right to access social security and public health care, whereas the Code has its principal focus on labour and health. These limitations arise in Article 4.5 of the WHO Global Code, which requires that member states ensure that under applicable laws migrant health personnel enjoy the same legal rights, and responsibilities as domestically trained health workforce in terms and conditions of employment. This reflects an overall weakness in the existing global governance system on health worker-migration and -recruitment, and specifically a disjuncture between global migration and labour rights regimes.

D IMPLEMENTATION MECHANISMS

There are two aspects to the scope of the implementation mechanisms. The first is that only governments were originally identified as having access to the implementation mechanism. Although non-state stakeholders were incorporated into the process in 2016 through ISRI this was only in relation to *monitoring* and even this has not yet been universally taken up. Indeed, the involvement of stakeholders other than governments remains limited (WHO 2016a). The second aspect is that there is no mechanism in the Code linking the international standards of conduct it outlines to other areas or initiatives in global policy. This means, for example, that donors and recipients in global health partnerships and global health development assistance are not required to sign up to the principles in the Code (Mackey and Liang 2013). The absence of a link between international agreements and national regulation was also raised as an issue in national reports submitted to the WHO-EAG (Campbell *et al.* 2016).

Even voluntary instruments can be strengthened by referring to them in binding international agreements (Sauvant 2015) so the absence of 'lateral' implementation mechanisms isolates the Global Code from global policies embedded in the UN normative framework, such as the UN Convention for the Protection of the Rights of All Migrant Workers and Members of their Families and ILO Conventions on labour migration and recruitment standards. Similarly, the failure to 'future proof' the Global Code in this way has become all the more apparent given the subsequent emergence of 'landmark' initiatives bearing upon health worker-migration governance. These include the WHO's Global strategy on human resources for health, the SDGs and the global financing agenda, and the 2018 UN Global Compact for Migration, the amongst others (see Chapter 7).

E JOINED-UP GOVERNMENT RESPONSES

There is a lack of clarity about which organisation or government department has the overall responsibility for implementing and monitoring the Code at the national level. Interviews we conducted in 2013 highlighted a concern that WHO had not sufficiently promoted better collaboration and shared responsibility for the implementation and monitoring of the Global Code between different Ministries (health, justice, finance, employment) in source and destination countries (Yeates and Pillinger 2013).

*4.2.2 Resources to support monitoring and implementation of the Code*

A DATA QUALITY

High quality data is an essential component of the Global Code's implementation. The joint submission to the WHO public hearing by Japan, Norway, Thailand and USA in 2011 (WHO 2011a) argued that the monitoring of the Code should be used not only to create momentum in support of implementing the Code but also to collate important global data and an evidence-base on health worker-migration, as well as to stimulate greater multisectoral coordination for better workforce policies and planning (WHO 2011a). The importance of health workforce information systems covering both public and private sectors in source and destination countries was also reiterated in the joint submission to the public hearing of 15-member governments under the Asia Pacific Action Alliance on Human Resources for Health (AAAH) (WHO 2011a).

Both rounds of reporting revealed a lack of standardised data on recruitment, migration and health workforces. Many of the national reports submitted for the WHO-EAG identified the absence of data systems for standardising, collecting and exchanging data (Campbell *et al.* 2016). The absence of such data systems is a major barrier to implementing and monitoring the impact of the Code (WHO 2013a, 2016a). A further challenge relates to the definitions of the types of data needed and the comparability of data. The Canadian submission to a public hearing urged greater clarity on migration vs recruitment data: 'While much of the data that will be collected is migration data, this data does not accurately reflect the intent of the Code, which was on recruitment and not migration' (WHO 2011a: 2). The quality of international data in this area is a long-standing problem, identified in Mejia's study during the 1970s and by many others since (Mejia *et al.* 1979; WHO 2006a; OECD 2008; Paina *et al.* 2016; Abugala and Badr 2016; Abadalla *et al.* 2016).

B WHO'S CAPACITY TO MONITOR IMPLEMENTATION

The WHO-EAG received evidence that many Member States were either unaware of the Code or its reporting obligations. It was also noted that some WHO country officials had never heard of the instrument (WHO 2015a). This points to the Global Code being insufficiently integrated into the work of WHO as a whole.[6] One issue here is that WHO did not prioritise the implementation of the Global Code within core WHO programmes, and that the leadership and policy direction from WHO head office on the WHO Global Code remains weak. This is linked in large part to the fact that WHO's capacity to monitor the Global Code was reduced shortly after the conclusion of the agreement. Internal restructuring led to the 35-person HRH team being disbanded in 2013, leaving just one policy officer with responsibility for monitoring the Code. This is an issue about which some member governments expressed their concerns to the WHO Executive Board (Yeates and Pillinger 2013). On the other hand, the integration of the GHWA within WHO and its role (in its reincarnation as the Global Health Workforce Alliance, GHWN) in jointly providing technical support to countries to implement the Code ensures GHWA is more strategically focused on health worker-migration and the implementation of the WHO Global Code in the future (GHWA 2014).

Under-resourcing of the implementation of the Code has been a major issue. These limitations include a lack of resources and staff capacity within WHO at the global and regional levels 'to effectively support countries in the implementation of the Code, follow-up and reporting' (WHO 2015a: 8). The need for greater resources for technical support in support of the continued implementation of the Code has been consistently highlighted by WHO (WHO 2015a). Campbell *et al.* (2016) found that many of the national reports submitted for the WHO-EAG called for greater levels of technical assistance than WHO could feasibly provide.

To date, the higher levels of technical support and resource at global, regional and country levels requested has only materialised in one project. The 'Brain Drain to Brain Gain' project[7] provides on-going support to five countries. It focuses on national data collection to support reporting and implementation of the WHO Global Code in three priority source countries (Uganda, Nigeria and India), one destination country (Ireland) and a country that is both a source and destination for migratory flows of health workers (South Africa). The aim is to support the development of improved data on 'stocks and flows' aimed at strengthening migration management. Despite apparently good outcomes, the restriction of the project to five countries is a limitation. The ability to scale-up such assistance is hampered by resource constraints within WHO and a reliance on donor financing.

## C NATIONAL COMPLIANCE: AN ISSUE OF POLITICAL WILL OR CAPACITY?

WHO's repeated emphasis on technical assistance and technical cooperation to support implementation raises the question of to what extent member states' failure to fully implement the Code resides in countries' lack of willingness or their lack of capacity. Complicating this is that implementation of the Code requires different responses from source and destination countries, bearing in mind that many countries are both simultaneously, and that they have very different resource (financial and institutional) bases available to them. Destination countries with health workforce shortages increasingly need to address policy coherence between domestic and global health policies, while most source countries (including those with critical shortages of health workers) have yet to implement the Code, despite the fact that implementation could assist in their efforts to scale up health workforce planning and retention.

For some, though, the key point is less the 'headline' provisions regarding international recruitment and countries' adherence to all aspects of the Global Code than one of actually dealing with the root causes of health workforce shortages (Buchan 2010). Low levels of health services funding, low pay, limited career opportunities, inadequate infrastructure, and economic and political instability all need to be part of the overall picture of workforce policy and planning that delivers adequate resources to train and retain health workers where they are needed (Buchan 2010; Abadalla *et al.* 2016; Poppe *et al.* 2016; Tomblin-Murphy *et al.* 2016). Nevertheless, this raises the question of whether countries actually have sufficient resources and capacity to implement the Code. Weak national capacity and weak health systems are key issues especially for lower-income countries which contribute to international migration (WHO 2013b, 2015a, 2015b). Pressures on national health systems from ongoing demographic and social changes were further compounded by the aftermath of the most recent (2008/2009) global economic crisis which disproportionately adversely impacted upon developing countries (Siyam and dal Poz 2014; WHO 2013).

## 5 The regulation of private enterprises: a neglected issue

Recruitment companies are an important part of the global dynamics of health worker-migration and although these companies are referred to in the Global Code[8] their adherence to its principles and provisions is not mandatory. At the same time, there have been calls for better regulation and monitoring of national and transnational recruitment companies in recent years as evidence has emerged of their role in unethical recruitment and unethical business practices. This need for stronger responses relates as much to the multilateral level as the national one.

### 5.1 Growth of the international labour recruitment and staffing industry

Growing international demand for health workers has been accompanied by globalising health labour markets in which private sector enterprises have flourished. Such enterprises span all parts of the migration 'industry': from training and education, through recruitment and relocation, to employment (Yeates 2009b: passim). This industry has undergone rapid expansion since the 1980s in both developed and developing countries (Jones and Pardthaisong 1999; Yeates

2009b; ILO 2014a). The growth of private sector agents in countries of origin and destination/employment has been phenomenal. Yeates' study showed that they have developed to increase their share in the overall provision of training and education for health workers (nurses especially), in overseas job placements and in employing health workers (Yeates 2009b). Furthermore, this increased share has been accompanied by a decline in the role of direct employer recruitment and public employment services as well as by a general shift in fee payment from employer to worker (although at these higher levels, employers often still pay some charges (Martin 2005; Yeates 2009b). Private enterprises have also established a presence across all segments of the health workforce sector, including increasingly in private educational institutions many of whose curricula are oriented towards 'export' overseas upon completion of training (ibid.).

This expansion has occurred courtesy of state policy aiming to increase the production of health workers, often as part of a generalised export-oriented development strategy, and it has attracted significant amounts of investment from domestic and overseas sources of private capital. This is the case in India, as it is across many Asian countries (Yeates 2009a, 2009b). The reasons for this growth are clear: health worker training and education, recruitment to work overseas, the relocation of workers abroad, and employment of migrant health workers are all highly profitable (ibid.). Private enterprises and corporations in this sector regularly report significant profits, while employers in recruiting countries save considerable costs in recruiting an already-trained health worker compared with having to educate and train one themselves. The use of temporary staffing agencies in the health labour industry enables health employers to reduce their staffing costs and commercial companies to share in the financial benefits of these reduced costs while charging fees to intending migrants (ibid.).

### *5.2 Unethical business practices and labour exploitation*

While individuals personally profit from migrating to work abroad through higher wages, either in the immediate term or over the longer-term by virtue of experience gained and enhanced career prospects, they often face significant costs associated with entering the international labour market and remaining in it. These costs take many forms including exploitative working conditions, de-skilling, abuse and trafficking (Wickramasekara 2002, 2011; ILO 2008, 2016a; Pillinger 2010, 2013, 2015; Pittman *et al.* 2014; Yeates 2009a, 2009b). Even where regulation has been introduced at the national level this has not prevented the proliferation of unlicensed subagents and brokers and collusion between agents and employers, or the abuse and exploitation of people migrating to certain countries to work in low- and high-skilled sectors (Agunias 2011). Countries that promote the migration of high-skilled health workers as part of their 'migration for development' objectives may be particularly vulnerable in this regard (Wickramasekara 2010).[9]

Malpractice and fraud by recruitment agencies is fairly common. One problem is that recruitment companies sometimes charge excessively high recruitment fees even though these fees are prohibited by international conventions on labour standards (see Section 5.3, this chapter and Appendix 3). Studies of migrant nurses have reported complaints where recruitment agencies misrepresent the pay and conditions that the nurses can expect to enjoy, a problem that has been reported internationally (Redfoot and Houser, 2005). Concerns about misinformation and exploitative recruitment practices were frequently reported by migrant health and social care workers in a PSI participatory research study involving interviews with over 4,000 health and social care workers who had migrated, returned or were planning to migrate in Kenya, Ghana, the Philippines, South Africa, Nigeria and Australia (Pillinger 2010, 2011a, 2011b, 2012, 2013, 2015). Given that the majority of interviewees were recruited through an agency, it is not surprising that ethical recruitment practices were of crucial importance to migration decisions and experiences. One-quarter of the interviewees said there had not been ethical recruitment, few were aware of existing ethical migration policies and practices, and many did not know if they could trust a recruitment agency – if it was legitimate or not.

The study uncovered unethical recruitment practices including: excessive recruitment and placement fees paid to recruitment companies and agents; lack of knowledge of what fees were for; contractual arrangements and agreements reneged upon, including lower levels of pay and different working time and shift arrangements than other workers; lack of information about contracts and working conditions; lack of practical support, including accommodation and food on arrival, and promises of information and support on arrival not materialising. In the Philippines, for example, recruitment companies have aggressively targeted health and social care workers through advertising and in some cases setting up recruitment fares in hospitals in return for a fee for the hospital (Pillinger 2013).[10] Workers were often paid at lower rates than home country workers and there was poor regulation and monitoring of pay and conditions, particularly in private care homes. In some cases, lower rates of pay existed because migrant workers were paid directly by a recruitment company. The South African study points to the vulnerability of health and social care workers to exploitative working conditions: one interviewee, a fully qualified and experienced nurse was recruited by a UK-based recruitment agency to work in a private residential home for older people. Instead of working as a nurse she discovered she was employed as a lower paid care worker, working a 47-hour week, living in accommodation provided by her employer and receiving payment of just £1 an hour. She found herself trapped in poverty in the UK and subsequently returned to South Africa (Pillinger 2011).

Such cases have been reported by the UK Royal College of Nursing which denounced some of them as a 'modern form of slavery' (Yeates 2009b). Forms of indentured labour arise when loans taken out to pay private agencies' fees make it difficult for migrants to leave unsatisfactory employment in the destination country until the debt has been repaid. Annuity models of payment used by recruiters whereby the recruiter receives a share of the salary earned as long as s/he stays with the hospital that the recruiter hired him/her also tie health workers to a single employer. The pressure to stay with one employer is especially acute when state employment permits given to a migrant are tied to a particular employer. Indentured labour contracts are forms of exploitation that may be compounded by the working conditions encountered in practice. Problems include deskilling and downward occupational mobility by virtue of discrimination a lack of opportunities for career progression and being channelled into non-career grades (Yeates 2009b: 107–119).

National and international labour standards require that migrant health workers receive the same pay and conditions as their colleagues, although evidence suggests that exploitative practices often start from the unethical recruitment practices of labour brokers and companies (Bach 2004). Entering unionised employment in a country of destination offers some protection against discriminatory pay and exploitative conduct that workers entering non-unionised private systems do not have (Yeates 2009b). Indeed, there is a significant difference between public and private sector employment and some of the worst abuses of migrant nurses documented are those taking place in private nursing (Bach 2004: 19). Some unions have established union informal networks or sections for migrant workers in countries of destination, an example of which is the South African nurses' network in the UK. Union-to-union bilateral agreements and sharing of information, including automatic union membership for a migrant worker arriving in a country of destination and information for migrant workers to enable them to make informed decisions about migration, have been advocated by global unions such as the PSI.[11]

### 5.3 Strengthening the global governance of recruitment and staffing companies

The call for global action from civil society and trade unions to more effectively tackle unethical business practices has had a strong labour advocacy base. The PSI has been especially active on these issues since 2012. A PSI Resolution addressed the use of 'labour brokers in the public sector globally, and their emergence as powerful multinational companies operating across national boundaries' that are often responsible for the 'manipulation of exploitative short-term contracts … in order to deny workers the benefits associated with full time employment' and the benefits of unionisation (PSI 2012a: 1). It highlighted that 'private recruitment and staffing agencies have helped to accelerate migration trends and contributed to the privatization of public jobs and services' and that they have found 'new ways to extract private profit from public systems by collecting exorbitant fees from employers and/or migrant workers themselves' (ibid.). The Resolution highlighted the need to:

> engage employers and governments to prevent privatisation in all of its forms, and to work towards the eradication of labour broking in favour of decent work and permanent employment, including the filling of all vacancies, and an expansion of public works to meet the needs of communities.
>
> (PSI 2012a: 1)

A key focus of the PSI's ethical recruitment campaign has been the need for stronger regulatory and accountability mechanisms as part of a shared responsibility between source and destination countries to uphold human rights and labour standards for health workers. One aspect of this campaign was a programme of training programmes for representatives of health care and nursing unions in Africa and Asia to ensure that trade unions understood the WHO Global Code, its applicability and potential for trade union advocacy for the implementation of the Code at the national level. According to the PSI this helped mobilise unions at the national level to engage in discussions with employers and ministries about ethical recruitment, including the monitoring of recruitment companies and the launch of a national and international campaign for the ending of illegal of excessive charging of fees.[12]

Still, as important as these advocacy initiatives are, the weaknesses of the global institutional architecture and their role as an 'upstream' source of such abuses are apparent. Although the Global Code makes several references to private recruitment companies, its provisions have generally been poorly implemented. From the perspective of the Code's concern with sustainable health workforces, given that private sector enterprises have permeated all corners of the global health worker labour market, that they have a direct economic interest in making provision where profits are greatest and the fact that it is in the private sector where the worst abuses of migrant health workers occur, the poor implementation and subsequent monitoring of private enterprises is at best a missed opportunity and at worst highly problematic.

There are a number of issues here. First, if Member States do not implement the Code then the activities of private enterprises in their jurisdiction are not legally subject to the Code's provisions. Second, among those Member States who do implement the Code, the efficacy of its provisions is in practice mediated by the quality of governments' actions to domesticate the Code's provisions into national frameworks. There is nothing in the Code itself which stipulates *how* the Code's provisions should be implemented, and states are entirely free to choose whether they do so by non-legally binding means of encouraging 'best practices' or through legally binding and enforceable means. Third, as Yeates (2009a, 2009b) highlights, although Member States' legal authority can be sufficient to regulate all forms of private enterprise activity within their jurisdictions, the territorial scope of state regulation on the one hand and business structures and practices on the other hand are not necessarily congruous. This latter issue has attracted a great deal of attention when it comes to health worker-recruitment. One problem in this regard is that migrant workers can be pressurised into signing a supplementary contract setting out requirements for additional fees to be paid (Martin 2005). Because they are outside the jurisdiction of the source country government

> this effectively leaves migrant nurses who have legitimate grievances about the terms and conditions of their work in a difficult situation, since their only option is to pursue the complaints with the recruitment agency based in their country of origin.
>
> (Yeates 2009b: 109)

In recent years there has been a great deal of attention given to improving standards and monitoring of international labour recruitment companies, for example, through registration and monitoring measures for assuring decent work, contracts of employment, integration, and clinical and cultural orientation programmes on arrival. While measures have been introduced at country level for the regulation, monitoring and enforcement of private employment agencies, they remain insufficient as mechanisms to regulate international recruitment agencies which operate on a transnational basis.

This is not to say that international standards have not been defined. International recruitment has been a recurrent theme in the policy instruments and programmes of work of ILO, starting with ILO Recommendation on Nursing Personnel (see Chapter 3) and continuing with various initiatives that are not sector or migration specific, but which nonetheless impact on international recruitment companies.[13] These include the ILO Private Employment Agency Convention, 1997 (No. 181) and Recommendation 1997 (No. 188), as well as the Employment Service Convention, 1948 (No. 88), all of which provide international standards for fair and decent labour recruitment practices (Appendix 3). The 1998 ILO Declaration on Fundamental Principles and Rights at Work set out key pillars for the prevention of abuses, including the abolition of forced labour (the latter of which resulted in the adoption of a Protocol to ILO's Forced Labour Convention, 1930 (No. 29), and a Recommendation on Supplementary Measures for the Effective Suppression of Forced Labour). The 2006 ILO Multilateral Framework on Labour Migration (ILO 2006), contains non-binding principles and guidelines for a rights-based approach to labour migration, including in relation to recruitment.[14]

All of these standards were in place at the time of the Code but it made no reference to any of them either in the body of the Code or in the implementation and monitoring mechanisms. Had it done so this would have helped to mobilise and raise awareness at an early stage about the applicability of existing standards and instruments, their obligations on governments and where gaps needed to be filled. Even if the Code could not reasonably have referenced ILO standards not yet in place, a clause governing all standards of private sector enterprises that prevail in the health services sector would have been a significant way of strengthening the provisions of the Code. As it is, the Code's failings on this front also missed the opportunity to link the definition of ethical recruitment by private sector companies to standard-setting activities by ILO and other bodies that include the regulation of recruitment.

This oversight is all the more astonishing given that the recruitment industry itself has taken a global approach to ethical recruitment and the Code of Practice of the International Confederation of Private Employment Agencies (World Employment Federation 2016) could have been embedded in the Global Code. This business Code prohibits the charging of fees to workers and includes compliance with the ILO Declaration of Fundamental Principles and Rights at Work, the UN Guiding Principles on Business & Human Rights and the UN Protocol to Prevent, Suppress and Punish Trafficking in Person. In addition, CIETT members are requested to encourage their governments to adopt the provisions of ILO Convention No. 181 on Private Employment Agencies and its accompanying Recommendation No. 188, on the basis that they 'provide a framework that allows for improved functioning of private employment services and protection of workers' (CIETT, 2015: 1). Also relevant in this regard is an initiative by the International Organization of Employers (IOE) and the IOM to promote ethical recruitment of migrant workers through a voluntary certification process (IOM/IOE 2014).

Despite the significant increase in initiatives aimed at ending abuses by recruitment companies, including whether international labour standards and human rights are comprehensive and specific enough to tangibly impact upon health worker-recruitment practices by those companies, their efficacy remains open to question. A major problem is that none of them are underpinned by statutory obligations or enforcement mechanisms. These issues are discussed further in Chapter 7 which discusses how fair recruitment has been propelled back onto the agendas of ILO and the UN as part of the Sustainable Development Agenda and the implementation of the SDGs. For now, suffice it to note that even though it was a major breakthrough that recruitment fees were included in the 2018 UN Global Compact on Migration, this initiative remains non-binding with minimal implementation or enforcement mechanisms. The 2017 proposal for a binding treaty on business and human rights made by the Human Rights Council, if accepted, could potentially provide strengthened frameworks for due diligence and respect for human rights in business operations, and would be applicable to transnational recruitment companies working across borders (see Chapter 7).

## 6 Conclusion

This chapter continued our in-depth discussion of the multilateralisation of ethical recruitment initiatives, with a specific focus on the WHO Global Code, during the first decade of the twenty-first century. These voluntary initiatives are the hallmark of what we identify as the second key historic phase in the development of the global policy field on health worker-migration and -recruitment. Their proliferation has already received considerable criticism not least because they are based on voluntarism and self-regulation, which 'render the Codes toothless and represent persuasive moral imperatives rather than obligatory statutory requirements' (Pagett and Padarath 2007: 46). Others have similarly argued that the voluntary nature of these Codes results in a lack of incentives and sanctions (Buchan and Dovlo 2004; Willets and Martineau 2004), resulting in problems in balancing an individual's right to migrate with international equity issues (Bach 2004; Mcintosh, Torgerson and Klassen 2007; Bourgeault *et al.* 2016).

In this context, we discussed how, on the one hand, the agreement for a Global Code represented a major breakthrough in establishing an additional global governance instrument on ethical recruitment of health workers. It was at the time a reflection of governments and global organisations' recognition of the need to strengthen global policy through a multilateral framework. The messages underpinned by the Global Code remain a powerful reminder of the responsibilities of governments to address the impact of recruitment on the health systems in source countries as part of their ethical recruitment strategies. On the other hand, the Code is institutionally weak, its provisions are variously ill-defined and implementation of the Code has so far been unspectacular as judged by our analysis of the published evidence and the additional data analysis we undertook for the purpose of this study. Indeed, since the Code came into effect WHO has continually highlighted challenges in sustaining momentum around it at both national and international levels. Our analysis has captured this, but we have particularly emphasised that the 'implementation gap' is at least partly the result of its original design. A key problem is that it is 'unanchored' in the wider global governance institutional architecture of labour and business regulation and development that could have buttressed the Code's implementation. We also identified failings in the organisational leadership of WHO whose efficacy in supporting implementation and monitoring has been constrained by severe resource restrictions. Such is the array of issues with the Global Code, from design to implementation, that its transformative potential has not been realised.

Ultimately, though, the overall lack of progress in strengthening the global institutional framework governing health worker-migration during this second phase reflects the unwillingness of destination country governments to engage in binding measures. This, as we discussed in earlier chapters (see Chapters 2–4) is a long-standing problem, particularly among the higher-income recruiting countries. In this respect, the Code reflects the growth of multilateral non-binding initiatives and consultative forums as well as continued enthusiasm for trade-based responses to health worker shortages and labour market 'liberalisation' measures (particularly temporary and circular migration). The failings of the Global Code are also attributable to a deep-seated reluctance by many governments to engage in global institution-building and regulation that surpasses what is minimally necessary to address some of the direst social consequences of labour market and services trade liberalisation.

The evidence we have reviewed in this chapter points to the need for more decisive and strengthened international action to regulate and monitor international labour migration and recruitment in the health sector. Non-binding agreements can exert significant leverage over time. They can generate a constituency and dynamic of their own, and their scope, content, implementation mechanisms and standing can all be increased (Sauvant 2015). In this vein, Dhillon (2015) argues that the Global Code's potential effectiveness remains fragile. Indeed, it will fail to achieve its desired effects, including the goal of universal health coverage unless there is concerted mobilisation around the Code's implementation. This conclusion can be taken as a 'call to action' addressed to diverse constituencies of the Code. Indeed, WHO's response has been to argue for greater levels of engagement by all stakeholders and more resources to be dedicated to overcoming problems associated with weak national capacity to address health workforce issues. It has continually emphasised that these issues can be addressed and rectified through technical cooperation and assistance (WHO 2013a). In this respect, a major challenge is to increase the level of donor support for health workforce issues. WHO needs donors behind it with secure, long-term funding (rather than ad hoc special projects) if it is to effectively monitor the implementation of the Code.

Bearing this in mind, we need to look at the wider perspective. The absence of a legally binding instrument backed up by a robust system of statutory monitoring and reporting as part of a comprehensive enforcement system is a fundamental problem. All the technical assistance in the world provided by WHO, or projects funded by the EU and ILO or others, cannot compel governments, recruitment agencies or employers to comply with any of the provisions of the Global Code. WHO's recommendation that the Code be incorporated into national policies and laws as a way to make it legally binding has been systematically ignored by most of its member states. This is a fundamental and inherent weakness of the Code and will remain so until such time as its legal status is changed, or binding obligations upon states and all other social actors involved in health worker-recruitment and -migration to adhere to its provisions can be instituted. In this light, the question must be asked why there is no global advocacy to strengthen the Global Code's institutional provisions through an updated Code, or to press for an alternative mechanism or set of instruments capable of effectively regulating the buoyant international trade in health workforce recruitment and migration that is set to be a major feature of the decades to come.

## Notes

1　WHO-EAG is made up of 20 members, comprising 12 member-state representatives (two from each WHO region) and eight representatives from ILO, IOM, OECD, along with experts from international NGOs and other non-affiliated (independent) experts.
2　The Third Round of Code reporting was launched in May 2018 and the findings were presented to the 72nd WHA in May 2019. The findings from the 3rd round of Code reporting will also inform the Second Review of Code Relevance and Effectiveness. At the time of writing it was too early to analyse the results of the third round of reporting.
3　The names of the 179 signatures from national and global NGOs and health organisations for the call can be seen at: www.healthworkers4all.eu/fileadmin/docs/eu/hw4 all_papers/HW4All-CTA-signatories.pdf. For further information see: www.health workers4all.eu/eu/contributions/hw4all-events/health-workers-migration-a-health-worker-for-everyone-everywhere-launch-event-of-the-european-call-to-action-madrid-5-june-2014/
4　This is important because, as Sauvant (2015) argues, in some countries voluntary instruments can potentially be used in courts, thereby turning 'soft' law into 'hard' law. He gives the example of the US, where soft law can be invoked by courts in action against firms.
5　Thus, Article 3.2 only refers to

> the setting of voluntary international principles and the coordination of national policies on international health personnel recruitment [which] are desirable in order to advance frameworks to equitably strengthen health systems worldwide, to mitigate the negative effects of health personnel migration on the health systems of developing countries and to safeguard the rights of health personnel.

Article 3.3 refers only to consideration for '... the countries that are particularly vulnerable to health workforce shortages and/or have limited capacity to implement the recommendations of this Code' and urges the provision of 'technical and financial assistance to developing countries and countries with economies in transition aimed at strengthening health systems, including health personnel development.'

6   The WHO-EAG argued that 'The Code and the WHO Secretariat's capacity should be integral elements of the forthcoming Global Strategy on Human Resources for Health' (2015a: 5). It also suggested the 'streamlining' of reporting requirements for member states, so that reporting on all relevant HRH-related resolutions be carried out in 'a single periodic monitoring linked to the accountability mechanisms of the Global Strategy on Human Resources for Health' (WHO 2015a: 5).

7   The project is funded by the EU and NORAD (the Norwegian international aid agency). For further information see: www.who.int/workforcealliance/brain-drain_brain-gain/en/.

8   The relevant Articles of the Global Code are Article 4.2

> (Recruiters and employers should, to the extent possible, be aware of and consider the outstanding legal responsibility of health personnel to the health system of their own country such as a fair and reasonable contract of service and not seek to recruit them),

Article 8.4

> (Recruiters and employers should cooperate fully in the observance of the Code and promote the guiding principles expressed by the Code, irrespective of a Member State's ability to implement the Code),

Article 8.5 (states should 'maintain a record, updated at regular intervals, of all recruiters authorised by competent authorities to operate within their jurisdiction') and Article 8.6 (states should 'to the extent possible, encourage and promote good practices among recruitment agencies by only using those agencies that comply with the guiding principles of the Code') (WHO 2010a).

9   Some source country governments have introduced national registration and accreditation measures to suppress unethical recruitment practices and bogus recruitment companies. Examples include Uganda, India, Sri Lanka (ADBI/ILO/OECD, 2016) and the Philippines. In the latter country, there continue to be many examples of exploitative and unethical recruitment practices operated by recruitment agencies. The Department of Labor and Employment (POEA) has a mandate to follow up investigations on unethical recruitment practices and in 2010, it handled 1,648 cases of illegal recruitment (Pillinger 2013) and it continues to strengthen its regulatory and implementation system (Pillinger 2013).

10   Examples of slogans used in advertising often create unrealistic expectations for migrant workers, and include, 'Provide a good future for your children!'; 'Why put up with a low salary when you can make millions'; 'Believe in yourself, Canada believes in you'; 'The Surest Way to Success' (Pillinger 2013). See also Yeates (2009b) on the advertising practices of recruitment agencies. In the Philippines, for example, recruitment companies have aggressively targeted health and social care workers through advertising campaigns. There have also been cases of direct recruitment whereby private recruitment agencies set up recruitment fairs on the premises of hospitals in the Philippines in return for a fee paid to the hospital (Galvez-Tan 2008). Such practices are not associated only with contemporary state or corporate globalisation. For example, British hospital employers engaged in forms of open recruitment strategies in Ireland for Irish nurses during the mid-twentieth century, travelling directly to Ireland to openly recruit to British hospitals, circumventing state regulation and authorised institutional channels and procedures (Yeates 2009b).

11  The PSI's web site contains a wide range of information resources drawn up with migrant health workers in trade unions in key source countries – these resources give up to date information about labour rights, ethical recruitment processes and channels, information about the legal rights on arrival and reintegration on return (for union members in the health and social in South Africa, Philippines, Kenya, Ghana, Sri Lanka and Nigeria; and resources for workers migrating to Finland, Norway, Germany, Denmark and Australia). See: www.world-psi.org/en/issue/migration-and-refugees. PSI programmes have grown since its 2012 Congress Resolution on ethical recruitment (PSI 2012b, 2). These include the 'Passport Card to Workers' Rights' initiative to promote portable union membership among PSI affiliates across the world.

12  Interview by Jane Pillinger with Genevieve Gencianos, PSI (10 September 2018)

13  For many decades, ILO has provided technical support for sound national policies to regulate recruitment, especially in Asia. Such activities include the adoption in June 2014 by the International Labour Conference of a Protocol to ILO's Forced Labour Convention, 1930 (No. 29), and a Recommendation on Supplementary Measures for the Effective Suppression of Forced Labour. Over the last five years, ILO has campaigned to address fraudulent and abusive recruitment practices. Its Tripartite Technical Meeting on Labour Migration recommended that the Office develop 'guidance to promote recruitment practices that respect the principles enshrined in international labour standards' (ILO 2013: 30). In particular, ILO called for strengthened laws, policies and enforcement mechanisms in line with ILO Convention No. 181 and other standards and the promotion of fair business standards and partnerships in the recruitment industry. In 2014 the ILO Director-General proposed a global Fair Migration Agenda, reflecting the 'growing international concern about abusive and fraudulent recruitment practices affecting migrant workers in particular and issues of human trafficking and forced labour' (ILO 2014b). In addition, ILO had been arguing for some time that fair recruitment needed to be firmly embedded in the ILO Fair Migration Agenda as part of the wider post-2015 development agenda and which emphasised both fair recruitment and rights-based approaches to international migration. The general principle that recruitment fees should not be charged, was one of the conclusions of the 2016 ILO Tripartite meeting of experts on fair recruitment guidelines which recommended that as a general principle 'No recruitment fees or related costs should be charged to workers or jobseekers, and the costs should be borne by the employer' (ILO 2016a: 19). The consequent establishment of the ILO Fair Recruitment Initiative (ILO 2014b), added greater momentum and urgency in ILO to implement the detailed guidance in Convention No. 97 on recruitment, placing and conditions of labour of migrants, including under government-sponsored arrangements and the provisions in Convention No. 181 to prohibit private employment agencies from charging fees to workers, directly or indirectly. In addition, this was a further opportunity for ILO to add to the requirements set out in Convention No. 97 for member states to conclude bilateral agreements to prevent abuses and fraudulent practices. For ILO, the need to strengthen efforts in this area, including technical assistance and guidance on fair recruitment practices, along with increased cooperation between governments arose because of the 'very extensive involvement of private agencies in the recruitment of workers for employment in other countries has all too frequently been associated with serious abuses' (ILO 2014b, 22), opening up a space for ILO global action in this area and country-level activities. ILO also succeeded in linking the Fair Recruitment Initiative to the work of the Global Migration Group (GMG), which was chaired by ILO in 2014 (under the auspices of its Task Force on Migration and Decent Work). ILO's adoption in 2016 of the non-binding General Principles and Operational Guidelines for Fair Recruitment, which apply to recruitment within or across international borders, firmly embedded human rights norms and standards into international recruitment (ILO 2016b).

14 The Multilateral Framework states that 'Governments in both origin and destination countries should give due consideration to licensing and supervising recruitment and placement services for migrant workers in accordance with the Private Employment Agencies Convention, 1997 (No. 181), and its Recommendation (No. 188).' In implementing this, the guidelines will give practical effect to this principle.

# 6 Bilateral agreements

## A resurgent feature of global policy

## 1 Introduction

Bilateralism is an inherent feature of the global governance of health worker-migration and -recruitment policy. Bilateral agreements[1] are among the earliest cross-border policy instruments in this field, and they are the most prolific types of inter-state agreement on international migration. More particularly, and most relevant from the perspective of this book, they have been actively promoted by multilateral organisations over the past 70 years as a means of regulating matters of common concern. ILO has been a major proponent of such agreements in matters of labour migration since 1949 (ILO Convention No. 97). Its Nursing Personnel Recommendation encouraged governments to enter into bilateral arrangements to manage international nurse migration, and its Programme of Action (ILO 1976a) highlighted bilateral agreements as a way of limiting the loss of education and training resources when skilled personnel emigrate. WHO also encouraged bilateralism as a way of ensuring 'a more mutually beneficial approach to regulating health manpower migration' (Mejia *et al.* 1979) (see also Chapters 2 and 3). Bilateral agreements continue to be actively promoted by the UN and its specialised agencies. ILO has taken active steps to promote bilateral agreements for well-regulated and fair migration between Member States (ILO 2014b), adding the prevention of abuses and fraudulent recruitment practices to the requirements of Convention 97 (Appendix 3). The UN's promotion of bilateral agreements has been echoed by the OECD and the GFMD as important mechanisms for managing migration, workforce planning, ensuring ethical recruitment and guaranteeing fundamental rights at work. As such, bilateral agreements are entirely consistent with multilateral ones – indeed, they have been co-promoted over the years by international organisations. Moreover, as we argue in this chapter, they are a fundamental and integral feature of the on-going multilateralisation of the global policy field that is the subject of this book.

This chapter examines this aspect of global policy in some detail. It situates the promulgation and use of bilateral agreements in relation to health workers in historical and contemporary periods. It reviews why they are supported by multilateral organisations (and others) as well as why there are mounting concerns about them. We bring into our review of this field original data analysis based on the WHO's National Reporting Instrument dataset. This enables us to elucidate as high a level of specificity and granularity as possible about the nature and range of bilateral agreements in relation to health worker migration that currently exist. We demonstrate that, despite the proliferation of such agreements, they are often devoid of the kinds of protections and compensatory mechanisms that ILO and WHO hold up as possible and desirable. In this context, we argue that most bilateral agreements in this field are little more than short-term agreements to provide quotas of health workers for temporary or circular migration.

By way of a prefix to the next stages of the chapter, it is important to clarify that bilateral agreements are international agreements concluded on a bilateral basis between two participating governments. International bilateral agreements typically take the form of Memoranda of Understanding, Agreement or Cooperation but in practice there are various bilateral mechanisms of differentiated levels of formalisation and institutionalisation. The content of such agreements reflects the priorities of the signatories. They may include information with regard to how recruitment will be undertaken, the nature and degree of financial contributions of each country, the nature of protection of recruited health workers under employment and social protection laws, support, further education and training of recruited health workers, support and encouragement of recruited health workers to return to their source country, monitoring of the agreement as it is working in practice, and the benefits to the participating countries (Pagett and Padarath 2007). However, there is an exceptionally high degree of variance in practice.

On a methodological note, this area is notoriously difficult to research. Data on bilateral agreements are notoriously inaccessible. This is not only because there is a proliferation of such agreements worldwide using different nomenclatures but, more pertinently, they are beset by a lack of transparency such that texts of agreements are mostly not made publicly available by governments. Most information on bilateral agreements in relation to the health sector is in the European context with a limited amount of information available on such agreements in the rest of the world (Plotnikova 2014; Dhillon *et al.* 2010). The only other significant study of such agreements outside of the EU is that undertaken by ILO which reviewed 76 BLAs in ASEAN countries. Of these, it identified only two BLAs specifically addressed to health workers (Wickramasekara and Ruhunage 2018).[2] Several agreements referred to skilled workers and cooperation on training, although they did not specify which skilled workers are included.

## 2   Bilateralist labour, migration and health strategies

Bilateral agreements have long been a feature of international relations, inter-state diplomacy and global governance in matters of trade and migration. Bilateral labour agreements date to the late nineteenth century, when early versions of state-sponsored recruitment programmes were initiated by the US through trade agreements on commerce and navigation that also allowed entry to foreign workers with a limited right of residence in the party countries (Plotnikova 2014:

327). In Europe, bilateral labour agreements were concluded after World War I and continued apace after World War II in response to significant labour shortages and displacement resulting from the wars (Plotnikova 2014). In the 1950s and 1960s these induced an intense period of overseas labour recruitment mainly from 'peripheral' countries in Europe (Ireland, Greece, Italy, Portugal, Spain, Yugoslavia, Turkey) and North Africa (Algeria, Morocco and Tunisia) countries towards Belgium, France, Germany, the Netherlands and Switzerland (ibid.). These agreements were not health-sector specific but nonetheless played an important role in staffing the post-war expansion of health systems in the recruiting countries. The UK drew copiously on its (then) present and former colonies for supplies of labour to work in its fledgling national health service as nurses and midwives and in ancillary hospital services (catering, cleaning, laundry) (Yeates 2004a, 2014b, 2009b).

Following a decline in the number of bilateral recruitment schemes concluded by European countries after the oil crisis in 1973, when restrictive measures on labour immigration were introduced, bilateral labour agreements re-emerged in Europe in the 1990s and early 2000s after the opening of borders between Western European countries and Central and Eastern European ones. More widely, they were part of the 'free trade' and trade liberalisation movements that became increasingly embedded, discursively and institutionally, in national and cross-border spheres of governance. Bilateral trade agreements were favoured by the US during the 2000s in response to the stalling of the Doha round of multilateral trade negotiations (Yeates, *et al.* 2010), but gained momentum among more countries since, when the use of bilateral labour agreement has been growing. ILO reports that 'labour-related clauses are increasingly included in bilateral free trade agreements' (ILO 2018c: 40), including recently signed agreements by the United States, Canada and the EU. By the end of 2015, 76 trade agreements with labour provisions had been agreed. Of potential impact also are investment agreements which increasingly are including social provisions (ILO 2016c; UNCTAD 2017).

Bilateral agreements in all their forms have, then, long been used by governments to realise their trade and labour policy objectives, but they incorporated the health sector and international migration only in a disjointed way, if at all. During the opening years of the twenty-first century, however, bilateral agreements that relate explicitly and specifically to health workers have emerged. It is worth quoting Dhillon *et al.* (2010) extensively on this point:

> In the past, the challenges associated with migration in general, and health worker migration specifically, have been addressed tangentially through piecemeal agreements in the sectors of education, labor, trade, and sometimes health. A body of bilateral agreements focused specifically on managing migration flows and addressing the negative effects of health worker migration has not fully developed. This is due both to the significant political sensitivities associated with the topic of migration and the fact that the issue cuts across various sectors. Rather, a disparate group of bilateral agreements exist

that touch on the various challenges associated with the international migration of health workers. These include bilateral labor agreements, bilateral social security agreements, bilateral health cooperation agreements, and bilateral economic integration agreements, including the associated mutual recognition agreements. Recently there has been a growing trend towards the development of bilateral migration agreements that incorporate the concept of shared responsibility and take advantage of the ability to address the cross-linkages inherent in the topic.

(Dhillon *et al.*, 2010: 15–16)

Dhillon *et al.* identify two 'generations' of approaches to bilateral agreements relating to health worker-migration. The first generation embodies what they call a 'twentieth-century' approach. Initially, bilateral agreements to address the challenges to migration were approached through piecemeal agreements, focused on labour recruitment, social security, welfare protection, and economic integration. Subsequently, and reflecting the growing focus on the migration-development nexus, bilateral agreements sought to 'comprehensively manage migration flows, with a particular focus on harnessing migration flows to maximise development in both countries of origin and destination and to address source country concerns regarding "brain drain"' (Dhillon *et al.*, 2010: 18). In this model, which remains prevalent, it is destination countries that usually drive the development of such agreements through which they pursue a wide range of goals (e.g. addressing labour shortages, protecting political and post-colonial relationships, promoting cultural ties, or facilitating services trade liberalisation and trade ties with the signatory country). Source countries, in this model, agree to enter into such agreements as a means of ensuring improving living and working conditions for nationals, addressing unemployment, and facilitating the acquisition of skills for their nationals (ibid.: 18). Many of the agreements into which the Philippines has entered into typify this approach.

The second generation, which the authors term a 'twenty-first century' approach, seeks to enable 'development-friendly' migration whereby the benefits and challenges of migration gain primacy alongside a focus on facilitating labour mobility and ensuring social protection for migrant workers. Central to this 'generation' of bilateral agreements is the concept of 'shared responsibility'. This places more emphasis on engaging with the various concerns of source countries and identifying the responsibilities of those countries and workers themselves (ibid.: 19). With this comes a de-emphasis on migration leading to permanent settlement and a greater emphasis on temporary and circular migration, mitigating adverse consequences of health worker-migration on source countries, and maximising the development benefits resulting from migration. Exemplars include agreements between France and Senegal, Spain with Morocco and with other West African states, the Philippines with Bahrain, and India with Denmark (ibid.: 21).

## 3 Global calls for bilateral action: institutions, rationales and limitations

Bilateral agreements result from government decisions to address matters of common concern to the two negotiating parties, but, such decisions are shaped by wider global regimes governing migration, labour, human rights, equality, social protection, health, trade and development. Multilateral organisations, especially the UN, have long called for governments to make greater and more effective use of bilateral agreements to achieve health workforce and wider development goals. In 2001 the Health Ministers of the Southern African Development Community (SADC) called for international action by the Commonwealth to promote bilateral labour agreements between governments in order to regulate the recruitment of health workers from developing countries (Pagett and Padarath 2007).[3] WHO's 'flagship' 2006 World Health Report (WHO 2006d) argued that bilateral agreements are vital elements of ethical and responsible policies when governed by multilateral principles.[4] The Pacific Code of Practice for Recruitment of Health Workers (WHO 2007) and the EU Green Paper on Health Workforce (CEC 2008) both urged governments to consider using bilateral agreements to regulate the recruitment of health workers from overseas. The WHO Global Code (WHO 2010) similarly calls for bilateral agreements and recommends that Member States use the Code when entering into bilateral arrangements.

The *2030 Agenda for Sustainable Development* (UN 2015) did not explicitly identify the scope for bilateral cooperation as a means of realising the Global Goals, but the Commission on Health Employment and Economic Growth argued in favour of bilateral agreements in achieving global health workforce goals (HEEG 2016). WHO (a member of this Commission) has also continued to press the case for bilateral agreements to achieve global health goals. The 69th World Health Assembly (2016) called on Member States to develop improved mechanisms for development partners to work together on a bilateral (as well as a multilateral) basis in assessing health workforce implications and drawing up effective assistance programmes that can be scaled up (Dhillon 2016). A year later, as part of WHO's High Level Dialogue on health worker-migration, a meeting between 29 senior representatives from national governments, regional organisations, and international organisations on the margins of the *4th Global Forum on Human Resources for Health* highlighted the role of bilateral policy measures as part of wider international cooperation efforts 'to better govern and advance mutual benefit from the international movement of health workers' (WHO 2017: 2). This work guides the work of the International Platform on Health Worker Mobility set up under the joint ILO-OECD-WHO Working for Health Programme (Chapter 7).

One reason for the growing interest in bilateral agreements is that they are recognised as important mechanisms for managing health worker-migration and -recruitment. Specifically, they have the potential to protect rights to decent work and social protection of migrant workers and mitigate the negative development impacts of emigration on the source country. They can do this by reducing a mismatch between supply and demand, specifying key labour rights to be protected and ethical recruitment processes to be followed. They can also strengthen accountability and collaboration between countries and promote technical cooperation and investment among them (HEEG 2016).

More generally, bilateral agreements have become more important in relation to health worker-migration and -recruitment as well as in relation to other policy fields such as social security, labour, trade and investment, because they afford a great deal more flexibility for the participating parties than other types of international agreements. Compared with multilateral agreements, they are easier to negotiate and quicker to conclude (Yeates *et al.* 2010). They offer governments more control and regulatory discretion, because they can tailor the agreement to the needs and circumstances of the two parties. The balance of power between negotiating parties is also a consideration here. The stronger party can exercise power over its negotiating counterpart: by entering into an agreement with just one other government it can bypass multi-state political blocs and alliances that emerge in multilateral negotiations and in which weaker states' voices can be amplified and can exert more leverage (ibid.; Yeates 2014b). In principle, bilateral agreements also have the potential to raise social and labour standards more rapidly as the two parties can go further in their agreement than what is usually possible in multilateral agreements (Yeates *et al.* 2010; Plotnikova, 2014).

It is important to recognise, however, that international agreements negotiated and concluded on a bilateral scale are far from unproblematic. A fundamental issue is transparency: accessing the text of agreements is notoriously difficult (Dhillon *et al.* 2010; Wickramasekara 2015). What databases that exist are far from comprehensive and tend not to include the text of the agreements. Furthermore, because such agreements are by definition negotiated one at a time, and they reflect the particular interests of the two negotiating parties, a patchwork of arrangements are instituted that inevitably offer incomplete and/or variable coverage. They also tend to generate discrimination between nationals, occupational groups and signatory countries (Yeates 2018b). EU social security agreements, for example, are negotiated by Member States, mostly in isolation from one another, and without reference to what other EU countries are doing (CEC 2012). Certain EU Member States deemed to be significant trading 'partners' may be pinpointed by other countries from outside the EU to enter into agreements, excluding other countries. Some countries may not be covered by bilateral agreements at all, yet have a significant overseas workforce (Yeates 2018b). Tellingly, as the European Commission argued, 'Migrants and businesses based in third countries not only deal with fragmented social security systems when moving between EU countries, but are also confronted with distinctive national bilateral agreements when moving into and out of the EU' (CEC 2012: 3). Even where these agreements exist, the process of moving from one place to another can result in a significant loss of entitlements because of the differentiated regulation of income maintenance and security provisions at the national and European levels (Meyer *et al.* 2013). In such cases, the results can be catastrophic, as migrants can lose acquired social security rights otherwise available for persons moving out of, or back into, the EU between countries that have concluded a bilateral social security agreement. This is just as likely to affect migrant EU citizens as migrants from third countries (CEC 2012: 3; Yeates 2018b).

Finally, bilateral agreements that emerge without reference to a common approach among states generate further problems. Once in place there is often no mechanism for harmonising states' approaches to solving the common problems they face. This is recognised as a problem even in the context of the EU, which has the most advanced multilateral institutional mechanisms for pursuing its common policy in relation to social security, migration and trade (CEC 2012: 3) and, increasingly, in relation to health worker-migration within its regional borders and with 'third countries'.

Like other bilateral agreements, those relating to health worker-migration and -recruitment encompass heterogenous policy and programmatic instruments, and they reflect different degrees of (in)formality and institutionalisation (Endnote 1), coverage and coherence. They encompass sector-specific agreements relating to labour recruitment, social security and welfare, general health cooperation, occupation/profession-specific agreements (e.g. mutual recognition agreements), as well as broader economic partnerships that may encompass health worker migration amongst other things (Dhillon *et al.* 2010: 17–18). The aims, duration, eligible occupations and policy approaches underlying them vary considerably. In the sections that follow, we examine further the international 'topography' of these agreements.

## 4 Global overview of bilateral agreements on health worker-migration and -recruitment

Better knowledge of what kinds of international agreements are likely to most contribute to strengthened governance of ethical recruitment and rights-based approaches to migration relies on the availability of high-quality data on the agreements in place and their effectiveness. A major issue, however, is the absence of readily-available data. ILO's database of member government's legal and regulatory instruments includes bilateral labour agreements but does not track which agreements have been implemented (and how) or whether they are still in operation. Dhillon *et al.*'s (2010) study of bilateral agreements on health worker migration estimated that there were over 100 inter-state bilateral agreements that intersect with the issue of health worker-migration. However, due to the piecemeal development of these, and national sensitivities in making available the text of such agreements, it was not possible to comprehensively ascertain their overall number or content, let alone their effects.[5] This point remains broadly applicable nearly a decade after their report.

### 4.1 WHO National Reporting Instrument reports database

Nevertheless, since Dhillon *et al.*'s report a WHO Reporting Instrument reports database has become available arising from the monitoring and reporting processes instituted by the 2010 WHO Global Code (WHO 2018b). The Code encourages information exchange on issues related to health personnel and health systems in the context of migration, and stipulates reporting by governments every three years on measures taken to implement the Code (Chapter 4). The database contains the self-assessment returns ('National Reporting Instrument' (NRI)) submitted by countries as part of their reporting obligations, including arrangements that take account of the needs of developing countries and economies in transition.[6] NRIs were introduced in Second Round reporting (2015–2016) to monitor progress in implementing the WHO Global Code; the most recent publicly available data is from 2015. As a result, we now have additional data on bilateral (and multilateral) agreements governing the international recruitment of health workers. In what follows we present original analysis of the WHO's NRI dataset.

The NRI database currently constitutes the single most comprehensive data source on bilateral agreements on health worker-migration. All WHO Member States are required to complete and return an NRI for their country. However, some qualifying comments first are needed regarding the limitations of this dataset. First, and most significantly, reporting rates are low. Just 74 out of 194 WHO Member States completed an NRI in the second round of assessment of the implementation of the Code, reflecting a return rate of only 38 per cent (Chapter 5). Second, the information provided in the NRI returns is of variable quality. Dates of agreements (start, duration, end) are not consistently provided. This was the case for Belize, Bangladesh, Bhutan, Canada, Bosnia & Herzegovina, Ireland, Finland, Zimbabwe, Djibouti, Qatar, Libya, Romania, Saudi Arabia and Morocco. Some returns (e.g. from Belize, Nigeria) did not provide full information on occupations covered, while the other signatory country to the agreement was not always identified (e.g. Morocco, Republic of Moldova). Inconsistencies are also evident at the level of reporting of agreements. Not all countries listed all agreements they had entered into. For example, Japan did not include its bilateral agreements with the Philippines or Indonesia in its NRI return whereas these countries included their agreements with Japan. Denmark did not include its agreement that was otherwise listed by Finland. The Russian Federation did not list its agreement with Namibia. France did not report its agreement with Canada (Quebec), while Canada did. Bangladesh did not include its agreement with Maldives which did report it. Bilateral agreements cited by other sources (notably Dhillon *et al.* 2010; HEEG 2016; Wickramasekara and Ruhunage 2018) confirm that this database is incomplete.

Third, a limitation of the database is that there is no evaluative data on the agreements. The wording of the NRI questionnaire only requests information about the content of agreements in relation to the occupational categories covered and does not require governments to provide any information about the implementation or impacts of the agreements. Thus, although the NRI database constitutes a significant advance over what was previously publicly available, it is by no means complete. Accordingly, supplementary research is needed to complete the information provided by governments to gain a fuller picture.

## *4.2 Overview of findings from analysis of the database*

Table 6.1 provides a summary overview of the information returned by each country, as supplemented by our additional research. It groups countries by their WHO regional affiliation. Countries are listed alphabetically within each regional grouping. The data presented relates to governments' responses to the question of whether they have entered into an international agreement. We distinguish between the bilateral and multilateral agreements they reported. The table provides summary details of the agreement(s), the country or countries with which the government had partnered, the date of the agreement, and the occupational categories covered by the measures.

Table 6.1 shows that of the 74 countries that made an NRI return, 34 declared at least one bilateral agreement. Broken down by WHO region, the proportions are as follows: AFRO 4 out of 9; AMRO 6 out of 9; EMRO 4 out of 7; EURO 12 out of 31; SEARO 5 out of 6; WPRO 3 out of 12.[7] Many of the agreements pre-date the WHO Code. The earliest agreement dates back to 1994 (Finland–Denmark), and this was followed in 1998 by two agreements involving South Africa, one with Tunisia, the other with Cuba. The increasing number of agreements since the mid-2000s is notable. There is great variability in these agreements, in terms of which countries enter into them and with which other ones, the forms the agreements take, their coverage, content and the approaches they take. These points are elaborated below.

Most countries have concluded more than one such agreement, although agreements listed by states in their returns are not necessarily in force presently. Only in a minority of countries – 19 – is there evidence that agreements are unequivocally 'live' at the time of the returns being made (i.e. in 2015): Burundi, Namibia, Zimbabwe, Bahamas, Brazil, Canada, Djibouti, Morocco, Qatar, Bosnia & Herzegovina, Finland, France, Germany, Ireland, Netherlands, Republic of Moldova, Maldives, Cambodia and Philippines. Many that were reported had already expired. The scope of coverage of health occupations in the agreements varies along a spectrum of inclusivity ranging at one end from the identification of one or more specific occupational categories to general statements that all health professionals are included at the other end. Doctors, nurses and midwives are the most frequently mentioned occupations covered by bilateral agreements.[8] Dentists, pharmacists, and allied health care professionals, including health administrators, physiotherapists and laboratory technicians, also feature.

Bilateral agreements reflect the positioning of countries within global and regional divisions of labour. Bilateral agreements actively channel health worker labour to overseas markets whether intra-regionally or extra-regionally. A major determinant of the distribution of risks, costs and benefits arising from health worker-migration is the terms on which international inter-state agreements are entered into (Yeates 2009a, 2009b). Agreements concluded with other similarly situated countries within the same region will be (all things equal) less lucrative to the source country government than those concluded with wealthier ones,

*Table 6.1* Summary overview of international agreements and arrangements on skilled health worker migration of NRI-returning countries, by WHO Regional Office

| WHO Regional Office | Country | International agreement or arrangement | Type of international measure | Partner country/countries, and date (where given), and occupations covered |
|---|---|---|---|---|
| African Regional Office (AFRO) | Burundi | Yes | Bilateral | Egypt, Cuba: 2010–2015: doctors and technicien de maintenance<br>Egypt, Cuba, China: 2010–2015: technicien de maintenance |
| | Cameroon | No | n/a | n/a |
| | Ghana | No | n/a | n/a |
| | Namibia | Yes | Bilateral | Kenya: mid 2000–2015: doctors, nurses, dentists<br>Cuba: mid 1990–2015: doctors, pharmacists, medical engineers<br>Ethiopia: from 2014: pharmacists<br>Zambia: from 2013: doctors, nurses, dentists, pharmacists<br>Russian Federation: since 2000: doctors |
| | Nigeria | No | n/a | n/a |
| | São Tomé and Principe | No | n/a | n/a |
| | South Africa | Yes | Bilateral | Cuba, Tunisia: 1998: doctors |
| | Uganda | No | n/a | n/a |
| | Zimbabwe | Yes | Bilateral | Cuba: since 2000 for an indefinite period: doctors, midwives<br>China: for 10 years: doctors<br>Democratic Republic of Congo: 10 years: doctors, pharmacists, physiotherapists<br>Democratic Republic of Korea: no date or duration given: doctors |

| | | | |
|---|---|---|---|
| Argentina | No | n/a | n/a |
| Bahamas | Yes | Bilateral | Barbados: 2015: doctors<br>Cuba: 2015–2017: pharmacists, allied health professionals<br>UK: 2015: National Institute for Clinical Excellence (NICE)<br>USA: 2015: stem cells |
| Belize | Yes | Bilateral | Cuba: for 2 years: doctors, nurses, midwives<br>Nigeria: for 2 years (no info on occupations) |
| Brazil | Yes | Bilateral | Uruguay: sub-national coverage, since 2002: doctors, nurses, midwives |
| Canada | Yes | Bilateral and multilateral | Multilateral: Canada, US, Australia, Ireland, UK: doctors<br>Bilateral: Manitoba–Philippines: 2008, 2010: doctors, nurses, midwives, all categories of the health workforce. The MoU is a labour mobility agreement for all occupations.<br>Bilateral: Saskatchewan–Philippines: 2006: all occupations that fall under the Saskatchewan Immigration Nominee Programme: all regulated health professions.<br>Bilateral: Quebec–France: 2015: doctors, nurses, midwives, dentists, pharmacists, includes many other health professionals.<br>Bilateral: Alberta–Philippines: 2008: cooperation in human resources: deployment and development. |
| Colombia | Yes | Bilateral | Portugal: 2008–2011: doctors |
| El Salvador | No | n/a | n/a |

*continued*

*Table 6.1* Continued

| WHO Regional Office | Country | International agreement or arrangement | Type of international measure | Partner country/countries, and date (where given), and occupations covered |
|---|---|---|---|---|
| | Trinidad and Tobago | Yes | Bilateral and regional | Bilateral: Cuba: doctors, nurses, midwives, dentists, pharmacists, health administrators.<br>Bilateral: Philippines: under negotiation: doctors, nurses, midwives, pharmacists<br>Regional: St Vincent and the Grenadines, St. Lucia, Grenada: under negotiation: doctors, nurses, midwives, pharmacists |
| | United States of America | No | n/a | n/a |
| Eastern Mediterranean Regional Office (EMRO) | Djibouti | Yes | Bilateral | Cuba, Egypt: unlimited valid period: doctors |
| | Iran | No | n/a | n/a |
| | Jordan | No | n/a | n/a |
| | Morocco | Yes | Bilateral | Cuba: date renewable: doctors, nurses, midwives |
| | Qatar | Yes | Bilateral, multilateral | Cuba: date renewable: doctors, nurses, midwives<br>Tunisia: date renewable: doctors, nurses, midwives, dentists, pharmacists, allied health care professionals<br>Multilateral: Gulf Cooperation Council: doctors, nurses, midwives, dentists, pharmacists, allied health professionals |
| | Sudan | Yes | Bilateral | Libya: 5 years: doctors, nurses<br>Kingdom of Saudi Arabia: 5 years: doctors, nurses, laboratory technicians |
| | Yemen | No | n/a | n/a |

*continued*

| | | | |
|---|---|---|---|
| Regional Office for Europe (EURO) South-East Asia Regional Office (SEARO) | | | |
| Armenia | No | n/a | n/a |
| Austria | No | n/a | n/a |
| Belgium | No | n/a | n/a |
| Bosnia and Herzegovina | Yes | Bilateral | Germany: 2013 onwards: nurses, midwives |
| Croatia | No | n/a | n/a |
| Cyprus | No | n/a | n/a |
| Czech Republic | No | n/a | n/a |
| Denmark | Yes | Bilateral | Finland: since 1994: doctors, nurses, midwives |
| Estonia | No | n/a | n/a |
| Finland | Yes | Bilateral | Denmark: since 1994: doctors, nurses, midwives |
| France | Yes | Bilateral | Six Gulf States [unnamed]: 2006–present: doctors |
| Georgia | No | n/a | n/a |
| Germany | Yes | Bilateral | Serbia: 2013–2016: nurses<br>Bosnia and Herzegovina: 2013–2016: nurses<br>Philippines: 2013–2016: nurses<br>Tunisia: 2013–2016: nurses |
| Hungary | No | n/a | n/a |
| Ireland | Yes | Bilateral | Bilateral: Pakistan: 2011: doctors<br>Bilateral: Oman: 2015: doctors |
| Italy | No | n/a | n/a |
| Kyrgyzstan | No | n/a | n/a |
| Latvia | No | n/a | n/a |
| Lithuania | No | n/a | n/a |
| Montenegro | No | n/a | n/a |
| Netherlands | Yes | Bilateral | Suriname: from 2013: doctors<br>Oman: January 2016–January 2021: doctors |
| Norway | No | n/a | n/a |
| Poland | No | n/a | n/a |

Table 6.1 Continued

| WHO Regional Office | Country | International agreement or arrangement | Type of international measure | Partner country/countries, and date (where given), and occupations covered |
|---|---|---|---|---|
| | Portugal | Yes | Bilateral | Cuba: 3 years [no start or end date given]: doctors |
| | Republic of Moldova | Yes | Bilateral | Following from EU–Moldova joint declaration on mobility partnerships between the EU and Republic of Moldova (2008); Germany: 2014: dialogue on priorities for cooperation in health personnel migration; invitation issued to Italy, Spain, Portugal and Israel to follow suit. |
| | Romania | Yes | Bilateral | Bilateral: from 2011: doctors, nurses http://lege5.ro/Gratuity/getz |
| | Russian Federation | No | n/a | n/a |
| | Slovakia | No | n/a | n/a |
| | Spain | Yes | Bilateral | Malta: 2014: nurses |
| | Switzerland | Yes | Bilateral | Le Protocole: since 2013: doctors, nurses, midwives. www.admin.ch/opc/fr |
| | United Kingdom of Great Britain and Northern Ireland | No | n/a | n/a |
| Western Pacific Regional Office (WPRO) | Australia | No | n/a | n/a |
| | Bangladesh | Yes | Bilateral | Middle Eastern Countries [no further information given] |
| | Bhutan | Yes | Bilateral | Cuba, Myanmar, India, Nepal: 2 years (no start or end date given): doctors |
| | Cambodia | Yes | Bilateral | Brunei Darussalam: 2015: doctors, nurses, dentists |
| | Cook Islands | No | n/a | n/a |
| | Japan | No | n/a | Japan: 2008: nurses |
| | Indonesia | Yes | Bilateral | Timor-Leste: 2010-2012: midwives |

| Country | | | |
|---|---|---|---|
| Kiribati | No | n/a | n/a |
| Lao | No | n/a | n/a |
| Malaysia | Yes | Regional | ASEAN: from 1997: doctors, nurses, dentists. |
| Maldives | Yes | Bilateral | Sri Lanka: 2014–2018: Bangladesh: 2014–2018: doctors, nurses, nurses/midwives, dentists, other paramedical. |
| Micronesia | No | n/a | n/a |
| Myanmar | Yes | Bilateral | Bhutan (2003–2004), Brunei (2003–2004): doctors. |
| New Zealand | No | n/a | n/a |
| Palau | No | n/a | n/a |
| Philippines | Yes | Regional, Bilateral | ASEAN: MRAs in 2006 and 2009: doctors, nurses, dentists.<br>Japan: 2009: doctors (training), public health professionals; 2015: nurses, caregivers.<br>Germany: 2013: nurses.<br>Canada: 2006, 2008, 2010: all skills.<br>Bahrain: 2007: *not implemented*: all health professionals.<br>Spain: 2006: health professionals.<br>UK: 2003: [*ceased*]: Nurses, other health care professionals.<br>Norway: 2001: health professionals. |
| Singapore | No | n/a | n/a |
| Thailand | No | n/a | n/a |

Source: Reporting Instrument (2015) reports database, World Health Organization, Geneva (www.who.int/hrh/migration/code/code_nri/reports). Accessed 12 April 2018. Moldova: https://nanopdf.com/queue/eu-moldova-partnership-joint-action-on-health-workforce_pdf?queue_id=-1&x=1524045303&z=ODYuMTczLjE0My4y MTg= Accessed 14 April 2018.

Notes
Some re-coding has been undertaken. Canada described its inter-provincial agreements as 'multilateral'. Because this description is inconsistent with the the meanings of multilateral used in this book, these agreements have accordingly been deleted from this table. Cambodia described its agreement with Brunei Darussalam as 'regional' but this has been re-coded in the Table as 'bilateral' as it involves just the two countries. Denmark described agreements amongst Danish regions as 'multilateral', and therefore these agreements have been eliminated from this table. Finland registered its bilateral agreement with Denmark as multilateral but this has been re-coded in the Table as 'bilateral' as it involves just the two countries. For the same reason, Ireland's description of its agreement with Oman as 'multilateral' is recoded as bilateral. Where only one signatory to an agreement was present, data is also recorded for the other signatory (e.g. Denmark/Finland) in this table.

whether within or outside of the region (Yeates 2009a, 2009b). In this regard we make the following observations.

Several European nations (Ireland, Netherlands, Germany, Bosnia & Herzegovina, Spain) have within recent years concluded agreements with neighbouring European countries (Serbia, Bosnia & Herzegovina, Malta) as well as some further afield (e.g. Oman (Ireland, Netherlands), Suriname (Netherlands), Cuba and Colombia (Portugal)). In the EMRO region, of the four countries declaring their bilateral agreements, three of the countries were supplied by Cuba. Otherwise, most agreements were with other North African and Gulf states. None were with countries outside the region.

In the Americas, Cuba has long been the principal supplier of health workers internationally through its bilateral relations with countries worldwide, although it did not complete an NRI return. The Bahamas – a high-income country – had entered into agreements with other high-income countries (Barbados, UK, USA), as did Colombia (with Portugal), and Canada (with France). Otherwise, most other agreements were concluded with lower-income countries. Outside of the region, these were the Philippines, Cuba, and Nigeria. Within the region, we note Trinidad and Tobago's negotiations (underway) of three bilateral agreements with other Caribbean countries as well as with the Philippines. Trinidad and Tobago's agreements with other countries regionally (i.e. in the Caribbean) are all with countries classified as a lower income than itself (Trinidad and Tobago is a high-income country; Cuba, St Vincent and the Grenadines, St Lucia and Grenada are all upper-middle income countries). Otherwise, Canada stands out for its plethora of agreements between its provincial states and the Philippines and France. The US is conspicuously absent from the field of countries reporting bilateral agreements with other countries. The absence of the US in this respect is all the more notable because of the extent to which its health workforce is comprised of overseas-trained health workers, and especially so given its propensity to enter into bilateral free trade and investment agreements (Yeates *et al.* 2010).

African countries forge agreements principally with each other from across the continent, with agreements also with Cuba, China, Egypt and Korea. Namibia and Zimbabwe stand out in the African continent as having a propensity to enter into bilateral agreements, followed by Burundi. Zimbabwe has a significant history of out-migration to higher-income countries regionally (South Africa, Botswana, Namibia) and beyond (UK, US, Canada, Australia, New Zealand) (Nepachem 2009; Chikanda 2004). All of its agreements are, however, extra-regional (Cuba, China, DR Korea), with the exception of DR Congo, another low-income country which is a leading regional supplier of health personnel, in particular to South Africa. Namibia, an upper-middle income country, has more agreements with other African countries than any other African country, all with lower-income countries than itself: Kenya, Zambia (lower-middle income) and Ethiopia (low income).[9] Outside of Africa, it had partnered with Cuba and the Russian Federation (both upper-middle income) countries.

Asian countries forge agreements with other Asian countries (e.g. Japan, Sri Lanka, India, Nepal, Myanmar) as well as those in the Middle East, Caribbean (notably Cuba), North America (Canada) and Europe (Germany, Spain, UK). The Philippines stands out as a serial signatory of bilateral agreements, with a long history dating back some two decades and several such agreements signed with countries in Western Europe, North America and the Middle East, as well as within the region (Japan). By 2014, the Philippines had signed bilateral labour agreements with 22 countries, the first of which was signed in 1968 with the USA (Pillinger 2013). Some agreements are for a specified period of between two and four years and others are indefinite. Some, but not all, include provisions on ethical recruitment in line with national legal and regulatory frameworks, protection of welfare of migrants, exchange of information, and exchange of expertise and training. In some cases, agreements have set a priority to reduce the numbers of health workers from the Philippines for ethical reasons, as was the case in an agreement made between Norway and the Philippines, which was terminated in 2002. Notably, lower-middle income countries entered into agreements predominantly with other lower-income countries within the Asia (SEARO) region. Only the Philippines and Indonesia were servicing high-income Japan; Sri Lanka and Bangladesh were servicing an Asia Pacific upper-middle income country (Maldives) (Table 6.1).[10]

Because the NRI reports database does not provide any further information on the qualitative aspects of the data, the next stage of this discussion draws on our re-analysis of data from extant research studies on bilateral agreements in this policy field. We identify examples of good practice as well as problematic issues relating to the content of the agreements and their implementation.

## 5 Qualitative aspects of bilateral agreements: raising social standards?

An objection to bilateral agreements is that they produce a variable patchwork of non-transparent arrangements and splinter common frameworks agreed for addressing global issues (see Section 4.2 above). Most attention focuses on the degree of inter-state variance, but the specific provisions and content of agreements signed by the same state can also vary considerably. This is illustrated by a comparison of two ostensibly similarly-purposed agreements entered into by the UK – one with Spain, the other with the Philippines. In the agreement signed between the United Kingdom and Spain (2000) on recruitment of nurses, the UK Department of Health played an active role in the coordination, administration and financial provision for the recruitment process in Spain. By contrast, in the agreement between the United Kingdom and the Philippines (2003) the Department of Health was not required to fulfil recruitment functions as the infrastructure of public and private agencies specialising in recruitment of Filipino nurses was deemed to be very well established and substantial financial and/or administrative assistance from the British Government was not seen as necessary (Plotnikova 2014: 333).

Not only do bilateral agreements vary hugely within and between states, but a strategy of managing health worker-migration founded on securing an array of bilateral agreements is administratively and financially burdensome for a country. As Bobeva and Garson (2004) note, the financial costs and organisational burden of recruiting health workers from overseas can be onerous. For each agreement, a multitude of agencies are involved and must follow the stipulations of the agreement. Even if recruitment is centralised, there are a range of administrative procedures that must be carried out and coordinated, including verifying the qualifications of overseas candidates, evaluating their professional abilities and integrating employees into sociocultural and institutional environments.

A key argument promulgated in favour of bilateral agreements is that they are legally enforceable and have the capability of instituting robust social standards governing the recruitment, settlement, and return process. Yet unless a bilateral agreement relating to health worker migration is comprehensive, clear and specific in its inclusion of rights to social protection, labour standards, and of measures mitigating adverse development impacts of enabling the movement of health workers from (usually) poorer countries to (usually) richer ones, then it can easily fail to fulfil its potential to uplift social standards and development outcomes. The potential advantages of bilateral agreements *only* hold if decent work and labour standards as well as specific re-investment provisions are written into the agreement. However, more often than not they are devoid of all but the minimum of obligations towards the migrant workers and their source country, paying little more than symbolic value to these obligations (Plotnikova 2014; Pagett and Padarath 2007). Moreover, the legal enforceability of bilateral agreements cannot be counted on (Dhillon *et al.* 2010; see also endnote 1).

## 5.1 'Good practice' exemplars: a widespread phenomenon?

Cognisant of these issues, especially those concerning lack of transparency and accountability, there has been an effort to highlight good practices as models for countries seeking to negotiate agreements with partner countries. PSI, the global trade union federation, identifies as good practice ethical recruitment and human resource development cooperation embedded in the BLA between the Philippines and Germany signed in March 2013 ('The Triple Win Programme'). A positive feature of this agreement is that Filipino health professionals may not be employed in the Federal Republic of Germany under working conditions less favourable than those for comparable German workers. An innovation of that agreement is its establishment of a Joint Committee made up of ministries of labour and health and trade unions representatives from Germany and the Philippines to monitor and evaluate the implementation of the agreement. This was the first of its kind enabling trade unions direct oversight of the work of a BLA (PSI 2017b). This agreement has also been commended by the Commission on Health Employment and Economic Growth (HEEG 2016).

The Global Forum on Migration and Development has done similarly, and its Compendium on bilateral temporary labour agreements (GFMD 2008) identifies good practice elements in bilateral labour agreements between national governments.[11] Equality of treatment has been embedded in some agreements, as in the example of an agreement between Spain and the Philippines which provides for nurses and other highly skilled Filipino workers to work in Spain with the same protection and rights as Spanish workers. In some cases, bilateral agreements are used as a basis for the recognition of qualifications. For example, a UK–Spain agreement gives recognition to Spanish nurses' skills in the UK. There are also examples of cooperation agreements for training, research and development that include provision of training for South African doctors in Cuba, Iran and Tunisia. The latter agreement covers the temporary recruitment of doctors and qualified health personnel from Cuba, Iran and Tunisia to fill labour shortages in the health sector in South Africa (GFMD 2008).

The Health Worker Migration Initiative (a joint initiative of WHO and the Global Health Worker Alliance) commissioned a Guidebook on bilateral agreements addressing health worker-migration that sought to identify innovative best practice agreements (Dhillon *et al.* 2010). The Commission on Health Employment and Economic Growth (HEEG 2016) similarly highlights exemplar agreements and their importance to increasing health workforce capacity. It highlights Cuba's contributions to expanding health workforce supply:

> Cuba has trained over 33,000 health professionals from 134 countries, including 26,000 graduates from the Latin American School of Medicine; Cuba's bilateral cooperation with 68 countries has supported education, training and health system strengthening.
>
> (HEEG 2016: 35–36)

The extent to which BLAs protect labour rights and mitigate the negative impacts of outward migration depends on the content of the agreement as well as its implementation and enforcement mechanisms. On the former, certainly, there are examples of 'best practice'. Amongst the most successful agreements are those which have the principle of equality of treatment embedded in them and which are benchmarked against international labour standards. This is the case of the agreements between the Philippines and Spain and Germany guaranteeing migrant health workers the same rights as Spanish and German workers. A further good practice in using ILO decent work standards and ethical recruitment principles is evidenced in a Memorandum of Agreement (MoA) between the Philippines and Bahrain on Health Services Cooperation (Republic of the Philippines and Kingdom of Bahrain, 2007) which is embedded in a framework of equal treatment. Article 2 on rights of workers specifies that:

> Human resources for health shall be provided equal employment opportunity in terms of pay and other employment conditions; access to training, education and other career development opportunities and resources; the right to due process in cases of violation of the employment contract.... Human resources for health recruited from the Philippines shall enjoy the same rights and responsibilities as provided for by relevant ILO conventions.

The agreement covers the exchange of health workers in recruitment, rights of workers, capacity building, sustainability of the development of health workers and mutual recognition agreements on qualifications. An ethical framework for the recruitment of health workers was established through a partnership between Philippine and Bahraini health care and educational institutions, designed to enhance international education and professional development, and includes scholarships, academic cooperation on health work and technology cooperation. The agreement also specifies the reintegration of health workers who return to their home country. The quality of this MoA is a reflection that the Philippines had ratified ILO's migration conventions (C97 and C143) and other core conventions, which was not the case with Bahrain. Unfortunately, this agreement has remained a 'model' in the sense that it has never been implemented (as reported by the Filipino government in its NRI 2015 return: see Table 6.1).

The participation of trade unions and employers in the public and private health sectors is essential to concluding effective BLAs. The former are particularly well placed to ensure that such agreements make reference to the ILO normative framework on equal treatment (Conventions No. 97 and No. 143) and labour migration (ILO Multilateral Framework on Labour Migration) and the UN Convention on the Protection of the Rights of All Migrant Workers and Members of their Families. If all relevant stakeholders are involved it will be easier for BLAs to be implemented within a framework of equality of treatment.

Not all bilateral agreements incorporate such principles. Indeed, there are many instances where bilateral agreements do not address decent work or labour market issues. Often these are negotiated and signed by the Ministry by Foreign Affairs, with no links to the Ministry of Labour or to representatives of employers' and workers' organisations. This is a problem not least because the latter can make significant contributions to providing data on labour dynamics in the health sector (Yeates and Pillinger 2013: 30). Coordination between Ministries of Health, Labour and Finance is essential to the successful conclusion of bilateral agreements (ibid.). A study by Makulec (2014) of BLAs in the Philippines found numerous challenges need to be overcome for BLAs to achieve their objectives. Foremost amongst its recommendations were the systematic inclusion of: normative standards on decent work and guidelines on ethical recruitment; portability of social protection; support for integration in destination countries; access to career and skills development, and support with return and reintegration.

BLAs signed on the basis of economic partnerships have been amongst the less successful and most exploitative of bilateral agreements in this area. The bilateral Economic Partnership Agreement signed between Japan and Indonesia (2008), for a quota of nurses and nurse specialists from Indonesia to work in Japan, is an example of this. Requirements were put in place for Indonesian nurses to take Japanese language lessons and during this time to work as caregivers or assistant nurses at hospitals or nursing homes for the elderly. A similar agreement, the Japan–Philippines Economic Partnership Agreement (JPEPA) led to nurses returning to the Philippines amidst complaints from the nurses about

exploitative employment practices, poor support and lack of facilities for integration (Pillinger 2013; Yagi *et al.* 2013).

In the light of this history, it remains to be seen whether the Japanese-
sponsored Asia Health and Well-being (2017) initiative in relation to nursing
care will be concluded on a different basis. There are certainly strong incentives
for Japan to make its recruitment process more productive and efficient to
address its domestic labour shortage problem. Despite resources put into training
and institutional support for foreign nurses and care workers, both in the source
country pre-departure and in Japan post-entry, to help them pass the licensing
examinations, applications from the Philippines and Indonesia for the positions
of EPA nurses and care workers have significantly declined in recent years,
partly due to the negative and discouraging images of the Japanese EPA system,
and partly because the supply pools in the Philippines and Indonesia are beginning to decline. Applications over the last couple years have not even come close
to the 1,000 annual quota.[12] However, the signs are that the new Japanese initiative is a scaling up of previous economic partnerships to the entire region,
driven by the Japanese state allied to corporate interests and with a possible aim
of becoming the hegemon in the regional market for health workers.[13] Unless
this initiative is also made fairer to health workers recruited under its auspices it
will also have failed in its quest to make the process more economically productive than its predecessor.

### 5.2 Promoting temporary and circular migration

A major problem with the present 'generation' of BLAs is that their increased
usage is associated with a global policy shift towards temporary and circular
migration.[14] Circular migration regularly surfaces in policy forums as a solution
to developing countries' development needs and as an alternative to permanent
migration. It is seen as conducive to facilitating 'brain gain' and 'brain circulation', such that specialist knowledge and experience gained from working overseas can be used as a tool for development and contribute to quality health
services when the individual migrant returns home after their right to reside
overseas expires (GFMD 2013). Circular migration is actively promoted by
many high-income countries and by international organisations such as the European Commission (CEC 2007) and the IOM. It has also regularly surfaced in
GFMD discussions which argued that 'bilateral or circular labour agreements;
including MRAs, in specific sectors ... are expedient, more targeted, mutually
agreeable, and cost effective' (GFMD 2012). An IOM research project concluded that, '[g]enerally, circular and return migration should be encouraged
instead of permanent migration' (Tjadens *et al.* 2013: 170).

In Europe, mobility partnerships with proximate 'third countries' have
become a much-used mechanism for addressing health workforce shortages, and
many of these incorporate the principle of temporary and circular migration.
Although involving a multilateral organisation (EU) and a 'third country', they
are in fact bilateral agreements in the sense that the EU acts as a single state

partner with another one. Mobility partnerships are viewed as a mechanism for promoting comprehensive measures for cooperation, transparency and ethical recruitment (Dhillon *et al.* 2010; Makulec 2014), as a well as part of a broader approach to migration management which includes developing or strengthening measures taken by the 'third country' to manage labour migration. So far, five such partnerships have been concluded, between the EU and Morocco (2013), Armenia (2011), Georgia (2009), Moldova (2008, 2018) and Cape Verde (2008).[15]

The EU–Moldova Mobility partnership arose from the EU-funded 'Better Managing the Mobility of Health Professionals in the Republic of Moldova' project. Under the EU–Moldova partnership, WHO has a role to implement a project on the 'Efficient management of the mobility of the health care staff of the Republic of Moldova', with a particular focus on minimising the negative impact of the migration of healthcare staff, through the promotion of programmes of circular migration schemes. Cooperation is being established with the University of Medicine and Pharmacy, Nicolae Testemiteanu Pharmacy College and the IOM Moldova Office. Financial assistance has been given from the European Commission, and bilateral assistance from Portugal, Sweden, Romania, Italy, Belgium, Germany and France. A dialogue has started with partners from Germany to determine priorities for cooperation in the field of health worker migration (Berzan 2014).

Despite the growth of BLAs promoting circular migration, there is no evidence that it is preferred by skilled health workers or employers, or that it fosters migration where there is continued connection with, and integration in, source and destination countries (Newland 2009). Indeed, temporary and circular migration may restrict migration choices and the right to enjoy permanent patterns of migration (Wickramasekara 2011; Pillinger 2014). Global trade unions (ITUC 2011; PSI 2010) have been critical of temporary and circular migration programmes as they can exacerbate precarious and exploitative work and diminish workers' rights to training, career development, decent work and family reunification. For the PSI circular and temporary labour programmes are *only* sustainable if they promote the development of skills and human resources necessary to strengthen public service delivery in both source and destination countries, *and* facilitate knowledge transfer and 'brain gain' in low income countries (PSI 2010). In other words, they need to have embedded a clear understanding of the migration-development nexus and include identified and substantial 'compensatory mechanisms' in order that source countries stand a reasonable chance of securing wider development benefits.

Agreements that meet these conditions are few and far between. Wismar *et al.* (2011) identify four types of bilateral agreements used in Europe according their aims.[16] Crucially, their study found no examples of compensation schemes that had been established with the explicit purpose of mitigating the loss of investment in training and human resources in source countries. The absence of in-built mechanisms to build the capacity of health workers and the health sector by, for example, reducing outflows of health workers from rural areas, reducing attrition and introducing incentives and policies to retain highly skilled workers, and putting in place policies for 'brain gain' and knowledge transfer, research and training between source and destination countries, means the potential of bilateral labour or trade agreements to contribute to economic and social development remains unrealised (PSI 2010).

### 5.3 'Thin' compensatory mechanisms

The WHO Global Code states that BLAs 'should take into account the needs of developing countries and countries with economies in transition through the adoption of appropriate [compensation] measures' (WHO 2010a). Compensation mechanisms can take various forms, ranging from financial recompense to scholarships to exchanges of experts, alongside joint ventures and investments in health care facilities. BLAs can provide source countries a means of recouping the cost of educational investment, as happens under the bilateral agreement between Germany and the Philippines – the 'The Triple Win Programme'. However, findings from research carried out by the ILO/EU Decent Work Across Borders project on skilled health worker-migration suggests that there needs to be a system for monitoring these provisions as there are examples of bilateral agreements that have contained clauses for destination countries to contribute back to the health education budget that have never been implemented. For example, some commitments to support health workforce development in the Philippines with Canada have not been implemented. Proper monitoring of implementation with the engagement of non-governmental actors is essential (Yeates and Pillinger 2013).

Our further analysis of the 2015 NRIs reports shows the variable quality of bilateral agreements in respect of compensation. Table 6.2 summarises the different types of measures that take account of the needs of developing countries (and economies in transition), as reported by governments having declared in their NRI report that they had entered into a bilateral agreement.

The most common types of compensation among these measures are training (18 countries) and educational programmes (12 countries), followed by measures for promoting circular migration (eight countries), twinning health facilities (seven countries) and, finally, retention strategies (four countries). Only Trinidad and Tobago reports that it generally recruits from countries which have indicated they have 'surplus staff'. No government reports that equality of treatment or decent work are a feature of the agreements they have entered into. Germany reports that overseas-recruited workers shall be entitled to salary and social insurance, but it does not indicate that this is based on equality or decent work principles. Notably, nine countries (Bhutan, Maldives, Netherlands, Portugal, Spain, Namibia, Zimbabwe, Canada and Bosnia & Herzegovina) state that their agreements do not take account of the needs of developing countries and/or economies in transition. These countries are among the most active in forging bilateral agreements (cf. Table 6.1) so this is indicative. However, it is unfortunately not possible to tell from the NRI responses whether these are statements about

Table 6.2 Of those countries that have declared having entered into bilateral or multilateral agreements in their NRI, stated types of measures that governments say take account of the needs of developing countries and countries with economies in transition

| WHO region | | Training | Twinning of health facilities | Promotion of circular migration | Retention strategies | Educational programmes | Other |
|---|---|---|---|---|---|---|---|
| AFRO | Burundi | ✗ | ✗ | ✗ | ✗ | ✗ | Prestataires de service dans les formations sanitaires [trans. health services training allowances] |
| | Namibia | ✗ | ✗ | ✗ | ✗ | ✗ | |
| | South Africa | ✓ | ✓ | ✗ | ✗ | ✗ | |
| | Zimbabwe | ✗ | ✗ | ✗ | ✗ | ✗ | |
| AMRO/PAHO | Bahamas | ✓ | ✓ | ✗ | ✗ | ✓ | |
| | Belize | ✓ | ✗ | ✗ | ✗ | ✓ | Training for technical skills; personnel to fill human resource gaps |
| | Brazil | ✓ | ✗ | ✓ | ✗ | ✓ | |
| | Canada | ✗ | ✗ | ✗ | ✗ | ✗ | |
| | Colombia | ✗ | ✗ | ✓ | ✗ | ✗ | |
| | Trinidad and Tobago | ✗ | ✗ | ✗ | ✗ | ✗ | Generally, recruit from countries that have indicated they have surplus staff |

| Region | Country | | | | | | | Notes |
|---|---|---|---|---|---|---|---|---|
| EMRO | Djibouti | ✓ | | ✓ | ✓ | ✓ | ✓ | |
| | Morocco | ✓ | | ✓ | ✓ | ✓ | ✓ | |
| | Qatar | ✓ | | ✓ | ✓ | ✓ | ✓ | |
| | Sudan | ✓ | | ✓ | ✓ | ✓ | ✓ | |
| EURO | Bosnia and Herzegovina | ✗ | | ✗ | ✗ | ✗ | ✗ | |
| | Finland | ✗ | | ✗ | ✗ | ✗ | ✗ | Immigration strategy 2020 will strengthen people's living conditions locally and provide them with better opportunities and capabilities to influence their own life. Competences and connections of immigration organisations are used for practical development cooperation in order to respect good governance and human rights. |
| | France | ✓ | | ✓ | ✓ | ✓ | ✓ | |

continued

Table 6.2 Continued

| WHO region | | Training | Twinning of health facilities | Promotion of circular migration | Retention strategies | Educational programmes | Other |
|---|---|---|---|---|---|---|---|
| EURO | Germany | ✓ | ✓ | ✓ | ✓ | ✓ | Support the selection of candidates/matching process; coordination of placement process between Germany and partner country (e.g. standards – workers shall be entitled for salary and social insurance as German workers); coordination of departure phase of the candidate; language training; coordination of family reunification; monitoring of nurses and employers and the process of recognition of competences in Germany; analysis of needs in the administration to engage the diaspora. |

| | | | | | | |
|---|---|---|---|---|---|---|
| Ireland | ✓ | ✓ | ✓ | ✓ | ✓ | 2010 HSE and Irish Aid signed a Memorandum of Understanding with the aim to contribute to the health needs of less developed countries. Explicit focus of this collaboration is to undertake measures to strengthen health workforces in other countries, working closely with Irish training institutions. Out of the MoU, Ireland joined the ESTHER Alliance (EEA) in 2012 aiming to strengthen HRH capacity in low- and middle-income countries through institutional health partnerships. |
| Netherlands | ✗ | ✗ | ✗ | ✗ | ✗ | |
| Portugal | ✗ | ✗ | ✗ | ✗ | ✗ | |
| Moldova | ✓ | ✗ | ✓ | ✗ | ✗ | |
| Romania | ✓ | ✗ | ✗ | ✗ | ✓ | |
| Spain | ✗ | ✗ | ✗ | ✗ | ✗ | |
| Switzerland | ✗ | ✗ | ✗ | ✗ | ✗ | |

*continued*

Table 6.2 Continued

| WHO region | | Training | Twinning of health facilities | Promotion of circular migration | Retention strategies | Educational programmes | Other |
|---|---|---|---|---|---|---|---|
| SEARO | Bangladesh | ✓ | ✓ | ✗ | ✗ | ✓ | |
| | Bhutan | ✗ | ✗ | ✗ | ✗ | ✗ | |
| | Indonesia | ✓ | ✗ | ✗ | ✓ | ✗ | |
| | Maldives | ✗ | ✗ | ✗ | ✗ | ✗ | |
| | Myanmar | ✓ | ✗ | ✗ | ✗ | ✓ | |
| WPRO | Cambodia | ✓ | ✗ | ✓ | ✗ | ✗ | |
| | Malaysia | ✓ | ✗ | ✗ | ✗ | ✗ | |
| | Philippines | ✓ | ✓ | ✓ | ✗ | ✓ | Investment to improve health facilities |

Source: Reporting Instrument (2015) reports database, World Health Organization, Geneva (www.who.int/hrh/migration/code/code_nri/reports. Accessed 12 April 2018).

Notes
This data is based on self-reporting by governments having entered into an international agreement on health worker migration. Reporting practises vary significantly between governments. 43 out of the 74 countries (58%) stating they had entered into an international agreement on health worker migration responded to this section of the NRI. For the purposes of this table, all responses are reported, including countries that state the international agreement(s) into which they have entered do not take the needs of developing countries and/or economies in transition into account. Stated types of measures are standard categories used in the NRI template. Entries in 'Other' column are taken from additional 'open text' information in governments' NRI. The NRI template (and responses) are insufficiently detailed to ascertain which agreements the development needs taken account of correspond with. As such, it is not clear how critical governments are being in their returns. For example, it is unclear whether developing countries and economies in transition that have responded to this question are referring to the terms of agreements that they have entered into with higher-advanced countries. It should also be recognised that these returns say nothing about whether and how they are implemented in practice.
Eight countries (Bhutan, Bosnia & Herzegovina, Canada, Namibia, Netherlands, Maldives, Portugal and Spain) report that the international agreements into which they have entered (see Table 6.1) do not take account of the needs of developing countries or economies in transition.

the absence of needs being taken into account or about the (in)adequacy of provisions written in.

Ireland's NRI report highlights its participation in the ESTHER alliance as evidence of its commitment to meeting the needs of source developing countries.[17] More than a third (36 per cent) of Ireland's doctors in 2014 were foreign trained, mainly originating from India, Pakistan, South Africa and Sudan (Brugha *et al.* 2015), and Ireland has one of the highest proportions of overseas trained nurses in the OECD (Yeates 2010), so ethical recruitment and compensation are salient issues for the country. Through two agreements (Ireland–Pakistan BLA (2011), Ireland–Oman MoU (2015)), it is involved in the twinning health care facilities and the development of retention strategies, while an MoU signed in 2010 between the Health Services Executive and Irish Aid aims to enhance Ireland's contribution to health needs in less-developed countries through 'collaboration to undertake measures to strengthen the health workforce in other countries, working closely with Irish training institutions'. Support for this is provided through Irish Aid's bilateral programmes in Ethiopia, Mozambique and Tanzania, while a programme on retention of surgeons in Africa is supported by the Irish Aid-funded RCSI COSECSA project. Also widely cited as a good practice is the International Medical Graduate Initiative adopted by the HSE and the Forum of Irish Postgraduate Medical Training Bodies (2014). The Initiative permits overseas doctors to undergo postgraduate medical training in the Irish health service, over a fixed period of time. The objective is to enhance access to training that is not available in their home countries. These are of course excellent initiatives, but they fall within a temporary and circular migration policy approach. Thus, recruits are trained in Ireland while also contributing to 'the overall productivity and effectiveness of health care services provided in Ireland' (HSE/Forum of Irish Postgraduate Medical Training Bodies 2014: 4), usually for a period of two years after which they are expected to return to their source countries. During this time, they receive not a wage but an allowance and cannot accrue any rights of residency or settlement. Their family have no right to join them, and any children they bear during this time will not have Irish citizenship.

## 6 Conclusion

Bilateral agreements are of great significance for the health sector. They are a key part of the global institutional architecture governing health worker-migration and -recruitment, health workforce management, the development of health systems and access to health. They have been promulgated by international organisations from the earliest days of the UN and more recently by an increasing number of organisations operating outside of the UN system. Indeed, such is the extent to which they are promoted as answers to health workforce and health care issues that we conclude they are an integral feature of the global policy field of health worker-recruitment and -migration. While there are (mainly isolated) exemplars of good practice, there are also clear tensions when we consider them from the perspective of the need for more robust international responses to a set of social issues that are global in scope and impact.

The evidence we have brought to this discussion clearly points to the conclusion that, as a means of managing migration flows, such agreements do not address underlying causes of outward migration such as low salaries, inadequate staffing levels to meet population needs and provide quality patient care, poor and stressful working conditions, limited opportunities for career development and poor access to medical technologies. They are a policy mechanism initiated by states to manage symptoms of underlying health workforce issues. They provide countries that have a 'surplus' health worker population with a 'spatial vent' and facilitate the directed export of health labour overseas. For countries with 'shortages' of health labour, bilateral agreements can channel a ready-made source of labour supply. There is little evidence that such agreements are being concluded in the interests of health workers, as they tend to exclude broad labour and social protection, and are weak on compensation provision.

It is clear that, in principle, bilateral agreements have the potential to mitigate some of the negative effects of migration if principles of ethical recruitment and decent work are embedded alongside rights-based approaches and compensatory measures addressing the migration/development nexus are included in bilateral agreements. They have the *potential* to contribute to a country's economic and social development in building the capacity of the health workers and the health sector, for example, by reducing outflows of health workers from rural areas, reducing attrition and introducing incentives and policies to retain highly skilled workers, and putting in place policies for 'brain gain' and knowledge transfer, research and training between source and destination countries. However, this is by no means common (let alone default) practice. Without such provisions, bilateral agreements have a tendency to become short-term agreements to provide quotas of health workers for temporary or circular migration. Furthermore, as a strategy for managing health worker-migration they are administratively and financially burdensome and generate significant complexity and needless discrimination.

Despite the enthusiastic calls in global policy for greater use of bilateral agreements to realise ethical recruitment, they 'fail' as judged by many hallmarks of 'good' agreements. They are non-transparent and inaccessible to those outside of the governments concluding them. There is uncertainty about their legal status and enforceability. Variability and inconsistency are also key considerations here: the forms they take, their scope of coverage, and content are as diverse as the motivations behind migration itself. Far from providing assurance of robust treatment of those who they cover, they are generative of discrimination on the basis of national origin amongst other things. While they are a key policy instrument in managed approaches to the migration of health workers, they are also associated with the ushering in of increased use of temporary labour programmes and the differentiation of labour and social rights in national institutional regimes.

The research evidence we have brought to the discussion based on our ana-lysis of WHO's NRI database leads us to conclude with Dhillon *et al.* (2010: 7) that heterogeneity and ambiguity on the role, form and content of bilateral agree-ments to serve a health-related purpose are a marked characteristic of these agreements, and that '[t]his lack of clarity poses a particular challenge for devel-opment countries, which have the most at stake'. Our survey of the compensa-tory measures reported by signatory governments testifies to the fact that bilateral agreements have failed to fully engage with the migration-development relationship (ibid.). There remains very limited evidence of whether bilateral agreements have benefited source countries, and if so how, not least because of the lack of clarity about whether they have been implemented and if so how. It is the responsibility of the signatory countries to ensure that the provisions of the agreement are upheld, but clear conclusions are confounded by the absence or inaccessibility of the monitoring and implementation mechanisms. As such, it may well be the case that a 'second generation' of bilateral labour agreements on health worker-recruitment and -migration are inflected by discourses on ethical recruitment (Dhillon *et al.* 2010) but what evidence exists about the agreements that are actually enacted point only to a loose adherence to well-specified inter-national standards on 'ethical recruitment' or 'fair treatment' of health workers.

We conclude that bilateralist approaches to health worker migration at once reflect and reinforce the fragmentary nature of global governance that character-ises this global policy field. The absence of comprehensive, legally enforceable agreements has the potential to undercut existing multilateral agreements and stall their institutional strengthening. Thus, it is not just that bilateral agreements mostly fall short of the highest standards on provisions for equal treatment, com-pensation or ethical standards, but they pose a serious threat to multilateral agreements whether based on the principle of the most favoured nation (MFN) or a socially-just notion of global ethics, including non-discrimination and non-depletion of other countries' resources. Far from being building blocks to more comprehensive and robust global governance of health worker-migration and -recruitment, bilateral agreements constitute a roadblock.

## Notes

1 Bilateral agreements can take many forms and include bilateral agreements, cooperative agreements, covenants, memoranda of understanding, memoranda of agreement, concerted management agreements, agreed minutes, inter-agency under-standings (IAU); protocols; and notes verbales (Dhillon *et al.* 2010; Wickramasekara 2015). Whether such agreements are legally-binding depends on whether the particip-ants intend to be so obligated and this can be inferred from a variety of factors, includ-ing the text and the status of the signatories (Dhillon *et al.* 2010: 14).
2 These were the 2013 MoU Concerning the Placement of Filipino Health Professionals in Employment Positions in the Federal Republic of Germany (19 March 2013), the so-called 'triple-win agreement', and an annex to an agreement MoU between Alberta (Canada) and the Philippines (2008), Annex A on 'Priorities for Collaboration and Cooperation' calling for partnerships between Albertan and Filipino institutions to train nurses in the Philippines to standards that are consistent with those recognised by Alberta.

3  The Health Ministers also recommended a greater role within SADC on south-south cooperation and intraregional staff exchange programmes alongside action by the Commonwealth (Pagett and Padarath 2007).

4  It argued that 'Richer countries receiving migrants from poorer countries should adopt responsible recruitment policies, treat migrant health workers fairly, and consider entering into bilateral agreements' (WHO 2006: xxii). It also argued that '[d]iscussions and negotiations with ministries of health, workforce planning units and training institutions, similar to bilateral agreements, will help to avoid claims of "poaching" and other disreputable recruitment behaviour' (ibid.: 103) and that "[b]ilateral agreements on health service providers can provide an explicit and negotiated framework to manage migration' (ibid.: 105) on the basis of responsible recruitment (WHO 2006).

5  This, as Dhillon *et al.* (2010) note, is despite the considerable work undertaken by the OECD and IOM supplemented by the authors' own secondary research and their personal outreach efforts. Wickramasekara (2015) similarly notes difficulties in obtaining full information, including texts of agreements, as do Pagett and Padarath (2007) in relation to eastern and southern Africa.

6  The NRI sought information from governments about national measures to support Code-consistent responsibilities, rights and recruitment practices; health workforce development and health system sustainability; partnerships, technical collaboration and financial support; and data gathering, research and exchange.

7  Four countries (Canada, Malaysia, Philippines, Qatar) report they are also party to a regional multilateral agreement (ASEAN, Gulf Cooperation Council, NAFTA) covering the international migration of health professionals.

8  The majority of agreements on health professions in Plotkinova's (2014) study predominantly refer to nurses. She notes that in the early some agreements that were initially negotiated to recruit overseas nurses were subsequently extended to doctors. This propensity to conclude agreements on nurses reflected increased demand for nurses as well as their increased international migration. As her study was confined to Europe, where data is most plentiful, it is not possible to say whether this finding is generalisable to other regions of the world.

9  In respect of the agreement with Kenya, Pagett and Padarath (2007) note that

> the agreement was formed as a result of Kenya's inability to employ all of its health workers in Kenya due to conditions of an IMF agreement that limit the number of health workers in Kenya. Kenya continues to produce a large number of health workers, even though many health workers continue to be unemployment. This arrangement [with Namibia] allows for Kenya health professionals to work in Namibia for a set period of time to gain employment, experience and skills, while providing needed health workers to Namibia.
>
> (p. 18)

The movement is unidirectional, from Kenya to Namibia. It is referred to as a 'tour of duty' of limited duration. Kenya is responsible for paying salaries during the tour of duty, while Namibia covers transportation, health coverage, living accommodation and living allowances (ibid.).

10  Classifications of countries as low, middle or high income are derived from the World Bank World Development Indicators (World Bank 2017).

11  It identifies three overarching 'pre-conditions': ensure legal access to labour markets; provide protection by improving working conditions and outcomes and skills of migrants; ensure temporariness of migration. The latter includes easing reintegration into the source country, providing possibilities for repeat migration, and ensuring that retirement pensions, social security and health benefits are portable.

12  We thank Professor Ito Peng for this insight.

13  The first meeting of the initiative took place in February 2017 agreed to establish a vocational training school for Asians to attain qualifications for care work in Japan.

Notably, the initiative aims to 'strengthen self-supported nursing care when Japanese corporations expand their nursing care business in Asian countries' (JIGH 2017).

14 Circular migration is 'a generic term which can apply to migratory movements between any groups of countries' (Wickramasekara 2011: 13–14).

15 EU Mobility partnerships do not involve all EU member states. The EU–Morocco Mobility Partnership involves Belgium, France, Germany, Italy, the Netherlands, Portugal, Spain, Sweden and the United Kingdom. The EU–Armenia Mobility Partnership involves Belgium, Bulgaria, the Czech Republic, France, Germany, Italy, the Netherlands, Poland, Romania and Sweden. The EU–Georgia Mobility Partnership involves Belgium, Bulgaria, the Czech Republic, Denmark, Estonia, France, Germany, Greece, Italy, Latvia, Lithuania, the Netherlands, Poland, Romania, Sweden and the United Kingdom. Ten years after the Joint Declaration on a Mobility Partnership between the EU and the Republic of Moldova (2008), the EU–Moldova Partnership came into existence and involved Bulgaria, Cyprus, the Czech Republic, France, Germany, Greece, Hungary, Italy, Lithuania, Poland, Portugal, Romania, Slovakia, Slovenia and Sweden. The EU–Cape Verde Mobility Partnership involves Spain, France, Luxembourg and Portugal (Source: www.europa.eu, Accessed 15 May 2018).

16 First, agreements to dissuade recruitment from countries with critical workforce shortages. Second, agreements to facilitate systems for mutual recognition of diplomas. Third, agreements to target specific categories of health professionals for recruitment. Fourth, agreements to temporarily open labour markets in EU accession states. Twinning arrangements and staff exchanges between medical schools or research institutions in source and destination countries have included programmes financially supported by the EU (Wismar *et al.* 2011).

17 The ESTHER Alliance describes itself as 'an alliance of governments and allied organisations' in Ireland, Switzerland, Norway, Germany, France, Spain and the UK engaging with 'effective and sustainable North–South partnerships [to] strengthen the capacity of the health workforce and institutions to provide quality health services for people in low and middle-income countries'. It promotes institutional health partnerships through knowledge generation, sharing best practice, collaboration and advocacy (ESTHER undated).

# 7 The global campaign for universal health coverage
## The SDGs and beyond

## 1 Introduction

The evolution of global governance regimes on human rights, migration, equality, labour, social protection, health and development since the end of World War II have laid firm institutional foundations on which to build the global health worker-migration and -recruitment policy field. Health worker-migration and -recruitment have become increasingly visible in global policy, with two multilateral policy initiatives (Nursing Personnel Recommendation (ILO 1977c) and the WHO 2010 Global Code (WHO 2010a)) flanked by a plethora of inter-state agreements and programmes of action and research. These foundations were the outcome of decades of cumulative efforts on a wide range of fronts by diverse advocacy actors to institute common frameworks to address universal responses to linkages between health workforce (un)availability, international migration, weak health systems, poor health outcomes and uneven development. Even as the worsening development context thwarted the realisation of these goals, such actions have nonetheless mainstreamed the issue of health worker-migration and ethical recruitment into global policy. Indeed, the 2030 Sustainable Development Agenda (hereafter 2030 Agenda) (UNGA 2015) marked an unprecedented global commitment to global health and universal health coverage (UHC) and incorporated health workforce issues as part of these.

This chapter turns to what we argue is the beginning of a third phase in the development of this global policy field. Formally starting in 2016 with the 2030 Agenda, but with a run up of 4–5 years since the WHO 2010 Global Code was agreed, we identify the significant emergent contours of this phase, and identify challenges to it as well as sources of its renewal and extension. The discussion focuses on the visibility and attention given to international migration of health workers in recent global policy and the role of health workforce policy actors in shaping this third phase. The chapter also considers the underlying imperatives driving this – notably the maldistribution of health workers globally – in the light of revised health workforce densities required to implement UHC which are calculated to rise to an unprecedented demand for 40 million health workers and a predicted needs-based shortfall of 18 million health workers by 2030 (HEEG 2016). We discuss how this is being tackled in global policy and what recent policy developments tell us about the wider global currents that are likely to shape how the migration and recruitment of health workers may feature in future global policy.

Earlier chapters discussed how the global governance framework developed incrementally, showing the complex and sometimes competing agendas of labour and human rights-based approaches and trade and corporate-led ones in global policy. This third phase has seen a significant increase in dialogue about, and a multi-stakeholder approach to, global governance on health worker-migration and skills, reflecting the urgency of finding common solutions and avert looming shortages. We argue that developments are already going further than the second phase not only in respect of the mainstreaming of health work-force issues into global policy but also in reinforcing a global governance rooted in voluntarism and ethical recruitment, while also emphasising bilateralism, global trade approaches and commercialism. Global skills partnerships, the work associated with the UN's High-Level Commission on Health Employment and Growth (HEEG), and the programmes of ILO and WHO are identified as exemplars of this. The structural incorporation of multi-stakeholder partnerships into the field of global health, embedded in the 2030 Agenda, has brought in an ever-greater range of social actors from the public, private (corporate), labour and NGO sectors into global policy formation. This has generated concerns about the role of the private corporate sector in global policy formation and implementation, the rise of selectivist rather than universalist responses, and the impacts this has on the capacity of governments (and the public sector) to achieve sustainable and high-quality public health services and adequate numbers of trained health workers essential for the achievement of UHC and other global health goals.

## 2 Global policy challenges

By the start of the second decade of the twenty-first century, the global policy field that had evolved had real strengths but also serious flaws, as well as a number of pressing problems to be dealt with. The most recent global mechanism to tackle the problems, notably the WHO Global Code, was in part a response to the need to mitigate the adverse development impacts of out-migration. Yet as an approach to ethical recruitment, the ambition in some countries to restrict migration from countries with critical shortages has had limited leverage (see Chapters 4 and 5). Typified in the UK's ethical code, banning 'active recruitment' from named countries with critical health shortages remains problematic precisely because it puts limits on the human right to migrate (Mensah *et al.* 2005). It also restricts some of the gains that can be made from research cooperation, skills sharing and learning between countries and globally, which have often been promoted through programmes of skilled worker migration contribution to 'migration for development'.

Furthermore, despite their surface appeal compensatory measures have had limited resonance as a way to mitigate the worst adverse effects. The more radical versions of such measures circulating during the first phase (see Chapters

2 and 3) failed to gain traction, while our assessment of the weaker versions of the measures instituted under the WHO Global Code showed that they have been hardly used and are difficult to implement (see Chapters 4 and 5). Because problems arise in compensating actual lost training revenues after a skilled health worker migrates, the approach has been more one of generalised development aid programmes. Examples of this are the linked aid and medical bilateral training programmes drawn up in Ireland under a 2010–2017 MoU between the Health Services Executive and Irish Aid and relevant source countries, which was revised in 2017 with the aim of strengthening partnerships with developing countries and improving Ireland's response to global health emergencies (Irish Aid 2017). By promoting circular and temporary migration, bilateral agreements have also combined graduate training programmes that can serve to cover health workforce shortages on a temporary basis, as in the case in Ireland's graduate training programme (see Chapter 6), but this fails to deal with the longer-term sustainability of health systems to ensure adequate staffing levels in both source and destination countries.

At the same time, health workforce availability and international migration have never been more salient global issues. Demographic changes, changed disease profiles and rising health expectations led to growing demands for health and social care, and with it, for health workers (ILO 2017a). Yet in many countries, government health expenditures had not been adequate to create or sustain robust health systems (WHO/GHWA 2013). For example, the Abuja Declaration by African Union (AU) Heads of State and Governments, which pledged at least 15 per cent of their annual budgets to the health sector in 2001, had not been achieved ten years later. Of the 26 countries that had increased the proportion of total government health expenditure only Tanzania had achieved the target, and 11 countries had actually reduced government health expenditure. Similarly, by 2009, only five international donor countries had made strategic health workforce planning priorities in their development cooperation programmes with low-income countries (WHO 2011a).

The economic and societal costs of lack of investment in health continue to be eye-wateringly high. An estimated eight million deaths per year occur in LMICs from conditions that are treatable, resulting in US$6 trillion in economic losses (Kruk *et al.* 2018). The outbreak of the Ebola virus epidemic in West Africa in 2014 was a further reminder of the costs of weak health systems (WHO 2015b). WHO and other global institutions are now very well aware that the devastating effects of the Ebola virus epidemic could have been mitigated if there had been robust public health systems and adequate workforces in Guinea, Liberia and Sierra Leone (WHO 2015b). The costs of building such systems is estimated to have been one-third the cost of the Ebola response (Save the Children 2015).

The lack of sufficient progress in global health, including in the implementation of the Global Code, became palpably clear in the closing years of the MDG era (2000–2015). Renewed efforts to link health workforce issues to global health and development became especially important at a time when the international community was preparing a new round of global goals from 2016 and further strengthening of the global migration framework. From the perspective of many IGOs and advocacy groups, the obvious place to start was with the implementation problems with the Global Code (see Chapter 5) while also ensuring that health workforce issues were fully embedded in what was to become the 2030 Agenda.

Efforts to strengthen the implementation of the Global Code began with the 2013 Global Forum on Human Resources for Health (WHO/GHWA 2013) which called for efforts to be stepped up to improve key determinants of access to health care. In preparation for the Global Forum, a major research project identifying progress made (Campbell *et al.* 2013) was flanked by political efforts through a meeting hosted by the Norwegian government, WHO and GHWA with some other high-income countries in advance of the Global Forum to consolidate a shift in thinking about the health workforce as an issue for all countries irrespective of their 'development' status. An increasing number of high- and middle- income countries were projecting health worker shortages in the next decade, adding extra urgency to the need to situate health workforce challenges in a global context, improve health workforce planning in high income countries and to implement fully the WHO Global Code. In this context, the 2013 Global Forum was an important marker of the gear-shift needed to align the health workforce retention with the broader goal of UHC. These discussions, along with other advocacy and civil society initiatives and the active role of GHWA, were critical to ensuring that both health worker-migration and a set of ambitious targets on health were included in the 2030 Agenda (Yeates and Pillinger 2013).

## 3 Landmark initiatives: the SDGs and the Global Compact

Two landmark initiatives structure this third phase. The first of these is the 2030 Agenda (UNGA 2015), the second is the UN Global Compact on Migration (UNGA 2018). The main features of these as they pertain to our study are summarily outlined in turn.

### 3.1 The 2030 Sustainable Development Agenda

The SDGs prioritise a range of challenges that impact on health worker migration, ranging from the implementation of UHC, new strategies on skills in the context of migration, and greater multi-stakeholder participation. Indeed, many of the SDGs are relevant to health worker-migration and -recruitment (see Appendix 4). SDG Goal 3 has a broad health agenda that includes UHC and makes reference to health workforce recruitment and retention, albeit only in relation to developing countries. Its inclusion of non-communicable diseases as well as communicable ones prompted upward revisions to health workforce requirements. The importance given to international migration in the SDGs reflect sustained global advocacy and recognition of the inter-connection of migration with other goals, such as on gender equality (Goal 8) and UHC (Goal 3). SDGs 4, 5, 8, 10, 16 and 17 recognise the benefits that migration bring and target 10.7 calls for the facilitation of 'safe, regular and responsible migration' and the implementation of 'well-managed migration policies'. The goals relating to poverty, education, decent work, inequalities, and to peace, justice and security, and partnerships also have a bearing on the health goals and how they will be realised. Perhaps of greatest significance is that the 2030 Agenda set an ambitious framework for action towards a life of dignity for everyone, striving for equality and social justice with the promise in the Preamble that 'no one will be left behind'. It emphasises an integrative approach with interdependent, indivisible Goals and interlinked targets that require extended collaboration across sectors, calling on a wide range of stakeholders to overcome 'silo-thinking' for achieving the transformative impacts needed.

This emphasis on the multi-stakeholder partnership approach is generally a positive development in its formal support for wide-ranging participation in policy formation. It opens up legitimate spaces for advocacy, dialogue and the participation of CSOs in SDG processes. At the same time, it also reflects a more pervasive influence of the corporate sector and of non-UN bodies gaining ground in influencing new discourses about international economic and social development, potentially crowding out ILO and WHO (Section 5) (see also French and Kotzé (2018) for a critique of the SDGs). Moreover, some of the most important developments involve increasing levels of joint working leading to multi-stakeholder multilateralism amongst UN and non-UN international organisations, which is unprecedented in UN history. This has resulted in greater efforts to strategically address key global concerns, bringing ILO, OECD and WHO (2017) into joint working in areas such as skills development and workforce data.

Further priorities were also established by WHO in 2016 calling on member states to implement policies to consolidate health workforce data including annual reporting to the Global Health Observatory and implement national health workforce accounts to support national policy and planning and WHO's monitoring and accountability framework (WHO 2016, 2016a). In 2017 its Five-Year Action Plan strongly focused on data, evidence and accountability through the use of National Health Workforce Accounts (NHWA) to monitor indicators to support achieving UHC and health-related SDGs.

### 3.2  *The UN Global Compact for Human Mobility and Migration*

The UN Global Compact for Safe, Orderly and Regular Migration (UN Global Compact) was concluded in 2018.[1] It followed the 2016 New York Declaration for Refugees and Migrants, where 193 UN Member States recognised the need for a comprehensive approach to human mobility and enhanced cooperation at the global level. The Global Compact is consistent with SDG target 10.7 and aims to improve coordination and cooperation on global migration governance. It incorporates 23 objectives promoting, amongst others, pathways for regular migration, ethical recruitment, decent work, labour rights, social protection for migrants, social security portability, access to services, skills recognition and skills partnerships, and addressing vulnerabilities related to migration. The recognition of the role of civil society and trade unions in several of its provisions, including in its implementation, is a breakthrough, as are provisions linking fair and ethical recruitment with decent work. The latter helps strengthen the leverage and importance of WHO's Global Code and ILO's fair recruitment initiatives (see Chapter 5, and Section 4.4 below).

Civil society actors and the Council of Global Unions had pushed for a strong focus on the human rights-based approach to migration, including migrants' access to public services (ITUC 2018; Global Unions/BWI 2018).[2] However, during the negotiations a number of provisions were watered down following objections from a large number of governments, resulting in a weakening of the language of the text in areas such as access to services, justice and labour rights. Of concern is that it established a major precedent that will guide future global policy reflecting the insistence by States of their 'national sovereignty' over and above their obligation to implement international human rights law. This outcome has significant implications for the principle of the universality of human rights as established in ILO and UN Conventions. It established a UN Migration Network, led by the UNSG, including UN Agencies with competencies in the field of migration, and coordinated by IOM. At the time of writing it is too early to assess how governments were interpreting the UN Global Compact, including whether and if they will implement its provisions.

## 4 Health workforces for universal health coverage: the emergence of coordinated leverage?

### 4.1 Universal health coverage: a state responsibility?

There is now a global consensus that UHC is an achievable goal, with increasing recognition that health is a human right and a public good that should be accessible and equitable. Global advocacy for UHC, such as the global Universal Health Coverage Coalition, the introduction of World Day for Universal Health Coverage, the signature by more than 360 economists in 53 countries of the Economists' Declaration on Universal Health Coverage, and the Lancet Commission on Investing in Health, *Global Health 2035* (Jamison *et al.* 2013), are some of the initiatives from civil society, economists, health professionals, amongst others, pressing global policymakers to prioritise UHC as an essential pillar of sustainable development, and to ensure that UHC ensures that everyone has access to health services of a high quality, without suffering financial hardship. Importantly, these recognise the neglect of global health investments from donors for development assistance that focuses on health as a public good, including supporting 'leadership and stewardship of global institutions' on this issue (Schäferhoff *et al.* 2015). The then Director General of WHO, Margaret Chan, described UHC as the ultimate expression of fairness (Chan 2012), while Amartya Sen (2015) described UHC as 'the affordable dream'.

UHC was formally endorsed by UNGA in 2012 which reaffirmed the right to health noting that for millions of people these rights remained out of their each and urged all governments to invest in health to ensure universal access to basic health services and protect from financial hardship (UNGA 2012).[3] In stressing the need for improved health system financing for UHC, WHO argued that 'countries must raise sufficient funds, reduce the reliance on direct payments to finance services, and improve efficient and equity' (WHO 2010c:10). The same year, ILO's Social Protection Floors Recommendation (R202) similarly advocated for a rights-based framework for achieving universal access to essential health care, but it did so in the wider framework of ensuring basic income security by building high-quality comprehensive social security systems as an essential part of a sustainable system for UHC. The importance of the quality of health care is underlined by a joint OECD/WHO/World Bank report arguing that 'high-quality, safe, people-centred healthcare is a public good that should be secured for all citizens' (OECD/WHO/World Bank 2018: 58).

Recognition that the achievement of UHC is dependent on strengthened health systems and workforces has been taken up by WHO, which acknowledges that the workforce is key to achieving UHC and depends on the availability, accessibility, and capacity of health workers to deliver quality people-centred integrated care, particularly in expanding the primary health care workforce (WHO 2018b). It argued that '[f]unctioning health systems require a qualified health workforce that is available, equitably distributed and accessible by the population' (WHO 2018a: 8) and emphasised the importance of financing health systems and the health workforce by 'ensuring equitable access to health workers within strengthened health systems' to be achieved through investment in 'both the expansion and transformation of the global health and social workforce' (WHO 2018a: 1).[4] Despite universal consensus for UHC as a goal, the Lancet Global Commission argued that UHC should be seen as a 'starting point for improving the quality of health systems', rather than an end in itself, along with 'expanding coverage and financial protection' (Kruk *et al.* 2018: 1). It further argued that quality in health care can only be achieved if there is the full realisation of the human right to health and that a new approach to improving effective, safe and quality health care through the financing of strong and sustainable health systems is needed.[5]

A key issue concerns the role of the private sector in realising UHC. There are plenty of high-profile supporters favouring its involvement,[6] even if they are divided about the balance between this sector and others. However, private sector finance and provision produce socially inequitable access to health care (Lethbridge 2014; PSI 2018). The involvement of the private corporate sector presents key challenges from a health workforce perspective. Private sector employers have worse track records on employment and social protection matters than public sector ones which is related to lower levels of unionisation in the private sector than the public one (Yeates 2010; see also Chapter 5). Greater involvement of sector employers is associated with lower staffing ratios and worse working conditions, and risks undermining social dialogue processes upon which the more successful health workforce sustainability initiatives have been based (PSI 2018).

### *4.2 WHO's global health workforce strategy*

Access to quality health care services and sufficient numbers of suitably quali-fied health workers with appropriate skill-mixes have long been recognised by WHO as the foundations of strong health systems. This understanding is carried through in relation to UHC. WHO has been taking a lead in implement-ing UHC to giving added impetus to the urgency of addressing projected short-falls of health workers (WHO 2016a) and, with it, implementing the Global Code (Chapter 5).[7] The *Global Strategy on Human Resources for Health: Workforce 2030* (WHO 2016c) puts health workforce planning centre stage. This is a major flagship initiative arising from the Recife Political Declaration (WHO/GHWA 2014) and the outcome of two years' work by GHWA (GHWN)[8] to develop a new agenda as part of UHC and the post-MDG frame-work. Focusing its advocacy on inter-sectoral action and at high political levels (GHWA 2012), and driven by SDG target 3 relating to health workforces, the strategy emphasises the importance of the health workforce to realising health and development goals. It pinpointed chronic underfunding of training and staffing in some countries as a key problem because it 'reduces the sustain-ability of the workforce and health systems' (ibid.: 11). This brought WHO firmly back to its role and purpose in global health policy, with recommenda-tions for health workforce financing and development on the basis that there needs to be a 'paradigm shift': 'a strong and effective health workforce, able to respond to the 21st century priorities, requires matching effectively the supply and skills of health workers to population needs, now and in the future' (ibid.: 12). The Strategy paved the way for complementary global policy meas-ures, including the UN's High-Level Commission on Health Employment and Economic Growth.

### *4.3 UN High-Level Commission on Health Employment and Economic Growth*

Further impetus to strengthen the WHO Global Code has come from the UN High-Level Commission on Health Employment and Economic Growth (HEEG) (HEEG 2016) led by WHO, OECD and ILO. HEEG was spurred by the need to upscale efforts to meet the SDG targets. By its own account, its agenda was to develop '… ambitious solutions to ensure that the world has the right number of jobs for health workers with the right skills and in the right places to deliver uni-versal health coverage' (HEEG 2016: 6). A specific objective was to '… inten-sify support for national, regional and international investments and intersectoral reforms' (HEEG 2016: 6) and to address the projected shortfall of 18 million health workers, mainly in low- and lower-middle income countries by 2030. Above all, HEEG was to 'rethink' the health workforce and health care as a matter of economic investment: a source of employment with the potential to generate new jobs, particularly for women, and stimulate growth in infrastruc-ture, equipment, suppliers and technology production, administrative and other services (Addati *et al.* 2018). Realising these objectives would depend, it argued, on expanding, transforming and creating a sustainable health workforce, to create 40 million new jobs in health and social care within an overall framework of strengthening health and social protection systems, good governance and economic growth with the latter in particular linked to investments in health services and in the health workforce (HEEG 2016). Accordingly, it argued that the resources to support the implementation of the WHO Global Code and relevant ILO Conventions and Recommendations should be made available, and that such efforts should be aligned with relevant international instruments, including the UN Global Compact.

The Commission's recommendations use the language of 'transformative change' to create sustainable health systems with a workforce that has the capacity to respond effectively to population health needs. Such transformation involves changes in health service delivery models, labour market policies, education and training, also taking account of technological advances. Further, it calls for investing in high quality jobs with decent working conditions, ensuring gender equality, rights-based migration policies and improved capacity to respond to emergencies. Enabling these changes requires adequate health financing from multiple national sources, including extending social protection floors (SDG 1), as well as international sources in support of countries in need (SDG 10). The Commission framed the discussion in terms of the increasing trends in international migration of health workers and the need for 'more responsible recruitment practices' (HEEG 2016: 45). On this basis it argued that:

> the international mobility of health workers may also bring numerous benefits to source nations, destination nations and health workers themselves if it is based on ethical norms and standards. The adverse effects of migration must be mitigated. Migrant health workers' rights must be safeguarded and unnecessary barriers to mobility and practice removed.
>
> (HEEG 2016: 49–50)

In this regard, two courses of action it considered are of notable interest. First, it advocated progress on 'international recognition of health workers' qualifications to optimise skills use, increase the benefits from and reduce the negative effects of health worker-migration, and safeguard migrants' rights' (HEEG 2016: 12). This recommendation continued a long line of action by WHO action (Chapter 2):

> The convergence of competencies and quality standards at the international level must be improved, and targeted support provided to source countries and their health systems. There is considerable potential to explore the development of 'transnational standards' for select occupations in the health sector.
>
> (Ibid.: 50)

Second, it advocated a 'win-win' approach based on 'mutuality of benefits' on the basis that international agreements on the ethical international recruitment of health personnel are 'increasingly important to ensure mutuality of benefits and mitigate negative effects' and that such agreements can support 'mechanisms for technical cooperation and investments' (ibid.: 50). For the latter, it raised the prospect of revising the Global Code and ILO instruments:

> These instruments could be made more effective by an updated broader international agreement on the health workforce, including provisions to maximize mutuality of benefit from socially responsible health worker migration.
>
> (Ibid.: 50)

As part of the continuing review processes for the WHO Global Code, HEEG envisaged that resource transfers, migrant remittances and other investments arising from health workforce migration could be embodied in dialogues between states (HEEG 2016: 51). In doing so it *seemed* to resurrect the prospect of earlier work on human resource flow accounting (see Chapter 2). However, as it turned out, this was no vista onto earlier debates about wholescale resource transfers from developed recruiting countries to developing source ones.

The ensuing Five-Year Action Plan (WHO 2018a) set out an agenda firmly located within the existing global policy framework characterised by non-binding agreements reached through policy dialogue and mutual learning.[9] The establishment of the International Platform on Health Worker Mobility set up in 2018 to realise the Plan thus stated its aim is: 'To maximise the benefits and mitigate adverse effects from health labour mobility through elevated dialogue, knowledge and cooperation' (International Platform on Health Worker Mobility 2018). This approach had been endorsed by the Dublin Declaration of senior health policy makers that had met on the margins of the 4th Global Forum on Human Resources for Health (WHO 2017b). Noticeably absent from the Plan was HEEG's original recommendation for 'an updated broader international agreement on the health workforce' (HEEG 2016).

As we write, it is still too early to judge which parts of the programme will be delivered let alone evaluate its success in terms of the transformational changes HEEG stated were necessary. Nevertheless, the Plan will review ILO instruments pertaining to social and health work in the health sector. In this light, our own analysis of their implementation, presented in Tables 7.1 and 7.2, helps illuminate some of the global policy problems to hand. Table 7.1 shows the ratifications record of 30 OECD recruiting countries for nine ILO Conventions pertaining to health worker migration. All of these Conventions specify rights of migrants (Appendix 3 summarises their provisions). The table distinguishes between OECD countries with above average overseas health personnel in their national health workforce (Group A) and those with below the OECD average (Group B), and identifies their track record of ratification for the Conventions.

*Table 7.1* Ratifications of ILO Conventions pertaining to health worker-migration for 31 OECD health-worker recruiting countries[1,2]

| | 1 Migration for Employment (C097) | 2 Social Security (Minimum standards) (C102) | 3 Discrimination (Employment and Occupation) (C111)[3] | 4 Equality of Treatment (Social Security) (C118) | 5 Employment Policy (C122)[4] | 6 Human Resources Development (C142) | 7 Migrant Workers (Supp. Provisions) (C143) | 8 Maintenance of Social Security Rights (C157) | 9 Private Employment Agencies (C181) | 10 Total Conventions (of 9) ratified, by country |
|---|---|---|---|---|---|---|---|---|---|---|
| **Group A: Countries having greater than the OECD average of foreign-trained and foreign-born health personnel in the health workforce (17 countries)** | | | | | | | | | | |
| Australia | ✗ | ✗ | ✓ | ✗ | ✓ | ✓ | ✗ | ✗ | ✗ | 3 |
| Austria | ✗ | ✓ | ✓ | ✗ | ✓ | ✓ | ✗ | ✗ | ✗ | 4 |
| Belgium | ✗ | ✓ | ✓ | ✗ | ✓ | ✓ | ✗ | ✗ | ✓ | 5 |
| Canada | ✗ | ✗ | ✓ | ✗ | ✓ | ✗ | ✗ | ✗ | ✗ | 2 |
| Chile | ✗ | ✗ | ✓ | ✗ | ✓ | ✗ | ✗ | ✗ | ✗ | 2 |
| Estonia | ✗ | ✗ | ✓ | ✗ | ✓ | ✗ | ✗ | ✗ | ✗ | 2 |
| Finland | ✗ | ✗ | ✓ | ✓ | ✓ | ✓ | ✗ | ✗ | ✓ | 5 |
| Ireland | ✗ | ✓ | ✓ | ✗ | ✓ | ✓ | ✗ | ✗ | ✗ | 4 |
| Israel | ✓ | ✓ | ✓ | ✓ | ✓ | ✓ | ✗ | ✗ | ✓ | 7 |
| Luxembourg | ✓ | ✓ | ✓ | ✗ | ✓ | ✗ | ✗ | ✗ | ✗ | 4 |
| New Zealand | ✓[5] | ✗ | ✓ | ✗ | ✓ | ✗ | ✗ | ✗ | ✗ | 3 |
| Norway | ✓ | ✓ | ✓ | ✓ | ✓ | ✓ | ✓ | ✗ | ✗ | 7 |
| Spain | ✗ | ✓ | ✓ | ✓ | ✓ | ✓ | ✗ | ✓ | ✓ | 7 |
| Sweden | ✗ | ✓ | ✓ | ✓ | ✓ | ✓ | ✓ | ✓ | ✗ | 7 |
| Switzerland | ✗ | ✓ | ✓ | ✗ | ✓ | ✓ | ✗ | ✗ | ✗ | 4 |
| United Kingdom | ✓ | ✓ | ✓ | ✗ | ✓ | ✓ | ✗ | ✗ | ✗ | 5 |
| United States | ✗ | ✗ | ✗ | ✗ | ✗ | ✗ | ✗ | ✗ | ✗ | 0 |
| Sub-Total 1: number of ratifications by Convention by Group A countries | 5 | 10 | 16 | 5 | 16 | 11 | 2 | 2 | 4 | |

Group B: Countries having less than the OECD average of foreign-trained and foreign-born health personnel in the health workforce (14 countries)

| | | | | | | | | |
|---|---|---|---|---|---|---|---|---|
| Czech Republic | ✗ | ✓ | ✓ | ✓ | ✗ | ✗ | ✗ | 5 |
| Denmark | ✗ | ✓ | ✓ | ✓ | ✓ | ✗ | ✗ | 5 |
| France | ✓ | ✓ | ✓ | ✓ | ✓ | ✗ | ✓ | 7 |
| Germany | ✗ | ✓ | ✓ | ✓ | ✗ | ✗ | ✗ | 6 |
| Greece | ✗ | ✓ | ✓ | ✓ | ✓ | ✗ | ✗ | 4 |
| Hungary | ✓ | ✓ | ✓ | ✓ | ✓[6] | ✓ | ✓ | 8 |
| Italy | ✗ | ✓ | ✓ | ✗ | ✓ | ✗ | ✗ | 4 |
| Mexico | ✗ | ✓ | ✓ | ✓ | ✗ | ✗ | ✓ | 7 |
| Netherlands | ✗ | ✓ | ✓ | ✓ | ✓ | ✗ | ✓ | 5 |
| Poland | ✓ | ✓ | ✓ | ✓ | ✗ | ✓ | ✓ | 7 |
| Portugal | ✓ | ✓ | ✓ | ✓ | ✗ | ✓ | ✓ | 6 |
| Slovakia | ✓ | ✓ | ✓ | ✓ | ✗ | ✓ | ✗ | 6 |
| Slovenia | ✓ | ✓ | ✓ | ✓ | ✓ | ✗ | ✗ | 5 |
| Turkey | ✗ | ✓ | ✓ | ✓ | ✗ | ✗ | ✗ | |
| Sub-Total 2: number of ratifications by Convention among Group B countries | 6 | 14 | 14 | 13 | 7 | 4 | 0 | 8 |
| Total (Sub-Totals 1+2) number of ratifications (31 OECD countries) | 11 / 24 | 30 | 25 | 29 | 12 | 6 | 2 | 12 |

Source: ILO Normlex, accessed 14 September 2018, and OECD (2015).

Notes
(1) Ratifications registered with the ILO. (2) Countries are identified on the basis of OECD (2015) Tables 3.1, 3.2, 3.3, 3.4 concerning foreign-trained doctors registered, foreign-born practising doctors, foreign-trained registered nurses and foreign-born practising nurses (respectively) as a share of the health workforce of the country. Countries in Group A sit above the OECD average on at least one of these measures, while countries in Group B sit below it. The OECD average for these are as follows: foreign-trained registered doctors 17.1% (2012–2014 data); foreign-born practising doctors 22.2% (2010–2011 data); foreign-trained registered nurses 6.1% (2012–2014 data), and foreign-born practising nurses 14.5% (2010–2011 data). Data for Mexico relates to 2000–2001. Countries are listed alphabetically in each section of this table. For Group A, Australia, Canada, Ireland, Israel, New Zealand, Switzerland, UK and USA are greater than the OECD average on all measures except foreign-born nurses. Sweden is greater than the OECD average on foreign-born and foreign-trained doctors, while Belgium and Luxembourg are so for foreign-born doctors and nurses. Finland and Spain are greater than the OECD average for foreign-trained doctors, while Austria and Estonia are for foreign-born nurses. For Group B, all countries are less than the OECD average on all four measures. (3) This ILO convention has the status of a 'fundamental' right. (4) This ILO Convention has the status of 'governance' (priority). (5) When ratifying this convention New Zealand excluded Annex 1 and the UK excluded annexes 1 and 3. (6) After ratifying the Convention in 1964 the government denounced it in 2004.

The country that contains the greatest number of overseas health workers in its health workforce stands out for being the only country not to have ratified any of the Conventions: the USA. Equally, no country has ratified all nine Conventions (Italy, Group B, comes closest with eight ratified). We also observe that Group B is much more likely to ratify these Conventions than Group A (with the exception of C143 and C181 for which ratification rates are similar), and that more Group B countries have ratified over 50 per cent (five or more) Conventions than Group A (11 of 14 Group B countries compared with seven of 17 Group A countries. The most ratified Conventions across all countries (Groups A and B) are those relating to employment (C111, C122), followed by human resources for development (C142) and social security (C102), while the migration-specific Conventions (C097, C143, C157, C181) are the least ratified. Group B countries are more likely to ratify C181 on private employment agencies (accounting for eight of 12 ratifiers), but least likely to ratify C157 (maintenance of social security rights upon migration) (0 ratifications, although only two Group A countries ratified this Convention).

Table 7.2 contextualises this data, showing overall differences in ratifications (absolute numbers and proportions) across all ILO member states worldwide (irrespective of the share of overseas health personnel in their health workforces). Row A shows ratifications for all ILO member states for the nine Conventions, showing that those designated 'core' (C111) or 'priority' (C122) have the highest ratification rates (41 per cent and 59 per cent, respectively). Rows B and C distinguish between OECD and non-OECD countries. Row B shows just four Conventions (C111, C122, C142) are ratified by over 80 per cent of OECD countries. Row C shows a generally lower rate of ratification, with only C111 (a 'core' Convention) ratified by over 80 per cent of non-OECD countries and is done so at about the same rate as OECD countries. Row D shows that for nearly all Conventions, OECD countries are more likely to ratify than non-OECD countries.

The overall conclusions we draw from this data are that, first, OECD countries are significantly *more* likely to ratify these Conventions than non-OECD ones. Second, OECD countries with the highest proportions of overseas health workers in their health workforces are *least* likely to ratify these ILO Conventions. Third, all countries are less likely to ratify migration-specific Conventions than those which pertain to employment and social security in general. This highlights the magnitude of the implementation gap of existing multilateral agreements on health-worker migration or -recruitment, whether they are ILO Conventions or the WHO Global Code (see Chapter 5).

### 4.4 ILO campaigns on fair recruitment and decent work

For ILO, the SDGs and the Global Compact have given additional leverage to the importance of fair recruitment across all sectors including health care. At a time of increased levels of precarious and non-standard work (ILO 2017b, 2018c), fair recruitment has been an important entry point for discussions

Table 7.2 Ratifications of ILO Conventions pertaining to health worker-migration distinguishing between OECD and non-OECD countries[1]

| | 1 Migration for Employment (C097) | 2 Social Security (Minimum standards) (C102) | 3 Discrimination (Employment and Occupation) (C111)[2] | 4 Equality of Treatment (Social Security) (C118) | 5 Employment Policy (C122)[3] | 6 Human Resources Development (C142) | 7 Migrant Workers (Supp. Provisions) (C143) | 8 Maintenance of Social Security Rights (C157) | 9 Private Employment Agencies (C181) |
|---|---|---|---|---|---|---|---|---|---|
| Total ratifications, all countries | 49 | 58 | 78 | 49 | 112 | 70 | 24 | 4 | 35 |
| Countries ratifying (%) | 26 | 31 | 41 | 26 | 59 | 37 | 13 | 2 | 18 |
| OECD countries (36 countries)[1] | | | | | | | | | |
| n= | 11 | 26 | 34 | 12 | 29 | 29 | 6 | 2 | 14 |
| OECD (%) | 31 | 72 | 95 | 33 | 81 | 81 | 17 | 6 | 40 |
| Non-OECD countries (154 countries)[1] | | | | | | | | | |
| n= | 38 | 32 | 44 | 37 | 83 | 41 | 18 | 2 | 21 |
| non-OECD (%) | 25 | 21 | 93 | 24 | 54 | 27 | 12 | 1 | 14 |
| Percentage point difference between OECD and non-OECD countries | OECD > non-OECD 6 points | OECD > non-OECD 31 points | OECD > non-OECD 2 points | OECD > non-OECD 9 points | OECD > non-OECD 27 points | OECD > non-OECD 54 points | OECD > non-OECD 5 points | OECD > non-OECD 5 points | OECD > non-OECD 26 points |

Source: ILO Normlex.

Notes

(1) This table includes all 36 OECD member countries. In addition to the countries in Table 7.2 this also includes Japan, Iceland, Korea, Latvia and Lithuania. Non-OECD countries are those included in the ILO Normlex database. The database enumerates 154 countries. Countries are not grouped or ranked in any other way beyond member/non-member of OECD. (2) This ILO convention has the status of a 'fundamental' right. (3) This ILO Convention has the status of 'governance' (priority). All other Conventions are 'Technical'.

impacting on health worker-migration. ILO's longstanding work on fair migration (ILO 2014a, 2014b, 2016b) (see Chapter 5) fed into the Global Compact, giving the issue a new global impetus while also reflecting the need for mechanisms on fair recruitment in the light of the trend in global policy towards temporary and circular forms of migration (see Chapters 4 and 6).

Although ILO's work on fair recruitment is carried out through non-binding agreements, it has drawn up guidelines on fair recruitment leading to a new tripartite agreement (General Principles and Operational Guidelines for Fair Recruitment) (ILO 2016b). The ILO Tripartite Meeting of Experts on Defining Recruitment Fees and Related Costs aims to define recruitment fees and related costs (ILO 2018a), building on ILO's Fair Migration Agenda and Fair Recruitment Initiative (ILO 2014b) and implementing guidance in Convention No. 97 on recruitment, placing and conditions of labour of migrants and Convention No. 181's prohibition on private employment agencies from charging fees to workers, directly or indirectly. Related to this is ILO's on-going work for decent work across all sectors (see previous chapters, passim). Here, its contributions lie firmly in the discursive rather than in proposals for new instruments or agreements. Echoing GHWA it concluded that:

> Decent work in the health sector is fundamental to ensuring effective and resilient health systems, a prerequisite to addressing health workforce shortages, and to achieving the goal of equal access to quality healthcare. The health sector is essentially about people; without health workers there can be no healthcare.
>
> (ILO 2014b:1)

More recently, ILO Tripartite Meeting on Improving Employment and Working Conditions in Health Services (Geneva April 2017) drew up conclusions on improving employment and working conditions in health services, including in international migration (ILO 2017c). This stressed the importance of 'ensuring the sustainability of the health workforce in source countries' by adhering to the Global Code, ensuring 'clear processes for the international recognition of skills and occupational qualifications, protection from unethical and unfair recruitment practices, and adequate social protection of migrant health workers, including those employed in home-based care' (ILO 2017c: 4).

The role of social investment in health care systems and in the health workforce has been an important item on global policy agendas, particularly in the lead up to the SDGs and the Addis Ababa Action Agenda on financing sustainable development. Indeed, the SDGs have made it possible to highlight the interrelationships between the critical role of investments in health and the health workforce. ILO wasted no time in acknowledging the significant challenges involved:

> Health worker migration has been one of the means of addressing health worker shortages in many countries, yet it poses further challenges, including

integration of migrant health workers, ensuring decent work and access to health services, and preventing the drain of skilled workers. This drain puts undue pressure on source countries which may have already spent the scarce financial resources available on their training and may have a shortage of trained skilled workers themselves. Auxiliary and volunteer workers can also be used to fill the health worker gaps, but regulations are needed to ensure decent work. Privatisation and outsourcing of health services have further diversified the sector, which could in some cases lead to challenges in effective social dialogue if not properly monitored and regulated.

(ILO 2017c: para. 2)

Although ILO points out that recruitment practices should be in line with ILO general principles and operational guidelines for fair recruitment and the WHO Global Code (ILO 2017c: para. 6), it missed an opportunity to advocate for a strong rights-based approach to migration and decent work, along with adherence to international labour standards and fundamental rights at work. However, it calls on itself to

... actively contribute to the implementation of the HEEG Commission's recommendations and immediate actions with a particular focus on: the recommendations on the promotion of decent health sector job creation; maximizing women's economic participation and empowerment; and strengthening fair and rights-based health worker migration governance.

(ILO 2017c, para. 15c)

A further recommendation calls on itself, working with WHO and OECD and other relevant organisations, to draw up a health workforce research agenda with a view to strengthening 'evidence, accountability and action to promote decent work and productive employment in the health sector', including 'international recognition and acceptance of health workers' qualifications and certification' (ILO 2017c, para. 15.e).

## 5  The shifting contours of global health: enlarging corporate policy space?

As we discussed in Chapters 4 and 5, the authority of WHO as the prime global health actor has significantly diminished over the past four decades. At a time when delivery of UHC requires strong institutional capacity and leadership, there are concerns that its authority will likely be further challenged by the implementation of the SDGs. This is because the SDGs envisage an increased role for multi-stakeholder health partnerships of governments and civil society. The issue is that these partnerships lever in the private sector (corporate providers and philanthropists) as well as not-for-profit social actors. This growth of corporate policy space, as seen in the Post-2015 Partnership Platform for Philanthropy (UNDP *et al.* 2014) for example, builds on an already-established role for the corporate sector in influencing, for example, the Global Financing Facility (GFF) (World Bank 2015).[10] There are some concerns about the operation of the GFF, including lack of transparency and absence of meaningful civil society participation (Bretton Woods Project 2017).

More generally, although corporate involvement provides much needed resources, it reflects a global health funding pattern increasingly located outside of the systems of democratic governance, and most importantly away from the traditional practice of standard-setting through inclusive multilateral decision-making within the UN and the notion of health as a public good provided by health care services in the public sector (Martens and Seitz 2015; Chan 2014). Aided by market approaches to solving global health problems, corporate-led solutions seeking 'quick wins', raise questions about how this will impact upon the role and capacity of governments working through multilateral frameworks to negotiate universal health responses. Because of the proliferation of global health actors which emphasise commercial (trade-led) and corporate-led approaches, health worker-migration is potentially also moved further away from the UN normative system which underpins human rights approaches to migration (PSI 2017a).

It is in this context that we now turn to assess the idea and prospective contributions of 'global skills partnerships' and initiatives to strengthen the regulation of business. The section concludes by reviewing the role of advocacy actors during this period as further sources of informal governance of states and business in relation to health worker-migration and -recruitment.

### 5.1 Global skills partnerships: a new impasse or an opportunity?

First proposed by Michael Clemens (2015, 2017), Global skills partnerships (GSPs) are bilateral agreements that put in place resources for the training of skilled health workers in source countries, equipping health workers with the relevant skills and visas to migrate to work for an agreed duration in the country of destination that funded their training. In this sense,

> A GSP is an up-front agreement between employers and/or governments in destination countries and professional training centres in origin countries. These parties agree on a practical and equitable way for the benefits of migrants' professional service at the destination to finance training at the origin – training for both migrants and non-migrants. Such an agreement allows mutual gains by taking advantage of large international differences in both professional earnings and training costs
>
> (Clemens 2017: 1)

Because GSPs would be formed on the basis of bilateral agreements where destination country governments directly fund training and skills development programmes prior to migration, according to Clemens they avoid the loss of resources from source countries when a trained health worker migrates to work abroad. In this, he cites the estimate by Mills *et al.* (2011) of a cumulative total training cost of US$2.2 billion for African-trained physicians residing in Australia, Canada, the United Kingdom, and the United States. Clemens argues that his case for GSPs is economically compelling:

> It likewise costs at least 5–8 times as much to train a nurse in Western Europe as it costs in North Africa. Skilled migration can thus create enormous economic value. Global Skill Partnerships share that value in a way that origins, destinations, and migrants can agree to.
>
> (Clemens 2015: 1)

As we discussed in Chapter 6, some BLAs already contain a skills or training component and in some countries certain 'ethical recruitment' processes involve pre-departure training which gives orientation, language or other skills.[11] However, GSPs aim to go further than existing bilateral agreements and the provisions in the Global Code in specifying destination country funding for concrete training and placement targets *pre-departure*, while also contributing to general training health workers in source countries.

GSPs open up an opportunity for private finance through, for example, public-private partnerships as a lever for private financing of training (PSI 2018). Clemens (2015) also suggests that the costs of training could be recouped through a 'student loan' type system on the basis that fees would be paid back from the higher salaries in the destination country (a smaller payback is required if they do not migrate) or from public or private-sector employers themselves. They are also advocated as a gateway into international trade in health services, including making 'it easier for people to purchase health services in countries where costs are lower', such as in medical tourism (Clemens 2015: 3).

The idea of GSPs has gained traction. They are favoured by OECD (2018) as a means of deriving mutual benefits. The rationale is 'that for the same cost as training one person in a destination country, governments and employers could afford to train several people to the same standard in the regions of origin' (OECD 2018: 1). In theory, all participants would receive high-quality training for occupations in demand, regardless of their decision to migrate, stay or return. Countries of origin would benefit from having more skilled people at home and abroad, while employers in countries of destination would gain access to a larger pool of workers with desired skills. Heralded as a 'win–win' solution, they promise to help countries of destination that are facing growing shortages of health workers to recruit overseas health workers without skilled migration adversely impacting on source countries' economic and social development (Hooper 2018; OECD 2018). GSPs are also flagged in the Global Compact (UNGA 2018) (Art.33(e) and implicitly under 5: 20(b)) as a way to link migration and skills development for the mutual benefit of migrants, source and destination countries. Under Objective 18: 'Invest in skills development and facilitate mutual recognition of skills, qualifications and competences', it is proposed to:

Build global skills partnerships amongst countries that strengthen training capacities of national authorities and relevant stakeholders, including the private sector and trade unions, and foster skills development of workers in countries of origin and migrants in countries of destination with a view to preparing trainees for employability in the labour markets of all participating countries.

(UNGA 2018: para.18.(e))

Despite seemingly widespread enthusiasm for the idea, GSPs have all the ingredients of a destination country-led initiative to provide themselves with a ready-trained cadre of health workers with skills and qualifications that match those needed in the destination country. And, as always, there is the issue of how they will be implemented. OECD argues that for GSPs to work in practice they need to be based on concrete measures, such as by 'involving employers in both programme design and validation of migrants' skills; acknowledging the diversity of approaches and situations across countries and sectors in how skills development and migration are combined; creating one-stop-shops for promoting skills mobility partnerships, supporting their implementation and conducting evaluation (OECD 2018: 1). Such helpful clarifications highlight how many issues there are to be resolved. These include many unanswered questions about *how* skills partnerships will actually contribute to a net creation of health workers in the source country, mitigate the effects of health worker migration and prove an effective mechanism for addressing health workforce availability. In this, GSPs are wholly untested. However, there *is* evidence from bilateral agreements which is equivocal about the extent to which these agreements ensure mutuality of benefits through, for example, meeting the training needs of source countries and especially those with shortages of health workers (see Chapter 6). For GSPs to work effectively, politically they will require new funding strategies and significant investment by destination countries. However, with no strong rationale for destination country governments to invest in them or evidence testifying to their effectiveness, their impacts may be limited.

A major question is how they will ensure ethical recruitment and rights-based approaches to migration. If GSPs are not to undermine the WHO Global Code they will need to be consistent with the normative framework on migration and labour rights and other principles on fair recruitment established by ILO. There is also a concern that GSPs may further embed temporary and circular health worker-migration schemes (and quotas therein) rather than promote permanent migration and other rights-based approaches to migration established by the UN and ILO. An important part of GSPs is the implementation of migration and visa arrangements through bilateral agreements that specify rights of entry into a country or territory, including right of entry for family members and family reunion. A serious concern is that health workers will be tied to an employer and will have limited rights to move jobs if they face problems of discrimination or exploitation. Unanswered questions also remain about the status of a health worker who, through illness, loss of job, work exploitation or other factors, breaks a contract of employment and leaves their job.

Nor is there any clarity about how GSPs will contribute to the broader objectives of health system sustainability. Potentially they will result in short-term attempts to fill workforce shortages, rather than longer sustained attempts to build health systems in source countries. As they will direct attention to training quotas of skilled health workers for international migration, they will also distract from the provision of adequate resources and ensuring education and training capacity for quality health care services in the source country. Indeed, Gencianos (2018) argues that little can expected from GSPs given that the dominant discourse is financial incentives, employability, skills transfer and mobility rather than health systems sustainability, health equity, decent work and social protection. With their promise to harness the private commercial sector, a further concern is that GSPs may open up further expansion of private training providers, including public–private partnerships. This would require government regulation and additional quality assurance mechanisms to guarantee their transparency and ensure they are actually adhering to ethical recruitment and rights-based approaches to migration. In this context, Gencianos argues that the only reliable way forward for GSPs in these terms is for their implementation to be on a government-to-government basis carried out via public-public partnerships (Gencianos 2018). In this instance, we would add that it would also be important to institute robust scrutiny mechanisms within the implementation instruments governing the partnership. Those that are accessible by key stakeholders supported by resources to participate in them will be capable of holding both governments in the partnership to account for its effectiveness.

### 5.2 Human rights and global capital: initiatives to regulate business practices

Developments in business and trade governance in the realm of human rights during this phase may be one means of ensuring that any eventual GSPs are effective and that private health sector employers adhere to universal principles of global corporate social responsibility (bearing in mind that supervisory frameworks to ensure signatories' adherence to these principles vary considerably in their robustness (see Chapter 4)).

With the UN promoting private sector involvement through international partnerships in realising the SDGs, the issue of responsible business practices has inevitably returned to the UN's agenda. For example, the UNSG report on global partnerships in 2013 affirmed that responsible business practices should be aligned with the practices of the UN (UNSG 2013). Reflecting this broad impetus, the 2016 Framework of Engagement with non-State Actors (WHO 2016d) is a step towards a set of transparent legal and ethical standards for UN-business interactions, which includes addressing risks and due-diligence in respect of human rights. However, it is founded on voluntarism, and the issue will be whether the UN will enforce it across all business contracts it enters into.

Additionally, OECD and ILO initiatives have both been revised and, to a degree, strengthened.[12] The introduction of human rights due-diligence has implications for how companies can detect, identify and prevent human rights violations and abuses (UNHRC 2018a). Emerging due-diligence frameworks reported by the UNHRC notes that there are 20 government national action plans on business and human rights (UNHRC 2018b). Some governments have begun to take their human rights due-diligence responsibilities seriously. French law requires companies to identify and prevent risks to human rights, health, safety and the environment (including sub-contractors) (ECCJ 2017). Similar legislation is being discussed in the Netherlands, in addition to existing Dutch agreements on international responsibility in business conduct, although CSOs are concerned that trade policies are taking a greater priority (mvoplatform 2018). However, these two countries remain the exception to the rule.

Strengthened due-diligence frameworks are elaborated in policy instruments that remain, ultimately, voluntary. This has led to heightened global advocacy by transnational civil society networks such as the global Treaty Alliance[13] for a legally binding instrument to regulate the activities of transnational corporations and to provide appropriate protection, justice and remedies for the victims of human rights abuses. The follow-up mechanisms on implementation of the UNGP, particularly in monitoring human rights due diligence by corporations, had been widely criticised by CSOs whose joint statement (Joint Civil Society Statement on Business and Human Rights 2011) was presented at the twenty-fourth session of the Human Rights Council in September 2013. There, the Government of Ecuador declared on behalf of 85 countries that: 'A legally binding instrument would provide the framework for enhanced State action to protect rights and prevent the occurrence of violations' (UNHRC 2013: 2).

Following on from this, in June 2014 a resolution drafted by the governments of Ecuador and South Africa was passed by the UN Human Rights Council in Geneva (Resolution 26/9) for the establishment of an open-ended intergovernmental working group (IGWG) with a mandate to draw up an international legally binding instrument on Transnational Corporations and Other Business Enterprises with respect to human rights. The IGWG, chaired by Ecuador, met three times between 2015 and 2018 and has drafted proposals for a framework for a binding treaty obliging member states to implement regulatory measures requiring businesses to adopt and apply human rights due-diligence policies and procedures set out in the UNGPs. In November 2017, the UN Human Rights Council (UNHRC 2017a) drafted a legally binding instrument on business and human rights, with the prime objective of making due diligence *mandatory* in order to prevent violations or abuses of rights, investigate and punish abuses, and provide for compensation. The first discussions took place in October 2018, generating a significant build-up of civil society and trade union advocacy for a binding Treaty.

During these discussions the ITUC and global unions (ITUC/IndustriALL/ ITF/IUF/PSI/UNI 2018) took a strong stand in arguing for a treaty to cover all internationally recognised human rights and fundamental rights at work in international labour standards, as well as regulating human rights due-diligence policies and procedures, alongside strong international monitoring and enforcement mechanisms. If agreed, the instrument could have important implications for all health workers, migrant or not. It would strengthen regulatory oversight of recruitment companies in the health and social care sectors, provide a potential counterbalance to bilateral and multilateral trade agreements devoid of labour and human rights protections, and institute robust mechanisms to hold public and private actors responsible for human rights breaches through due-diligence frameworks. Support for such a Treaty has also been growing. In October 2018 the European Parliament passed a Resolution supporting a UN Binding Treaty to 'effectively address the issue of corporate liability for human rights violations and related challenges' (ibid.: para.19) and urged the EU and its Member States to take a constructive approach in supporting the Treaty.

### 5.3 Global advocacy and civil society mobilisation

Global advocacy and civil society mobilisations have been critical in realising better intersections between the right to health, UHC and health worker-migration in global policy. They have sustained campaigns for broad-ranging SDGs supportive of the right to health and health workforce strategies as integral to UHC, and of rights-based approaches to the international migration of health workers. CSOs in this field include NGOs and migrant advocacy organisations as well as workers' organisations (principally independent trade unions) at the national and global levels. ITUC and PSI have been the most active on the right to health, the role of the public sector in delivering quality health care services, and rights-based approaches to health worker-migration.

Annual 'Civil Society Days' that have run in parallel to the GFMD process have been instrumental in helping civil society and workers' organisations to develop common strategies to improve global migration governance. The Days enabled the creation of the global Migration and Development Civil Society Network which drew up the civil society transformative vision and priority issues for inclusion in the UN Global Compact (MADE Network 2017). The ten Acts in its 'Now and How TEN ACTS for the Global Compact' intersect with cross-cutting themes of gender-responsive public services and the rights of the child. Act 4 (Decent work and labour rights) includes recommendations on ethical recruitment and employment, strengthening the role of ILO in standard-setting, and better implementation of rights-based global migration governance (MADE Network 2017).

In relation to UHC and health workers specifically, civil society and workers' organisations have stressed the importance of the right to health and sustainable health systems. 'Health workers for all and all for health workers' (HW4All) is a European civil society project funded by the EU campaigning for sustainable health workforces worldwide, with a focus on the implementation of the WHO Global Code.[14] Analysis of the case studies submitted under the second round of reporting on the Code show how it helped promote a public health approach to health worker-migration amongst civil society actors and trade unions (Van de Pas *et al.* 2016). For example, in the Netherlands, ethical and fair recruitment initiatives have been inspired by civil society organisations and trade unions, working closely with recruitment agencies, labour inspectorates, the Ministry of Health, the Ministry of Social Affairs and Employment and local municipalities. The civil society-led *Call to Action: A Health Worker for Everyone, Everywhere* has gained wide support across Europe for urging EU institutions and Member States to step up their support for strong health workforces and sustainable health systems around the world and to take responsibility for the impacts of their recruitment policies on source countries (see Chapter 5).[15]

Such advocacy has also been firmly embedded in the migration programmes on health and social care workers of EPSU and PSI. These have taken union actions into new areas, particularly in connecting health worker-migration to the right to health, sustainable public health care systems and ethical recruitment. Not surprisingly, they have been highly critical of the socialisation of the financial costs of the global financial crisis and the privatisation of the financial windfalls accruing from quantitative easing, privatisation and public–private partnerships in health. As a global union representing public sector workers, PSI identified at an early stage the need for global action on the rights of migrant health workers, particularly women. It has been at the forefront of training and capacity building for unions on rights-based approaches to migration and ethical recruitment of health and social care workers in Africa, Asia and Latin America to ensure that there are strong and well-resourced public health services in source countries and that migration is an informed and real choice for health workers. Its *Global Campaign for Ethical Recruitment* (2015) brought public service unions into discussions about how to effectively monitor the WHO Global Code and to raise awareness about the need for reciprocal arrangements. A key objective was to integrate these activities into union organising and through this to pursue union-to-union bilateral cooperation to facilitate transportable union membership, twinning by health facilities/unions on specific initiatives, campaigning for quality health services and pay equity. Its 'Support Fair and Ethical Recruitment: #NoRecruitmentFees' campaigned to end the practice of charging recruitment fees to migrant workers. This PSI campaign was instrumental in getting the issue included in the UN Global Compact and the ILO Fair Recruitment Guidelines.

Recently gaining observer status at WHO, the PSI's 'Human Right to Health Campaign' (PSI 2017a) has advocated for the public provision of health care, on the basis that the state is responsible for the provision of quality health services. Its campaign slogan 'My health is not for sale' is a response to the growing commercialisation and privatisation of health and the influence of multinational corporations on the private health care and insurance markets.[16] Health workforce issues have occupied a core part of that, and the campaign advocates for mandated staff-to-patient ratios in the health sector as a basis for setting minimum standards for safe health care. UHC, it argues, will be impossible to deliver without health workers who have decent and safe working conditions, the right to freedom of association and collective bargaining, and gender equality. It highlights the inextricable connection between improvement in labour standards and the attainment of UHC, inasmuch as the 'migration of professionals who leave their countries due to low wages and poor working conditions threatens guaranteed health delivery around the globe' (PSI 2017a: 1).

Trade union advocacy on health workforces has also been on a regional scale. It has done so through the European social dialogue process using the EPSU-HOSPEEM Code of Conduct (see Chapter 4), the importance of which was reinforced in a joint statement by EPSU and HOSPEEM renewing their commitment to the Global Code's ethical recruitment principles in order to 'promote, guarantee and defend decent recruitment and working conditions for migrant workers, from the EU and from outside the EU, in hospitals and health care facilities across Europe' (EPSU/HOSPEEM 2018). Using the Code of Conduct, there has been good collaboration between EPSU and its affiliates to advocate for good conditions of employment to be included in the content of bilateral agreements, for example, between the Philippines and Germany. The German trade union confederation, DGB, initiated a 'Fair Mobility' project with multilingual information on fair wages and working conditions for migrant workers from CEE countries on the German labour market. The German services union Ver.di and the Spanish health worker trade unions (FES-CCOO and FSP-UGT) also used the Code to raise awareness about 'social dumping' after migrant Spanish nurses working in Germany were given inferior working conditions than existed under the collective agreements in Germany.

These initiatives give examples of the growing global advocacy and campaigning for global social justice, ethical recruitment and the human right to health, underpinned by decent work and adherence to labour standards. However, as the advocacy movement for a binding treaty on responsible business conduct demonstrates, the increasing privatisation and corporatisation of key areas of public life are driving unprecedented change. This needs to be tackled through business responsibility established at national and regional level (in the European Union), and on the basis that 'getting your house in order', for example, through laws on due diligence and through European Union policies, is an essential step to reducing global inequalities and ultimately unequal globalisation leading to health worker-migration.

## 6  Conclusion

This chapter has discussed the third and most recent phase in the development of the global policy field on health worker-migration and -recruitment. At the time of writing we are still in the early years of the SDG period and much can still evolve. However, there is good evidence showing that these issues are now much closer to the centre of global debates about global health and the universalisation of health care. Building health system sustainability and providing good quality healthcare are widely accepted as foundational to achieving good health outcomes for all. These developments alone show a mainstreaming of health worker-migration into global policy in ways that have spurred efforts to strengthen the implementation of the WHO Global Code and ILO Conventions and Recommendations regarding decent work, gender equality, social protection and migration. These are welcome developments because, as Chapter 5 showed, implementation of the WHO Code is faltering, while ratification data on ILO health worker-migration instruments also shows there is much ground to be usefully gained.

The process for agreeing the SDGs saw the surfacing of sustained global advocacy around global inequalities, migration, health, gender equality and decent work, amongst other areas. In addition, recent global initiatives for strengthening health systems and the health workforce share '… the call for transformative action, changing mindsets, and partnerships at all levels to seize the opportunities at hand and address the immense challenges ahead' (ILO 2017c, para. 1.1(7)). This phase has so far seen higher levels of public discourse about implementing high quality health systems in the context of UHC, and the implementation of measures to promote fair migration, gender equality and decent work for health workers. Closely connected to this is the need to ensure that the health workforce is adequate, well-trained and motivated through good conditions of employment and pay, adequate health facilities and equipment at work, with sufficient time for patient care, and career opportunities. Such measures would help to retain health workers in their countries of origin, while protecting health workers rights to migrate in circumstances that are not driven out of poverty or poor living and working conditions. In particular, there is a recognised need to shift international donor funding programmes towards longer-term universal health care improvements and strengthening of health systems, including provision of high-quality training facilities.

The 2030 Agenda has spurred an unprecedented amount of policy activity to renew efforts to address health workforce issues and, relatedly, migration and recruitment. Key themes are the upscaling of resources to meet rising health needs and the demand for health care and institutional health strengthening. WHO initiatives on health workforces and UHC have a high profile, but by no means are all the initiatives within the purview of WHO, though many of them are UN-led. Amongst these are the extension of UN global migration governance (UN Global Compact), social protection and labour governance (ILO Social Protection Floor, fair recruitment) and business and trade governance (human rights due-diligence mechanisms), all of which tangibly bear on employment and recruitment across health supply chains stretching worldwide.

We see continuing differences between the principal IGOs in this field. ILO still comes to the issues from a labour and migration rights perspective, the IOM from a circular migration and diasporic approach, and WHO from a 'human resources for health' and health systems strengthening perspective. Nevertheless, there is significant cross-organisational collaboration among them including with non-UN IGOs such as WB and OECD. Beyond specific collaborative projects, there seems to be a consensus on two axes. The first axis is strengthening the implementation of the WHO Code rather than fortifying its institutional provisions or even introducing new (stronger) global regulatory instruments.

The second axis is accepting the voluntary non-binding nature of multilateral frameworks on social (and health) standards. The only proposal for a legally binding global governance instrument relates to the UNHRC's initiative for a global treaty on business and human rights which has so far drawn support from just two countries in the Global South and the European Parliament. Despite the rightly ambitious 'transformative agenda' of the SDGs, there is so far little evidence of the kinds of robust initiatives that would inspire confidence in the international community attaining the global health and health-related goals to which it aspires.

Nevertheless, the initiatives have brought international organisations into new dialogues and thinking about global policy responses. In this respect, we highlight the importance within the SDGs not only of multi-stakeholder responses but of multisectoral partnerships. We commented critically on how these lever structural openings for corporate and private sectors in health financing and provision, and bring market-led and piecemeal approaches which risk distracting from addressing long-term planning, sustainable financing and institutional strengthening or capacity building, and undermining accountability in domestic and global spheres of governance that is essential for providing quality health care under UHC. Indeed, the further enhancement of the private commercial sector in achieving UHC risks compromising respect for and implementation of UN normative framework of standards and Treaty obligations and the importance of solidarity for health as a public good. This has potentially far-reaching consequences for strengthening health systems and for the achievement of human rights, health, social protection, decent work and equalities goals. Despite cross-organisational collaboration, there is far from a global consensus amongst IGOs about how to achieve UHC, and particularly the broader role of the public and private sectors in strengthening health systems more generally. This will be a continuing point of tension.

WHO seems so far to have sustained momentum from the 2010 Code with the support of other IGOs (notably ILO) as well as GHWA, health and migration NGOs and trade union organisations. The global commitment to UHC under the SDGs brought WHO back into its core work of health workforce training and health system strengthening. However, it will have to face up to further risks to the normative basis for rights-based approaches to international migration and the principle of equality treatment. Temporary and circular migration have become even more firmly embedded and WHO and others will need to be alert to the implications of this for achieving health workforce goals.

## Notes

1 Agreed by all UN Member States except USA and Hungary on 13 July 2018, and UNGA in December 2018 following a year of consultations and negotiations.
2 ITUC argued this results in a 'serious risk of a two-tier migration policy framework existing alongside two-tier labour markets' (ITUC 2018: 1). The Council of Global Unions' argued that 'This approach, contradicts protections in international human rights treaties and labour standards and a step backwards from well-established ILO doctrine and human rights principles' (Global Unions/BWI 2018: 1).

3  Universal health has been a stated global policy objective since the 1940s and has evolved since. The WHO Constitution recognises that 'the enjoyment of the highest attainable standard of health is one of the fundamental rights of every human being without distinction of race, religion, and political belief, economic or social condition'. The Alma-Ata Declaration (1978) stated that health is a fundamental human right and that health care should be available for all. WHO Resolution WHA58.33 (WHA 2005) identified sustainable health care financing as a key element of this, defining the UHC as providing 'access to key promotive, preventive, curative and rehabilitative health interventions for all at an affordable cost, thereby achieving equity in access'.

4  WHO made UHC a priority in its 13th General Programme of Work (WHO 2018c) which refers to the 'triple billion' targets: one billion more people benefiting from UHC; one billion more people better protected from health emergencies; and one billion more people enjoying better health and well-being.

5  The Lancet Global Health Commission argued that global development partners should support this agenda 'by aligning with each country's priorities, not funding flotillas of small-scale interventions over short project-cycles, and instead selectively investing in a few health system reforms over a longer time period' (Kruk *et al.* 2018: 45).

6  WB has argued that UHC can only be achieved if the private sector takes a role while the Bellagio Declaration holds that 'these reforms will not succeed without including the private health sector and other sectors' (Al-Janabi *et al.* 2018: 3).

7  See: www.who.int/workforcealliance/brain-drain_brain-gain/en/

8  Global Health Workforce Network (GHWN, previously the Global Health Workforce Alliance, GHWA) operates within WHO as a global mechanism for multi-sectoral collaboration and dialogue on health workforce policies. www.who.int/workforce alliance/en/

9  The Action Plan is a joint intersectoral programme of work among ILO, OECD and WHO to support governments to implement the recommendations of the High-Level Commission in line with WHO's Global Strategy (WHO 2018c: 5). It commits to '[f]acilitating policy dialogue, analysis and institutional capacity-building to maximize mutual benefits from international labour mobility' (ibid.: 8). Notably, it includes the social care workforce in the delivery of health care, marking a move away from a sole preoccupation with skilled health workers.

10  The GFF (2014) is a finance mechanism for reproductive, maternal, newborn, child and adolescent health (RMNCAH) programmes and policies, and is run through a multi-stakeholder partnership with support of the UNSG's Global Strategy for Women's, Children's and Adolescents' Health. GFF is the financing mechanism for Every Woman Every Child, linking UNAIDS, UNFPA, UNICEF, UN Women, WHO, and WB.

11  Examples of this are the mandatory government-run pre-departure orientation seminars in the Philippines (PDOS), Pre-Departure Orientation in Nepal, Final Pre-Departure Briefing in Indonesia, and the Canadian Orientation Abroad Initiative (delivered by IOM in over 40 countries of origin). Training is provided pre-migration (e.g. in the Philippines) and through training programmes developed between source countries and recruiting ones (a good example of this is the bilateral agreement between Alberta (Canada) and the Philippines 2008). The German–Philippine 'triple-win' programme has also facilitated health sector employers to fund professional training, language training, and integration assistance in the country of origin pre-migration, but it remains an isolated example (see Chapter 6).

12  OECD Guidelines were updated in 2011 following the adoption of the UNGPs to strengthen risk-based due diligence and responsible supply chain management. There is now a built-in grievance mechanism accessible by CSOs. Revisions to the ILO MNE Declaration in 2017 add principles relating to decent work, including new

guidance on 'due diligence' processes in line with the UN Guiding Principles on Business and Human Rights.

13 Transnational civil society networks formed a global Treaty Alliance to advocate for a binding Treaty that addresses the consequences of corporate abuse. The Alliance is made up of approximately 1500 individuals and 1100 CSOs worldwide. See: www. treatymovement.com

14 The project is EU-funded and implemented by the African Medical and Research Foundation (Italy); Center for Health Policies and Services (Romania); Humanitarian Aid Foundation Redemptoris Missio (Poland); Health Poverty Action (UK); Medicus Mundi International Network; Memisa (Belgium); Federation of Associations of Medicus Mundi (Spain); terre des hommes (Germany); and the Wemos Foundation (Netherlands).

15 The call for action seeks improvement in five areas: planning and training for a long-term, sustainable health workforce, investment in the health workforce, respecting the rights of migrant health workers, thinking and acting coherently at all (national, regional, and global) levels (HealthWorkers4all 2014).

16 The Manifesto of the PSI Human Right to Health Global Campaign argues that:

> This is having a devastating impact on universal access to quality healthcare for patients, on working conditions for health workers and on the financial sustainability of the health systems. The related increase in liberalisation and trade in services gravely undermines guaranteed public health services.
>
> (PSI 2017a: 1)

# 8 Conclusions

## Towards a new world order for health

## 1 Introduction

This final chapter of the book briefly summarises key arguments and findings from our study of the contemporary history of global governance and global policy on health worker-migration and -recruitment. We draw together insights from the study covering 70 years and consider what this means for a globalist analytics of global governance and policy more generally. In this, we reach 'beyond' the specific realm of health worker-migration and -recruitment to reflect on the implications of the study for future research, advocacy and policy. We consider what the findings mean for how we construct research fields examining the 'global condition' of health and welfare in ways that are theoretically robust *and highly engaged* with the global policy challenges which the international community must face. We also consider the implications of the book's findings for the future development of the global policy field, including the global leadership urgently required from IOs, states and advocacy groups.

Central to this discussion is the recognition that addressing key global health and social inequalities require more robust global governance responses for long-term sustainable solutions. In this sense, our conclusions are framed through a global *transformative* social policy lens (UNRISD 2016). They are rooted in the understanding that there is much scope for strong global leadership to steer turning global objectives into concrete programmes of action that: go beyond mitigating approaches to substantively address the root causes of health worker-migration and -recruitment, including ending dependence on overseas-trained health workforces to staff national health services; are grounded in evidence and normative values of global social justice and social sustainability; are integrated across different social and economic sectors (including but going beyond health) and policy-driven; and are informed by inclusive multi-stakeholder, multi-level partnerships.

The chapter begins by very briefly recapping on the three phases of the global policy field that we identified (Section 2.1), and then turns to consider some overall conclusions from the study as a whole (Section 2.2). Here, we focus on the combined effects of institutions, policy processes and material conditions shaping the global policy field under historical circumstances that have changed over time, where we highlight the unsatisfactorily slow incorporation of measures to address gendered inequalities in the health workforce and health care economy into global policy-making. Section 3 addresses concrete questions about the efficacy of global-level action to reduce global inequalities in health and related critical health worker-shortages. It identifies a range of measures and possibilities for key policy strategies, within a framework that understands the requirement for global responses to be proportionate to the scale, nature and urgency of the challenges. Such challenges, we emphasise, are trans-border and have extensive international reach and significant impact and so require policy responses capable of addressing them robustly and comprehensively. We emphasise the critical significance of prioritising actions for a better global governance of health worker-migration and -recruitment that are capable of enabling SDG health goals to be realised in a way that satisfies the conditions for a transformative approach to global social policy (Section 4).

## 2 Analysing global governance and global policy formation

### 2.1 Critical junctures: review

This book has discussed and charted policy and institutional developments in global governance as they relate to health worker-migration spanning seven decades, from the early establishment of dialogue and policy embedded in the UN's nascent global governance framework in the 1940s to present-day developments that reflect multi-stakeholder responses to international health worker-migration and -recruitment within an extensively pluralistic global institutional and organisational field in which the UN is but one global actor. Over this time, international health worker-migration and -recruitment have long been understood as issues of direct concern to global policy and governance and they have moved more towards the centre of global goal-setting on health, migration and development. This is not, however, an uncomplicated set of developments. This is because the overall trend has been a shift in the regulatory approach *away* from more radical forms of progressive redistribution from destination to source countries and *towards* global 'ethical recruitment' to try and ensure that health worker-mobility becomes a 'win–win' international trade benefiting all countries involved (those that continue to 'export' trained health workers *and* those that rely on them to staff their health services). In this sense, the multilateralisation of policy and governance has overseen the significant increases in levels of health worker-migration and -recruitment, especially from poor to rich countries. These levels have increased over time, with important consequences for the extent to which many poorer countries can realise major health goals, be it universal health coverage or improvements in health outcomes. In charting these (and other) developments, we identified three distinct phases of development, or critical junctures, since the earliest days of the global policy field. These are highly summarily described in Section 2.1 below prior to considering broader themes and conclusions arising from the study as a whole in Section 2.2.

## 2.1.1  The origins of global health worker-migration and -recruitment policy

During Phase 1 that stretched from the mid-1940s to the late 1970s, the global policy field was initiated and underwent rapid development. Its roots were firmly implanted in the nascent normative system developing under the global steward-ship of the UN. UNESCO, ILO and UNCTAD all played leading roles during the 1950s and 1960s by identifying the global dynamics of highly skilled labour migration, framing policy debates in *global* terms and identifying key priorities. Together, they established the normative and institutional bases for a radical global policy to 're-engineer' the distributive dimensions of gains and losses that were unequally shared by source countries, destination countries and migrants them-selves (see Chapter 2). The major advances in global human rights, equality, health, migration, labour and social protection institutional regimes, as well as in international trade and development, during this period beneficially impacted upon the rapid institutionalisation of this early phase in the global policy field of health worker-migration.

It was not until the 1970s, however, that a clear focus on migrant health workers in the global policy field became apparent (see Chapter 3). ILO's activ-ism on the new international economic order initiative, migration, labour stand-ards and equality combined with WHO's entry into the field through its 'landmark' study of international health worker-migration, bringing these two agencies into an alliance to institute the first global policy instrument – the ILO Nursing Personnel Recommendation (1977). Although the Recommendation was non-binding and suffered from monitoring and implementation failures, it none-theless formally brought a focus on health worker *recruitment* into the equation for the first time. Notably, Article 67 of the ILO Recommendation set out con-ditions for 'ethical' international recruitment that were far stronger than those agreed under the WHO Global Code nearly 40 years later.

## 2.1.2  The rise of the 'ethical recruitment' paradigm in global governance

Phase 2 saw the resumption of global policy activity in the late 1990s after a largely dormant period lasting more than two decades since the ILO Recom-mendation had been passed. Neo-liberal globalising forces had wreaked havoc on the material contexts of health worker-migration and -recruitment and weak-ened the material capabilities of many national governments and global organi-sations (in particular WHO) to address them. Nevertheless, the twenty-first century opened with a series of sub-global state and non-state 'ethical recruit-ment' initiatives. The platform that these initiatives provided combined with global advocacy initiatives increasingly focused on the relationship between the global mal-distribution of the health workforce and poor health outcomes, to help generate momentum in support of a new multilateral instrument. It was decided from the outset that this instrument would be framed in terms of ethical recruitment, 'homed' in WHO and be non-binding.

These calls, and the work culminating in the WHO Global Code in 2010, took place in a context scarred by the neo-liberalisation of global policy. Heightened dominance of 'free' trade in global policy making, an increasingly hostile environment to robust global social regulation 'with teeth', and re-energised global migration and development governance agendas engendered ideational and discursive shifts in the global policy field. The relatively weak non-binding Global Code was acceptable to all destination countries, as it was to source countries which believed it to be a step towards greater recognition of their needs (see Chapter 4). The chief beneficiaries of this process were rich destination countries because although the Global Code placed some (non-enforceable) constraints on the conduct of recruiting countries, its palliative provisions did not threaten the continuation of high levels of international health worker-recruitment. Indeed, it sanctioned such recruitment, including from poorest to richest, *so long as* source countries were not identified as having critical health worker-shortages.

The WHO Global Code suffers from similar shortcomings to the ILO Recommendation in terms of monitoring and implementation (see Chapter 5, Chapter 3). Shortcomings originating in the text of the Global Code were exacerbated by weak resourcing commitments and by destination country governments' systematic resistance to incorporating the Code's provisions into their national policies and laws. This resistance blocked a path to making the provisions of the Global Code legally binding. In addition, powerful corporate and commercial interests, often allied with states, have continued to exercise an influential role in the on-going globalisation of health care and health worker-migration and -recruitment. In this context, questions arise as to whether the Global Code is fit for purpose. At the same time, advocacy actors have looked outside WHO for stronger (enforceable) regulation of business conduct. The proposed binding treaty of the UN Human Rights Council (UNHRC 2018a) emerges as a potential means to enforce business' social responsibilities for human rights-led ethical recruitment and employment (see Chapter 5).

An important feature of Phase 2 was the growing significance of bilateral agreements as an emerging policy priority (see Chapter 6). Although bilateral cooperation has been promoted by ILO since 1949 and later by WHO (see Chapter 3), bilateral agreements of various kinds were heavily promoted by IOs during this phase as means of mitigating the impacts of losses of health workers borne by source countries. However, there are so few promising examples of cooperation that attain international standards or even promote good practices on ethical recruitment, labour rights, rights-based approaches to migration or building sustainable health systems, that we are led to conclude that these instruments are far from a source of inspiration. Their 'light-touch' approaches to sharing the costs of investment in training and education are especially dismal. In this sense, they have worked primarily to the benefit of destination countries seeking to alleviate their own domestic shortages of health workers.

Unfolding in tandem with and through this bilateralist approach to global governance is a further shift in focus. Global migration and development policy is increasingly lauding the benefits of circular migration on the basis that it can enhance the development dividends of health worker-migration for source countries and enhance migrants' skills. However, its promotion in global migration policy has contributed to elevating temporary migration as the 'new norm' for unilateral (national) policy. This detrimentally impacts on migrants' rights to permanence and citizenship. Overall, the track-record of bilateral approaches and agreements leads to the conclusion that they are at best short-term, palliative solutions to structural problems in health systems. Furthermore, they distract attention and resources from work needed to enable *sustainable* health systems in ways that address the root causes of international migration and recruitment in the health care sector.

### 2.1.3  Universal health coverage and achieving sustainable health systems

A theme running through this book is the necessity of simultaneously addressing health worker-migration and -recruitment and health system-strengthening while taking into account the need to tackle social inequalities and uneven development. These issues, and the connections between them, moved centre-stage in Phase 3 of the global policy field. This phase, we argued, is in its early stage of development. It is marked by a step-change in global policy. The 2030 Sustainable Development Agenda's bold and welcome commitment to 'leave no one behind' and tackle inequalities integrates rights-based approaches to migration and ethical recruitment processes into the raft of complementary measures for realising universal health care and sustainable healthcare systems. Even so, its identification of health workforce recruitment and retention as an issue *especially* for poorer countries evidences the legacies of WHO's long-standing 'look south' approach to global health systems. The Global Compact for Migration agreed in December 2018, spurred by Agenda 2030, also brings migration into the centre of global governance, but reflects the preference for non-binding global regulatory approaches. In some respects, it actually hardens state's sovereignty claims on migration management.

Agenda 2030's mobilisation of global action has been accompanied by the involvement of a much wider range of organisational actors, especially non-UN ones, in the 'implementation' of the SDGs. This potentially further undermines the UN normative system and the body of international human rights law on migration, health and fundamental rights at work. The inscription of partnerships for implementation in the SDGs brings a much greater role for multi-stakeholderism. Multi-stakeholderism has been important in widening debates and perspectives, particularly in recognising the voice and agency of civil society and trade union organisations, though the problem of how to achieve the SDG targets remains as contested as ever. In the context of UHC, support for the role of the private sector and public-private partnerships as solutions to reduced or limited possibilities for health service-funding has intervened in debates about the need for long-term sustainable investments in health systems. This has, in turn, translated into controversial proposals for Global Skills Partnerships in global health worker-migration and -recruitment policy. Given the track-record of bilateral agreements (see Chapter 6), there is little prospect of these bringing the kinds of lasting solutions required.

### 2.2  Reflections on findings

The consistent efforts by global organisations over the 70 years to 'tame' the dynamics of the global political economy of health worker-migration and -recruitment demonstrate the magnitude and complexity of the circumstances and interests that global policy makers have needed to respond to and negotiate. Charting the contours, characteristics and dynamics of this global policy field, we have shown how global policy initiatives are addressing (or are attempting to address) the causes and consequences of health worker-migration in source and destination countries worldwide and the efficacy of the initiatives. Our findings show that interconnected issues of health worker-migration and -recruitment, realising universal health coverage and attaining optimal health workforce availability have featured unevenly in this global policy field over the course of this period. There have been notable achievements in securing two global (non-binding) agreements to regulate health worker-migration and -recruitment, plus a substantial body of flanking international agreements governing business and state conduct in relation to recruitment, employment, social protection and health on the basis of equality and human rights. However, and crucially, global governance and policy have been neither sufficiently attuned to the scale and urgency of health workforce and health systems crises nor treated these crises sufficiently well as trans-boundary issues connected global capitalist dynamism. The efficacy of this legally significant body of international agreements has been undermined by implementation failures, such that despite formal acceptance that health workforce sustainability is a 'shared global responsibility', this is yet to be realised in practice.

In this sense, the 'thickening' of global governance over time cannot be characterised as a linear trajectory reflecting the increased influence of progressive social forces, even if these have been able to carve out 'spaces' within it. Nor can it be depicted as a wholly regressive set of developments, even if social forces in favour of maintaining copious supplies of health labour for import or export have secured the future of this trade as having a legitimate part to play in domestic and global development strategies. Yet for all that is to be commended in the ILO Recommendation, the WHO Global Code and the SDGs, and the numerous flanking treaties, Conventions, agreements and accords, global health goals will remain aspirational until and unless all these instruments are rigorously implemented in full. We discuss these 'practical' aspects of global policy development at further length in Section 3.

## *2.2.1 Revisiting the materialist analytics of global governance and policy*

Our study has been concerned with the combined effects of institutions' inter-actions and configurations of organisations, actors and ideas shaping global policy under different historical circumstances, as well as with their interplay with the material contexts that condition them. Our findings lend credence to an overtly materialist analytics of global governance and policy. We have shown how the multilateralisation of governance and policy on health worker-migration and -recruitment has taken place in material contexts which: are the outcome of past and present globalisations; have systematically depleted resources from those countries least able to afford losses; produced uneven development within and between countries, and adversely impacted upon the material capabilities of countries to reverse these impacts unilaterally and pursue redress. This apprecia-tion of the material realities of the globalising political economy health care illu-minates the highly unequal as well as varied health contexts and circumstances underpinning the historical processes of global governance and global policy formation. In particular, these materialities strongly condition unequal participa-tion in constructing the institutions of global governance and determining the pace, content and direction of global policy.

At the same time, the widespread impacts of health worker-migration and -recruitment, coupled with the overall weakness of global governance in this area, raise major questions about the contemporary global system. They require greater attention to geo-political and -economic power, the forces and institu-tions of global governance and the role of states. They especially require critical scrutiny of the collective power and extent of hegemony of rich destination countries in global policy formation. Furthermore, although global governance is not a state, it is nevertheless largely the result of past statist globalising strat-egies. This suggests that how states engage with each other and work through cross-border spheres of governance needs to be given more attention in this global policy field as well as in social, health and public policy analysis. Despite three decades of social policy scholarship (Townsend 1993; Deacon *et al.* 1997; Yeates 2001, 2007), these spheres of governance, and their modes of governing and their impacts, are *still* all too often relegated as 'contextual' factors in most contemporary histories of health care, labour and employment and welfare state restructuring. In this respect, we reaffirm that a globalist materialist analytics of the state, the welfare state, and different social and economic sectors can sub-stantially help better connect 'cross-border' and 'domestic' governance in ways that bridge heuristic separations in coding between what is 'national' and 'global' social policy.

The global institutional regimes that underpin global policy formation are characterised by multiplicity and interactivity; they are not static or 'complete', and have changed over time. They will continue to change. Over the period we looked at, we identified seven different such global regimes that have succes-sively and continually shaped the formation of global health worker-migration and -recruitment policy. Thus, although this global policy field most obviously sits at the intersection of global migration governance and global health governance, these two fields are insufficient in themselves to explain why it is, for example, that perspectives and approaches anchored in trade and business, social protection or international development have featured so strongly and influentially throughout the course of this policy field's history. Indeed, it is *only* by looking at the broad institutional canvas of global governance in terms of not one or two but the interplay between *several* regimes that it is possible to elucidate the diverse and competing sources of influence shaping the evolving contours of this global policy field. This field is, then, the outcome of historically situated complex institutional intersectionalism. This intersectionalism structures agency, both constraining and creating possibilities for global organisations and other global policy actors (including states) to leverage reform.

This recognition of institutional pluralism does not assert that all institutions of global governance are equally significant, however. They are clearly not. Some are more important than others. But the point is that different global institutional regimes combine in various ways at different points in time and under different circumstances to produce different outcomes. In particular, we found a closer association between major initiatives and spurts in global labour migration and development governance than with global health governance. This was certainly the case in relation to the timing of initiating global policy instruments in this field. Thus, the ILO 1977 Recommendation was possible precisely *because* of ILO's significant activism from 1974–1975 to strengthen international social standards on labour migration and recruitment as well its prior history of building international labour standards in a broader UN-led process to define fundamental human rights and its encouragement of its specialised agencies to actively exercise their mandates. The WHO 2010 Global Code benefited from the wave of major initiatives in the UN in the early 2000s to stimulate better global migration governance and to put development at the heart of international cooperation through the Millennium Development Goals. The impacts of major global initiatives in spurring global policy development are also seen in the present period. Thus, the 2016 SDGs were a significant global process that resulted in a better integration of health worker-migration and -recruitment into the global health agenda. Although this step-change was not preceded by major global initiatives on global migration governance (as the ILO Recommendation and WHO Global Code were), the SDGs did incorporate significant commitments to promote 'orderly, safe, regular and responsible' international migration. These were reflected almost word for word in the Global Compact on Migration agreed in 2018.

Power relations not only between states but other kinds of organisation and social actors are integral to global policy formation. Our study suggests this is a complex organisational field comprising many IOs and other transnational policy actors whose range, composition and mix has changed over time. Phase 1 was a UN-dominated policy field with a wide range of UN agencies involved in setting agendas on highly skilled labour migration. Although there were differences between UN agencies in terms of their perspectives and missions, this was largely a state-dominated sphere. Indeed, governments needed to formally negotiate only with organised labour and employers in ILO as other agencies' governance structures were statist. By Phase 2, the range of UN agencies had narrowed to ILO and WHO in a transformed organisational field. In particular, global health actors were far more diverse: they included non-UN IOs as well as civil society coalition campaigning groups drawn from outside the organised labour movement such as business and corporate groups as well as NGOs. Phase 3 saw advances in the institutionalisation of multi-agency and multi-stakeholderism in global policy-making and -implementation. This seems to have significantly further expanded the policy space for non-UN global health actors – notably business groups and the commercial interests they represent – in global policy formation. This can be expected to have significant future impacts on the ability to realise the health SDGs (see Section 4). None of the global policy actors involved has an exclusive or even primary mandate on global migration governance. However, the mandates of all of these organisations bear on health worker-migration and/or -recruitment to some degree and in different ways. As statist organisations, however, they at least have legitimacy and authority and a direct connection to democratic governance and accountability.

Besides the sheer diversity of global policy actors, questions also arise about which ones have access to and presence within the field. Questions also arise about whose voices are present in proposing or vetoing, campaigning or negotiating, and which of these is most influential at particular points in time. In this respect, as striking as the variety of IOs involved is how important the internal structures and policy governance processes of the different IGOs are in conditioning their ability to frame the policy field, pursue global institutional development, and negotiate global agreements. The contrast between ILO and WHO is revealing. ILO's tripartite governance structure has proved more conducive in framing and propelling global policy than WHO's governance structures that are formally restricted to member states. Equally, UNCTAD's governance structure, with its grouping of countries into negotiating blocs, is notable for having strengthened the voices of those seeking to advance understanding of the wider economic development impacts of (human) capital mobility and redress by pressing compensatory approaches.

If these internal organisational features of IGOs matter in terms of their ability to influence the global policy field, then so does well-organised and resourced activism within them. Well-resourced secretariats backed by strong and strategic leadership within the organisation seem to be especially important. UNCTAD's agenda-setting in the 1970s and 1980s that bolstered redistributive forms of global policies on highly skilled migration was in large part the result of its secretariat's activism. WHO's demonstration of greater leadership during the 2000s to date owed much to the work of a more assertive secretariat and a Director-General under pressure to assert the organisation's continued convening power in global health. The strategic alliance it constructed with civil society groups (GHWA in particular), some destination countries and international politicians and diplomats during phases 2 and 3 is a stark contrast with its previous efforts. Indeed, in the 1970s it failed spectacularly to capitalise on international political momentum for greater regulation of health worker-migration and -recruitment, and even failed to forge connections between international health workforce issues and universal primary health care in its own programmes. It could only secure some kind of agreement through ILO as a junior partner after which it withdrew from the policy field for two decades. ILO, on the other hand, has consistently been able to generate as well as teach global norms. In fact, it has been the single most important IO influencing the course, pace and direction of the global policy field. Its tripartism and its labourist and social protection approaches to health have been supported by strong constituencies outside ILO as well as within it. Indeed, of all the IGOs, ILO has proved the strongest and most enduring influence in global policy formation in this area. It has gained far more authority than WHO, which, despite its essential health needs approach and health workforce constitutional mandate, has taken a non-labourist health resourcing position. It has only very latterly – within the last couple of years – forged a strong strategic connection between universal health coverage issues and health workforce-migration and -recruitment ones.

Across the period examined, we found a plethora of commitments, projects and programmes giving tangible meaning to global policy as realised in practice. These have been, and continue to be, underpinned by diverse ideational drivers, social forces, political imperatives and material circumstances orienting global-level action. We conclude, in support of Orenstein (2008), that ideational and material (resourcing) sources of influence and authority of social actors pressing for policy reform are inseparable. Generating ideas, promoting them, and securing support for them costs money. Furthermore, if implementation is not resourced then the corpus of social 'law', however coherent and relevant, will not be given tangible expression let alone have an impact. This insight is perhaps best illustrated by the roll-out of the WHO Global Code. WHO's severely squeezed financial footing was a significant factor undermining implementation of its Global Code. It has to be said, however, that ILO also did not resource oversight of the implementation of its Nursing Personnel Recommendation. Overall, this suggests that analysis of global policies that is restricted to policy discourses without attention to whether and how policies are implemented is insufficient. Attention to the material and institutional resources (dis)invested in making policy 'real' is vital for understanding the nature of global governance and its impacts on national social systems.

As far as policy ideas are concerned, the fundamental ideas circulating within the policy field have actually changed very little since being first articulated in the 1960s. Although they have since been elaborated and permutated into many different proposals, the basic ideas developed during this era are still recognisable. At opposite ends of the spectrum sit, on the one hand, self-sufficiency and financial restitution proposals and, on the other hand, Global Skills Partnerships based on PPPs. Other kinds of trajectories in the enduring influence of ideas can be detected, though. Of note is that the more radical proposals for global redistribution and global regulation in support of universal health care and health system-strengthening have been largely replaced by conservative ones. If fully implemented, the latter would at best leave existing international relations among 'partner' countries intact and at worst entrench short-termism at the expense of prioritising long-term health systems sustainability.

Weaker versions of palliative approaches blunting the harsher edges of global recruitment dynamics are especially conspicuous because these emerged precisely at a time when WHO had finally integrated health workforce-migration and -recruitment into its UHC strategy, progress had been made on global migration governance, inter-IO cooperation had advanced, and more permissive multistakeholderism and international partnerships had been institutionalised. Whether or not this might be characterised as a 'paradox', some answers can nevertheless be found when we scratch the 'surface' of these developments in global governance to reveal a range of less socially progressive, highly problematic, currents. These include the normalisation of temporary migration, restrictions on migrants' rights to permanency, and the increased influence of commercial interests in sustaining high levels of international migration and recruitment.

Conducive configurations of material circumstances, mutual self-interest, pressure and political have always been, and are still necessary for successfully concluding international agreements (Sauvant 2015). That said, it seems that 'ethical' recruitment, like 'sustainable health systems' or 'sustainable development', can still be very widely interpreted to accommodate initiatives which appear to be at odds with landmark global commitments such as the SDGs. The permissive tolerance for a widely interpretable central concept of 'ethical recruitment' is what makes it an attractive and in many ways successful choice. Indeed, it was one that all WHO Member States could sign up to in the Global Code. However, the failure to clearly specify an international standard for 'ethical recruitment' in the WHO Global Code is a major oversight and stands as one of its enduring major weaknesses. This omission is especially conspicuous given the clarity of the 1977 ILO Recommendation in defining the conditions under which international nurse recruitment should not occur. The Global Code's omission was also a major foregone opportunity that could have significantly strengthened the extant provisions and standards encoded in the Recommendation.

### 2.2.2  Gendering global governance: analytics and policy

We reserve this final part of this section to reflect on the gendered nature of global social governance and policy. The gendered nature of this global policy field has been apparent since the outset. The early focus by UN agencies on 'brain drain' debates was on male occupational domains (physicians, engineers, technicians) and excluded female occupational domains (see Chapter 2). The feminisation of the global policy field started to emerge in the 1970s when ILO took up the cause of gender equality at work and in social protection (ILO 2011) and, later, when WHO initiated its international study of health worker-migration that included nurses as well as physicians (Mejia *et al.* 1979; Chapters 2 and 3).

This marked a shift in global regulatory attention that increasingly focused on feminised health (and other) occupations, and paralleled the growing numbers of women within expanding highly skilled international labour streams within and outside of the health sector, including lone female migration to take up paid work abroad.

Although there are signs of a shift taking place, our study found limited systematic analysis of the gendered nature of high-skilled health worker-migration in global policy or the unique experiences of skilled women health care workers. The overall neglect of this systematic gender analysis of high-skilled migration is wholly unacceptable given that women comprise more than 70 per cent of the global health workforce and that their unpaid care-work represents half of women's annual $3 trillion contribution to global health (WHO/GHWN/WGH 2018). As the joint report of the WHO, Global Health Workers Network and Women in Global Health rightly affirms, 'resilient health systems and universal health coverage (UHC) cannot progress without consideration of gender-related trends and dynamics in the health and social care workforce' (WHO/GHWN/ WGH 2018: 5).

Studies show that existing structural gender equalities are usually replicated and may even widen during labour migration (Reichenbach 2007; Yeates 2009b; WHO/GHWN/WGH 2018) and that gender is largely neglected as a key determinant in human resource planning and in the production of health care (Standing 2000). A crucial component of a gendered approach is understanding the multiple discriminations faced by women, based on their gender, their migrant status and their ethnic minority status. Notwithstanding the importance of addressing these structural and intersecting inequalities, women's agency is important in the context of skilled health worker-migration. Working abroad can be a positive experience for women, contributing to new and positive forms of empowerment and independence for them, shifting gender perspectives and gender relations between women and men, and contributing to women's roles as agents of progressive economic and social change (Pillinger 2007).

To date most research on the gendered nature of migration has justifiably focused on the inequalities faced by women in lower-skilled health and social care work, an issue which WHO has very belatedly begun to turn its attention to. The gender equality focus in the SDGs – particularly SDG 5 on gender equality, which is closely connected to achieving SDG 3 on health and well-being and SDG 8 on decent work and inclusive economic growth – has helped shine a light on the enduringly gendered nature of health worker-migration (Langer *et al.* 2015; Newman 2014). While the WHO Global Strategy on Human Resources for Health Workforce 2030 (WHO 2016a) and the UN High-Level Commission on Health Employment and Economic Growth (HEEG 2016) acknowledge the opportunities for, and importance of, increasing women's labour participation to achieving SDGs on health, including UHC, they largely exclude a detailed analysis of how structural and intersecting gender inequalities can be tackled and how a transformative approach can be achieved beyond increasing women's labour market participation in overcoming health worker-shortages.

Of relevance also is that although the *Working for Health Five-Year Action Plan* (OECD/ILO/WHO 2017) identified the need for actions for gender-transformative global policy guidance, it appears to go no further that giving broad recommendations for better capacity to overcome gender biases and inequalities in the education and health labour market. These issues were discussed in OECD/ILO/WHO *Working for Health*, which, together with the Global Health Workforce Network Gender Equity Hub, identified a clear 'gender dividend' of the SDGs in the transformation of the health and social workforce (WHO/GHWN/WGH 2018). These discussions about the need for a *transformative social policy approach* are of utmost importance but are largely relegated to issuing 'guidance'. There is an urgency in ensuring this gender perspective is integrated into global policy on skilled health worker-migration, particularly in the light of concerns about the lack of progress in achieving gender equality across different SDGs (UN Women 2017). In particular, further research is needed on this neglected area of how the gender dimension in skilled health worker-migration can be fully incorporated into global policy. Pushing this point even further, we would also emphasise the importance of recognising and integrating the value of an intersectional approach to global policy on skilled health worker-migration and -recruitment.

## 3  Shared global responsibility in health

Health worker shortages, including having workers with the correct skills/skill mix, continue to dominate global discourses about access to health and provision of quality health care services. In this context, achieving the SDG Index of 4.45 (midwives, nurses and physicians) per 1,000 population remains way out of the reach of many countries, many of which have low capacity and critical shortages of health workers, making it extremely difficult for them to meet essential health needs and UHC. Some of the consequences of these trends leading to widening inequalities, along with the projected shortage of 18 million health workers needed to achieve the SDGs, has helped to shift attention in some global organisations. This is expressed in WHA Resolution WHA69.19 – 'recognizing that health workers are integral to building strong and resilient health systems' – while the WB, WHO and OECD have argued the case for better quality health care, declaring 'that high-quality, safe, people-centred healthcare is a public good that should be secured for all citizens' (WHO/OECD/World Bank 2018: 58). Although there appears to be agreement and a basis for global cooperation to ensure that skilled health worker-migration can take place, including expanding legal opportunities for skilled migration (Hooper 2018), the way to achieve this in practice is less certain.

The question remains what role can and should global governance play in addressing the problem of significant global inequalities in health (and related critical health shortages) as a global issue that brings within its realm the international migration and recruitment of health workers, while also ensuring the implementation of UHC and the SDG health goals – and how can a strengthened system of global governance needed to realise this be achieved?

The challenges are considerable but eminently achievable providing the right level of investment is made. Recent global health UHC monitoring reports that 50 per cent of the world's population still do not have access to UHC and over 100 million people fall into poverty when they are forced to pay out of pocket expenses for health care (WHO 2016f). The costs of meeting the SDG targets in low- and middle-income countries (Stenberg *et al.* 2017) require an additional $274 billion spending on health per year by 2030 to make progress towards the SDG health targets. An ambitious scenario estimates the need for $371 billion per year to actually reach universal health system targets by that date. An estimated 75 per cent of costs are for health systems relating to the health workforce and infrastructure in particular. Achieving a minimum of UHC for populations in low- and middle-income countries will require better planning and human resource development, improvements in staffing levels, pay, specialist training and deployment of staff, and improved working lives and career development opportunities. In particular, countries with severe health care personnel shortages should be supported to strengthen their health workforce and to give particular support to enable the poorest people to access quality health care, along with strategies to retain and train skilled health workers (GHWA 2013). Doing so would potentially save 97 million lives, significantly increase life expectancy in these countries and dramatically affect the course of social and economic development. However, a funding gap of $20–54 billion per year is projected (Stenberg *et al.* 2017). There is little evidence to date showing that there has been sufficient progress made to upscale health financing.

WHO's *Global Strategy on Human Resources for Health: Workforce 2030* (WHO 2016a), the UN's High-Level Commission on Health Employment and Economic Growth (HEEG 2016) and the recently established International Platform on Health Worker Mobility (2018) are a reflection of the greater global urgency to find solutions and promote more coordinated and strategic global governance responses. However, turning calls for action into concrete long-term programmes of action requires multi-dimensional, multi-scale, intersectoral strategies to ensure that source countries with the weakest health systems can ensure long-term public health care on the basis of universalism. Essential to this is ensuring sufficient resources for long-term recurrent public health expenditure needed to support the health workforce and health infrastructures. UHC can be a starting point for building sustainable health systems (Kruk *et al.* 2018) but UHC will fail unless much greater attention is given to improvements in the quality and accessibility of health care, and particularly for the additional structural and financing mechanisms that are needed to meet universal health needs through universalist provision under democratic control.

Policy frameworks rooted in a shared global responsibility for ending the health workforce crisis and changes in global economic policies, including lifting of debt burdens and fair health financing mechanisms will go a long way to ensuring there is sufficient capacity and resources for the implementation of the SDG health goals, including UHC. However, without a step change in global financing for the ambitious agenda for national and global health underpinned by the right to health, the SDGs goals will remain aspirational. More persuasive and effective mechanisms are needed, including political agreement, to ensure this financing gap is fully bridged and that global obligations promoting the right to health are translated into concrete, durable programmes of action.

So what kind of global governance mechanisms are needed? Is there a need for new global norms and instruments or can existing mechanisms be strengthened? What are the key issues to be addressed as a matter of priority? Below we outline some possible ways ahead.

### 3.1 Strengthen the implementation of existing mechanisms

Strengthening the Global Code can help to ensure better training and retention opportunities for skilled health workers in countries facing critical shortages of health workers, by addressing access to quality health care, tackling staff workloads, workplace stress, salaries and career opportunities in particular in underserved or rural areas (Tjadens *et al.* 2013; Pillinger 2013). For this to be achieved, WHO will need to actively exercise its mandate to the fullest extent to require that all Member States not only report on the implementation of the Code but actively implement the main articles of the Code. Strengthening the global social responsibility obligations upon Member States under the Code would help to promote a shift from the dominance of self-interest of destination countries in global health worker-migration and -recruitment policy towards one of shared responsibility. Equally, amendments to the Code to strengthen its 'lateral' implementation mechanisms would forge strong connections with global policies embedded in the UN normative framework, such as the UN Convention for the Protection of the Rights of All Migrant Workers and Members of their Families and ILO Conventions on labour migration and recruitment standards.

Multi-stakeholderism, first enshrined in the WHO Global Code and more recently in the 2030 Sustainable Development Agenda, recognises the importance of the voice and agency of vulnerable groups and CSOs. Different 'stakeholders' bring different perspectives into policy formation and they have the potential to hold multilateral organisations and governments accountable for their actions. Having these checks and balances written more strongly into global policy makes it possible for civil society to play a much greater role in the future monitoring of the WHO Global Code, the negotiation of bilateral or multilateral agreements, and negotiation of social and labour clauses in trade agreements. The global alliances, networks and advocacy, notably the HWMI and GHWA, that propelled the Global Code have the potential to lead to better engagement with and between government departments, civil society, NGO, employers, trade unions and recruitment companies. Greater mobilisation of civil society and trade union organisations has already demonstrably promoted critical dialogue on the need for sustained campaigns for the right to health, socially-responsible trade and business conduct, amongst other areas. Trade unions in particular have advocated for better working conditions. Under ILO's mandate to build the social dialogue in the health sector it will be important in the future to ensure that this work engages with debates about health worker-migration in source and destination countries, and how governments can engage with ILO Convention 151 to improve industrial relations in the public sector and in the health care sector. In relation to the WHO Global Code, future monitoring should require multi-stakeholder consultations, building on the good examples of this by the WHO-Europe region and under the ILO/EU Decent Work Across Borders project.

This is only one part of a strengthened compliance regime, however. A binding agreement that is codified into international policies and programmes to promote health systems sustainability, including a duty upon states to become self-sufficient in respect of their health workforces, will help avoid reliance on overseas health workforces to solve domestic staffing crises. Several states have already adopted self-sufficiency as a matter of policy and IOs should play a stronger leadership role in norms-teaching, knowledge generation and mutual education on this front. This could open up possibilities for the WHO Global Code to tangibly move in the direction of promoting shared global responsibility by supporting the targeting of resources, including compensatory arrangements, between source and destination countries, and provide for reciprocal arrangements to support resources for training for health workers, the upgrading of health facilities, scholarship, research and job creation according to the principles of decent work.

A persistent issue is the absence of globally comparable data on international-migration and -recruitment of health workers in source, transit and destination countries. Health policy makers in all countries also need to institute better cooperation to jointly collect statistics on health worker mobility and develop strategies to forecast health workforce needs and better workforce planning. Although better data systems are evolving, it is still not possible to track international health worker mobility and commonly-agreed definitions and indicators are lacking. OECD, ILO, WHO, and WB have all argued that this absence impedes effective health workforce planning and capacity to systematically address global health worker shortages. Health worker mobility has become increasingly difficult to map owing to the proliferation of circular and temporary migration programmes. Global data and information systems being developed establish indicators to link data on workforce planning in individual countries, based on common indicators on stocks, flows and trends. However, accurate data is also needed on the numbers of health workers currently abroad, their living and working conditions and the skills and experience gained while working abroad. In particular, data on the gendered nature of health worker-migration would assist in identifying specific gender inequalities faced by skilled women health care workers, including how and why occupational segregation shapes women's employment opportunities, resulting in the systemic undervaluing of women's skills, the gender pay gap and women's unequal representation in senior and decision-making positions. Data systems improvements need to ensure that registration systems used by professional health councils can also ascertain whether a health worker took up a job that was offered to them, stayed in the job, moved on elsewhere or returned home. Recommendations made for a centralised EU-wide data and information collection (WHO/OECD 2010; Tjadens *et al.* 2013) are relevant here but the challenge will be to roll out such centralised data collection systems in other parts of the world, particularly in low-resource settings.

### 3.2 Global health governance renewal: new instruments

The WHO Global Code, UHC and the health-related SDGs bring much-needed attention to the urgency of reducing global inequalities and promote the view that migration should be mutually (and economically) beneficial for source and destination countries. However, global health governance renewal is needed to underpin the realisation of global goals. As Gostin *et al.* (2010) argue, collaborative and shared approaches are needed as '[f]raming the global health endeavor as Health Aid provided by the affluent to the poor is fundamentally flawed' (Gostin *et al.* 2010: 10). Moving away from an approach based on dependency and inequality inherent in 'aid' and 'charity' models, which tend to be based on short-term projects and targeted funding programmes, towards a model of shared responsibility and partnership in global health governance aimed at building sustainable health systems in the long-term is essential to collaborative and shared approaches. Such approaches position 'essential health goods and services [as] global public goods' (ibid.: 15). Others have argued that multilateral action similarly needs to have a renewed emphasis on equity, social justice and the right to health alongside a better understanding of transnational care relations. This includes global redistribution of resources as a global policy objective and ensuring that governments in high-income countries are supported in promoting the right to health and global justice for low and middle-income countries (Shah 2010) and through policies to promote transnational justice (Eckenwiler 2009). In this context, a strengthened WHO Global Code could form one part of a renewed global health governance wherein health is promoted as a 'public good' and the right to health is matched by binding commitments.

Despite adverse global developments towards conservative popularism, global inequalities and neo-liberalism, a global focus on social justice, equity and the right to health which already feature in global governance and in global advocacy campaigns need to be strengthened. Institutional strengthening is one key element of this. WHO's leadership, normative role and resources in global health that it has begun to develop with greater confidence and authority in recent years needs supporting.

> Such leadership is required to mobilize, coordinate, and focus the large and diverse set of global health actors around a clear mission, common objectives, effective approaches, sustained action, and mutual accountability. WHO has the unique authority and legitimacy to assume this role, including with its constitutional power to adopt conventions and promulgate binding regulations.
>
> (Gostin *et al.* 2010: 20)

It also requires a more engaged debate about the global responsibility for health and the possibilities for 'shared health governance' between governments and global stakeholders (O'Brien and Gostin 2011; Ruger 2012). The creation of a sustainable global health funding mechanism might be one answer to this. Mackey and Liang (2013) propose a Global Health Resource Fund coordinated by WHO and World Bank, with the capacity to create a global governance mechanism for sustainable health systems funding. Van de Pas *et al.* (2016) also propose a global fund with obligatory payments into it from high-income countries and private sector organisations which would reimburse countries for health workforce losses arising from health worker migration. These global fund proposals have much in common with those circulating in the UN system during the 1970s (see Chapter 3). Despite superficial attractions, however, such funding mechanisms may be too consistent with the 'Health Aid model' (Gostin *et al.* 2010) and it is easy to imagine that destination governments, which also tend to be health donors, would reduce their overseas aid budgets by the amounts they contribute to a global compensation fund. On the other hand, it could be a means to coordinate the disbursement of funds according to shared priorities rather than according to the preferences of individual donors. It may be, however, that Mackey and Liang's proposal for WB control (albeit shared with WHO) resurrects too many concerns given WB neo-liberal health care reforms of the 1980s and 1990s. World Bank and WHO support for universalist public health care systems is not yet sufficiently evident or robust to warrant the confidence that such a mechanism would require to sustain support.

One of the issues discussed at length in the early drafts of the WHO Global Code, and frequently raised by source countries, is the role that destination countries can play in compensating source countries for their losses. Standalone global funds are too reminiscent of Global Health Aid models, but compensatory arrangements duly contextualised within a renewed global health governance framework embodying global health equity and a social justice approach emphasising redistribution of resources and substantial shifts in priorities to increase public investment in health care funding could find support. This would, for example, make financial restitution to source countries for their lost investments in education and training, linked to supporting health systems strengthening including increased public expenditure to meet the goals for quality health services and adequate levels of health workers (Pillinger 2013; Agwu and Llewelyn 2009; Mensah *et al.* 2005).

### *3.3 A socially-progressive trade agenda*

One of the key findings from the book is that the entry of non-UN bodies into discussions about health worker-migration and -recruitment has arisen precisely because of the links between globalisation, trade and mobility in health. While non-UN bodies (OECD, World Bank, IMF) came to the issue from a trade perspective and economic development perspective, ILO came to the issue from a labour rights perspective and WHO from a human resource management and health systems perspective. These overlapping but very different perspectives are relevant to current global governance. This is reflected in the fact that global health and international health worker-migration appeared on early trade policy agendas of UNCTAD in the 1970s, while the intersection of international health worker-migration with trade and economic development has increasingly become part of the agendas of the World Bank, WIPO, WTO, and the OECD. In particular, ILO and WHO are now working more closely and in partnership with these wider agendas on trade and economic development, giving ILO and WHO an entry point into influencing global policy reforms that effectively link trade and economic development to global health, human rights, ethical recruitment and fundamental rights at work.

While there is much greater cooperation and multi-stakeholderism leading to participation of government ministries, employers, trade unions, health professional regulatory bodies, recruitment companies and international organisations in policy dialogues, this has come with a greater role for the private sector, an economic model based on privatisation and increasing use of PPPs, and the leverage that comes from trade agreements. In particular, the supply of services through the migration of workers in trade agreements (under WTO General Agreement on Trade in Services (GATS) Mode 4 provisions, introduced in 1995) has prompted calls by civil society and trade union organisations for better adherence to social and labour standards protecting migrant workers against exploitation and unethical recruitment. At the same time, legacies of the global 'free' trade agenda can be seen in the Trade in Services Agreement (TiSA), which represents the first plurilateral trade agreement focusing on trade in services since the GATS in 1995. It remains on the table today. For these calls for the 'socialisation' of international trade agreements to be effective, they need to go beyond the introduction of binding social clauses in international trade agreements and *require* actual adherence to fundamental rights at work, ethical recruitment and fair migration. These are highly pertinent issues for international health worker-migration, particularly as the emphasis in many trade negotiations favours the provisions enabling the privatisation of public services over and above the enforcement of international labour and migration standards and a progressive trade agenda. Better transparency of trade negotiations and stronger enforcement measures are needed to ensure rights-based approaches to migration and ethical recruitment, including ensuring their adherence to principles set out in the WHO Global Code. These developments should not be immune from the global commitments and goals made under the SDGs – in this sense trade negotiations should take into account global standards on sustainable development as a basis for the testing, checking and framing of future trade negotiations. This framing could also help to further mobilise the growing advocacy movements in civil society organisations and trade unions, linking trade agendas towards realising the SDGs.

The influence of global trade and the increasing roles of multinational companies in the global economy are significant challenges working against global equity, social justice and the normative base of the UN system. The inter-relations of globalising production, finance, trade and migration are leading to growing income inequalities between countries (ILO 2017a), which impede the ability of governments (and the public sector) to provide resources to meet growing demands for quality health care (Kruk *et al.* 2018) and further impact on socially just responses to health worker-migration. This is a time when the private sector is being given greater prominence for its contribution to UHC, and PPPs increasingly are being promoted as a solution to health care funding for training and infrastructure. This is despite a significant body of evidence showing the failures of PPPs and the enormous unnecessary additional cost burdens PPPs put on public finances. Suggestions for the private sector and PPPs to be instruments for funding UHC reflect increasing influence of the corporate sector in global health but are likely to work against global social justice approaches for redistribution and sustainable health care systems. Instead of social clauses in international trade agreements, much greater attention needs to be given to global social justice and the right to health as core principles of state policy, whether on a national or international scale, accompanied by sustained programmes of resourcing and implementation.

### 3.4 Fair treatment of migrant health workers

We have argued that the need for an equitable distribution of health workers across the world in order to meet the SDGs on health, and particularly UHC, are a redistribution of resources, a global policy approach rooted in global equity, and international cooperation to mitigate the harmful effects of outward migration and sustained investment in health care systems in low-income countries. But global social responsibility also means mobilising international development partners and high-income countries that recruit health workers to engage in more serious efforts to mitigate some of the factors that push health professionals to migrate, including through more effective and socially (and environmentally) responsive measures in future trade regimes. It also means strengthening provisions for prospective and actual migrant health workers to enjoy fair and ethical treatment throughout all stages of the migration and settlement process.

The principles guiding fair and ethical treatment are already established in provisions on ethical recruitment, decent work and fundamental rights at work but they need to be constantly reiterated. This will require transparency underpinned by the negotiating parties' commitment to accessibility (for example, through consultation on and scrutiny of proposed agreements prior to conclusion). Better monitoring of the concluded agreements is essential. Thus, ethical recruitment initiatives and bilateral agreements should be systematically benchmarked against international 'best practice' standards and norms prior to formal agreement, and their implementation monitored, especially in relation to pay, working hours, training, working conditions, grievances, recognition of skills, and responsibilities of recruitment agencies. Reciprocal arrangements should be put in place to ensure that if a migrant worker returns to their home country there is information, training or assistance prior to departure and reintegration into work in their home country. ILO has a key role to play in ensuring that national and international migration policies and bilateral and multilateral agreements adequately recognise migrant workers' skills, portability of social security benefits, access to social protection, protection against exploitation and improved work conditions, so that migration can take place in 'conditions of freedom, dignity, equity and security' and decent work. In the age of temporary and circular migration temporary visa holders should have access to social protection, including public health care, childcare, education and schooling for children and other public services.

The stronger leadership role of IOs in promoting self-sufficiency in health workforces should extend to the systematic uptake of good practices on ethical recruitment, including how source countries may take greater responsibility for ensuring that prospective emigrant health workers understand their rights and obligations, the labour and contractual conditions existing in countries of destination, and recourse to remedies in case of violation of their rights. In addition, there needs to be a commitment to sharing responsibility for monitoring global and regional trade negotiations, trade and economic partnership agreements and regional integration processes where these refer to cross-border migration of skilled health workers. Countries that have participated in these agreements and measures should be required to report on their implementation, a model for which exists under the WHO Global Code.

## 4 Mobilising research and advocacy for a new world order for health

International migration of health workers and the cross-border provision of health and social care services are significant features of the contemporary global economy that is increasingly typified by the marketisation, commercialisation and privatisation of public services. The developments underway at this current point in time risk further widening the doors to deeper intersections of capital (whether domestic or transnational) with public services financing and provision. In health, this will undermine the public sector as a provider of health care and the state as a guarantor of the right to health, as well as the achievement of universal health coverage and socially transformative global health governance.

If we need a reminder that this is not just an 'academic' subject or a non-urgent general concern, to do with other countries than our own and populations which are not 'ours', then learning from the West African Ebola outbreak crisis during 2014–2015 is a good place to start when thinking about the kinds of actions needed to tackle the consequences of health worker shortages and the global mal-distribution of health resources. The devastating outbreak in parts of West Africa is not a West African 'problem' any more than it is only an issue for low-income countries with weak health systems. Outbreaks have the potential to spread rapidly within and between countries under conditions of highly mobile goods and people, and unless all countries have robust health care systems with strong lines of democratic accountability built into them then the health security of none is assured. Worryingly, despite the intense scrutiny (and soul-searching within WHO) of what went wrong in the West African 'case', and for all the increases in resources for the health sector and for 'global health' in particular over the last decade, or the spate of UN resolutions on global health security over the last three years (see Appendix 1), limited capacity in the health care system when the outbreak of the Ebola crisis took hold continues today. If rich donor countries, most of which are also overseas health worker-recruiting ones, cannot find higher motivation to press for and support transformative social policy reforms through global institutions to secure global health on the basis of social justice as a priority of the first order, then self-interest should be sufficient.

Four years into the SDGs, and with little tangible sign of the increased investment required, it is time to integrate these insights into campaigns for public policy reforms across multiple scales, sites and processes of global governance. This book has aimed to make a modest contribution to that process. The laser beam it shines onto the contemporary histories of global policy and governance on health worker-migration and -recruitment underlines that we already have many of the tools and knowledge bases that can power the world to achieve better health outcomes for everyone. However, we still have some way to go. The imperfect system of global governance that we have inherited can – and must – be made to work better in the interests of all of us, and particularly for the benefit of the 97 million lives that will be needlessly lost by failure to invest $3,800 per year in each of them to realise UHC by 2030.[1] A genuinely globally-transformative social policy agenda will be central to successes in attaining these global health goals and to sustaining these achievements. Future programmes of action can be usefully informed by the kinds of globalist Social Policy analytics of governance that we have demonstrated and argued for in this book.

## Note

1 Authors' calculation derived from Stenberg *et al.* (2017) who calculate that $371 billion per year would reach universal health system targets by 2030 and this would potentially save 97 million lives.

# Appendix 1

*Appendix 1.1* UN General Assembly and ECOSOC Resolutions directly relevant to international health worker-migration and -recruitment (1948–2018)

| Date | Reference | Title |
|---|---|---|
| 1948 | A/RES/200(III) | Technical assistance for economic development |
| 1948 | A/RES/201(III) | Training for apprentices and technical workers |
| 1948 | A/RES/209(III) | Economic development and migration |
| 1948 | A/RES/217(III) A | Universal Declaration of Human Rights |
| 1949 | A/RES/306(IV) | Economic development of under-developed countries |
| 1949 | A/RES/315(IV) | Discriminations practised by certain States against immigrating labour and, in particular, against labour recruited from the rank of refugees |
| 1949 | A/RES/331(IV) | International collaboration in regard to economic, social and educational conditions in Non-Self-Governing Territories |
| 1952 | A/RES/527(VI) | Living standards of the working population |
| 1952 | A/RES/624(VII) | Migration and economic development |
| 1952 | A/RES/642(VII) | Integrated economic and social development |
| 1952 | A/RES/645(VII) | Educational, economic and social policies in Non-Self-Governing Territories |
| 1953 | A/RES/732(VIII) | Programme of concerted practical action in the social field of the United Nations and the specialized agencies |
| 1957 | A/RES/1161(XII) | Balanced and integrated economic and social progress |
| 1958 | A/RES/1283(XIII) | International Health and Medical Research Year |
| 1958 | A/RES/1331(XIII) | Offers by Member States of study and training facilities for inhabitants of Non-Self-Governing Territories |
| 1959 | A/RES/1392(XIV) | Interrelationship of the economic and social factors of development |
| 1960 | A/RES/1515(XV) | Concerted action for economic development of economically less developed countries |
| 1962 | A/RES/1824 (XVII) | The role of the United Nations in training national technical personnel for the accelerated industrialisation of the developing countries |
| 1965 | A/RES/2083 (XX) | Development and utilisation of human resources |
| 1965 | A/RES/2084 (XX) | United Nations Development Decade |
| 1965 | A/RES/2090 (XX) | The role of the United Nations in training national technical personnel for the accelerated industrialisation of the developing countries |
| 1967 | A/RES/2259 (XXII) | The role of the United Nations in training national technical personnel for the accelerated industrialisation of the developing countries |
| 1967 | A/RES/2320 (XXII) | Outflow of trained personnel from developing countries |

| Date | Reference | Title |
|---|---|---|
| 1968 | A/RES/2417 (XXIII) | Outflow of trained professional and technical personnel at all levels from the developing to the developed countries, its causes, its consequences and practical remedies for the problems resulting from it |
| 1969 | A/RES/2528(XXIV) | The role of the United Nations in training national technical personnel for the accelerated industrialization of the developing countries |
| 1969 | A/RES/2542 (XXIV) | Declaration on Social Progress and Development |
| 1970 | A/RES/2626(XXV) | International Development Strategy for the Second United Nations Development Decade |
| 1972 | A/RES/3017(XXVII) | Outflow of trained personnel from developing to developed countries |
| 1974 | A/RES/3224(XXIX) | Measures to improve the situation of migrant workers |
| 1974 | A/RES/3201 (S-VI) | Declaration on the Establishment of a New International Economic Order |
| 1974 | A/RES/3202 (S-VI) | Programme of Action on the Establishment of a New International Economic Order |
| 1975 | A/RES/3509(XXX) | Tripartite World Conference on Employment, Income Distribution, Social Progress and the International Division of Labour |
| 1976 | A/RES/31/127 | Measures to improve the situation and ensure the human rights and dignity of all migrant workers |
| 1976 | A/RES/31/176 | Tripartite World Conference on Employment, Income Distribution, Social Progress and the International Division of Labour |
| 1977 | A/RES/32/120 | Measures to improve the situation and ensure the human rights and dignity of all migrant workers |
| 1977 | A/RES/32/192 | Reverse transfer of technology |
| 1978 | A/RES/33/135 | Role of qualified national personnel in the social and economic development of developing countries |
| 1978 | A/RES/33/151 | Reverse transfer of technology |
| 1979 | A/RES/34/58 | Health as an integral part of development |
| 1979 | A/RES/34/172 | Measures to improve the situation and ensure the human rights and dignity of all migrant workers |
| 1979 | A/RES/34/200 | Development aspects of the reverse transfer of technology |
| 1980 | A/RES/35/56 | International Development Strategy for the 3rd United Nations Development Decade |
| 1980 | A/RES/35/198 | Measures to improve the situation and ensure the human rights and dignity of all migrant workers |
| 1981 | A/RES/36/43 | Global Strategy for Health for All by the Year 2000 |
| 1981 | A/RES/36/140 | United Nations Conference on an International Code of Conduct on the Transfer of Technology |
| 1981 | A/RES/36/141 | Reverse transfer of technology |
| 1981 | A/RES/36/160 | Measures to improve the situation and ensure the human rights and dignity of all migrant workers |
| 1982 | A/RES/37/169 | Question of the international legal protection of the human rights of individuals who are not citizens of the country in which they live |
| 1982 | A/RES/37/170 | Measures to improve the situation and ensure the human rights and dignity of all migrant workers |
| 1982 | A/RES/37/207 | Development aspects of the reverse transfer of technology |
| 1982 | A/RES/37/228 | Role of qualified national personnel in social and economic development of developing countries |
| 1983 | A/RES/38/86 | Measures to improve the situation and ensure the human rights and dignity of all migrant workers |

| Date | Reference | Title |
|------|-----------|-------|
| 1984 | A/RES/39/211 | Development aspects of the reverse transfer of technology |
| 1984 | A/RES/39/219 | Role of qualified national personnel in the social and economic development of developing countries |
| 1985 | A/RES/40/130 | Measures to improve the situation and ensure the human rights and dignity of all migrant workers |
| 1985 | A/RES/40/184 | International code of conduct on the transfer of technology |
| 1985 | A/RES/40/191 | Reverse transfer of technology |
| 1986 | A/RES/41/151 | Measures to improve the situation and ensure the human rights and dignity of all migrant workers |
| 1986 | A/RES/41/180 | Net transfer of resources from developing to developed countries |
| 1987 | A/RES/42/140 | Measures to improve the situation and ensure the human rights and dignity of all migrant workers |
| 1988 | A/RES/43/146 | Measures to improve the situation and ensure the human rights and dignity of all migrant workers |
| 1988 | A/RES/43/184 | Reverse transfer of technology |
| 1988 | A/RES/43/195 | International co-operation for the eradication of poverty in developing countries |
| 1989 | A/RES/44/55 | Achievement of social justice |
| 1989 | A/RES/44/155 | Measures to improve the situation and ensure the human rights and dignity of all migrant workers |
| 1989 | A/RES/44/212 | International co-operation for the eradication of poverty in developing countries |
| 1989 | A/RES/44/213 | Developing human resources for development |
| 1990 | A/RES/45/86 | Achievement of social justice |
| 1990 | A/RES/45/158 | International Convention on the Protection of the Rights of all Migrant Workers and Members of Their Families |
| 1990 | A/RES/45/191 | Developing human resources for development |
| 1990 | A/RES/45/199 | International Development Strategy for the Fourth United Nations Development Decade |
| 1990 | A/RES/45/213 | International co-operation for the eradication of poverty in the developing countries |
| 1991 | A/RES/46/17 | International Forum on Health |
| 1991 | A/RES/46/114 | International Convention on the Protection of the Rights of All Migrant Workers and Members of Their Families |
| 1991 | A/RES/46/141 | International cooperation for the eradication of poverty in developing countries |
| 1991 | A/RES/46/143 | Developing human resources for development |
| 1992 | A/RES/47/96 | Migrant women workers |
| 1992 | A/RES/47/110 | International Convention on the Protection of the Rights of All Migrant Workers and Their Families |
| 1992 | A/RES/47/134 | Human rights and extreme poverty |
| 1992 | A/RES/47/176 | International Conference on Population and Development |
| 1992 | A/RES/47/197 | International cooperation for the eradication of poverty in developing countries |
| 1993 | A/RES/48/148 | International Convention on the Protection of the Rights of All Migrant Workers and Members of Their Families |
| 1993 | A/RES/48/184 | International cooperation for the eradication of poverty in developing countries |
| 1993 | A/RES/48/186 | International Conference on Population and Development |
| 1993 | A/RES/48/205 | Developing human resources for development |
| 1994 | A/RES/49/110 | International cooperation for the eradication of poverty in developing countries |
| 1994 | A/RES/49/127 | International migration and development |
| 1994 | A/RES/49/128 | Report of the International Conference on Population and Development |

| Date | Reference | Title |
|------|-----------|-------|
| 1994 | A/RES/49/173 | Comprehensive consideration and review of the problems of refugees, returnees, displaced persons and related migratory movements |
| 1994 | A/RES/49/175 | International Convention on the Protection of the Rights of All Migrant Workers and Members of Their Families |
| 1995 | A/RES/50/105 | Developing human resources for development |
| 1995 | A/RES/50/123 | International migration and development |
| 1995 | A/RES/50/124 | Implementation of the programme of action of the International Conference on Population and Development |
| 1995 | A/RES/50/151 | Comprehensive consideration and review of the problems of refugees, returnees, displaced persons and related migratory movements |
| 1995 | A/RES/50/169 | International Convention on the Protection of the Rights of All Migrant Workers and Members of Their Families |
| 1996 | A/RES/51/85 | International Convention on the Protection of the Rights of All Migrant Workers and Members of Their Families |
| 1996 | A/RES/51/176 | Implementation of the Programme of Action of the International Conference on Population and Development |
| 1996 | A/RES/51/178 | First United Nations Decade for the Eradication of Poverty |
| 1996 | A/RES/51/202 | Implementation of the outcome of the World Summit for Social Development |
| 1997 | A/RES/52/115 | Convention on the Protection of the Rights of All Migrant Workers and Members of Their Families |
| 1997 | A/RES/52/189 | International migration and development |
| 1997 | A/RES/52/196 | Developing human resources for development |
| 1998 | A/RES/53/137 | Convention on Migrant Workers |
| 1998 | A/RES/53/169 | Development in the context of globalization and interdependence |
| 1999 | A/RES/54/23 | World Social Summit outcome |
| 1999 | A/RES/54/158 | International Convention on the Protection of the Rights of All Migrant Workers and Members of Their Families |
| 1999 | A/RES/54/165 | Globalization and its impact on the full enjoyment of all human rights |
| 1999 | A/RES/54/166 | Protection of migrants |
| 1999 | A/RES/54/211 | Developing human resources for development |
| 1999 | A/RES/54/212 | International migration and development |
| 2000 | A/RES/55/2 | Millennium declaration |
| 2000 | A/RES/55/46 | World Summit for Social Development outcome |
| 2000 | A/RES/55/88 | International Convention on the Protection of the Rights of All Migrant Workers and Members of Their Families |
| 2000 | A/RES/55/92 | Protection of migrants |
| 2000 | A/RES/55/102 | Globalization and its impact on the full enjoyment of all human rights |
| 2000 | A/RES/55/162 | Follow-up to the outcome of the Millennium Summit |
| 2000 | A/RES/55/210 | Implementation of the 1st UN Decade for the Eradication of Poverty (1997-2006), including the initiative to establish a world solidarity fund for poverty eradication |
| 2000 | A/RES/55/212 | Role of the UN in promoting development in the context of globalization and interdependence |
| 2001 | A/RES/56/165 | Globalization and its impact on the full enjoyment of all human rights |
| 2001 | A/RES/56/189 | Human resources development |
| 2001 | A/RES/56/203 | International migration and development |
| 2002 | A/RES/57/201 | International Convention on the Protection of the Rights of All Migrant Workers and Members of Their Families |
| 2002 | A/RES/57/218 | Protection of migrants |
| 2003 | A/RES/58/3 | Enhancing capacity-building in global public health |

| Date | Reference | Title |
|------|-----------|-------|
| 2003 | A/RES/58/166 | International Convention on the Protection of the Rights of All Migrant Workers and Members of Their Families |
| 2003 | A/RES/58/190 | Protection of migrants |
| 2003 | A/RES/58/207 | Human resources development |
| 2003 | A/RES/58/208 | International migration and development |
| 2004 | A/RES/59/27 | Enhancing capacity-building in global public health |
| 2004 | A/RES/59/241 | International migration and development |
| 2004 | A/RES/59/262 | International Convention on the Protection of the Rights of All Migrant Workers and Members of their Families |
| 2005 | A/RES/60/35 | Enhancing capacity-building in global public health |
| 2005 | A/RES/60/152 | Globalization and its impact on the full enjoyment of all human rights |
| 2005 | A/RES/60/169 | Protection of migrants |
| 2005 | A/RES/60/206 | Facilitation and reduction of the cost of transfer of migrant remittances |
| 2005 | A/RES/60/211 | Human resources development |
| 2005 | A/RES/60/227 | International migration and development |
| 2006 | A/RES/61/165 | Protection of migrants |
| 2006 | A/RES/61/208 | International migration and development |
| 2006 | A/RES/61/228 | 2001–2010: Decade to Roll Back Malaria in Developing Countries, Particularly in Africa |
| 2007 | A/RES/62/156 | Protection of migrants |
| 2007 | A/RES/62/207 | Human resources development |
| 2007 | A/RES/62/270 | Global Forum on Migration and Development |
| 2008 | A/RES/63/33 | Global health and foreign policy |
| 2008 | A/RES/63/184 | Protection of migrants |
| 2008 | A/RES/63/199 | International Labour Organization Declaration on Social Justice for a Fair Globalization |
| 2008 | A/RES/63/224 | Towards a New International Economic Order |
| 2008 | A/RES/63/225 | International migration and development |
| 2009 | A/RES/64/108 | Global health and foreign policy |
| 2009 | A/RES/64/166 | Protection of migrants |
| 2009 | A/RES/64/209 | Towards a New International Economic Order |
| 2009 | A/RES/64/218 | Human resources development |
| 2010 | A/RES/65/1 | Keeping the promise: united to achieve the Millennium Development Goals |
| 2010 | A/RES/65/95 | Global health and foreign policy |
| 2010 | A/RES/65/167 | Towards a New International Economic Order |
| 2010 | A/RES/65/170 | International migration and development |
| 2010 | A/RES/65/273 | Consolidating gains and accelerating efforts to control and eliminate malaria in developing countries, particularly in Africa, by 2015 |
| 2010 | A/RES/65/277 | Political Declaration on HIV/AIDS: Intensifying our Efforts to Eliminate HIV/AIDS |
| 2011 | A/RES/66/115 | Global health and foreign policy |
| 2011 | A/RES/66/172 | Protection of migrants |
| 2011 | A/RES/66/215 | Second United Nations Decade for the Eradication of Poverty (2008–2017) |
| 2011 | A/RES/66/217 | Human resources development |
| 2012 | A/RES/67/81 | Global health and foreign policy |
| 2012 | A/RES/67/172 | Protection of migrants |
| 2012 | A/RES/67/217 | Towards a New International Economic Order |
| 2012 | A/RES/67/219 | International migration and development |
| 2013 | A/RES/68/4 | Declaration of the High-Level Dialogue on International Migration and Development |
| 2013 | A/RES/68/98 | Global health and foreign policy |
| 2013 | A/RES/68/179 | Protection of migrants |

| Date | Reference | Title |
|------|-----------|-------|
| 2013 | A/RES/68/228 | Human resources development |
| 2014 | A/RES/69/132 | Global health and foreign policy |
| 2014 | A/RES/69/167 | Protection of migrants |
| 2014 | A/RES/69/227 | Towards a New International Economic Order |
| 2014 | A/RES/69/229 | International migration and development |
| 2014 | A/RES/68/300 | Outcome document of the high-level meeting of the General Assembly on the comprehensive review and assessment of the progress achieved in the prevention and control of non-communicable diseases |
| 2014 | A/RES/68/308 | Consolidating gains and accelerating efforts to control and eliminate malaria in developing countries, particularly in Africa, by 2015 |
| 2015 | A/RES/70/220 | Human resources development |
| 2015 | A/RES/70/183 | Global health and foreign policy: strengthening the management of international health crises |
| 2015 | A/RES/70/147 | Protection of migrants |
| 2015 | A/RES/70/6 | Human resources for health and implementation of the outcomes of the United Nations' High-Level Commission on Health Employment and Economic Growth |
| 2015 | A/RES/70/1 | Transforming our world: the 2030 Agenda for Sustainable Development |
| 2015 | A/RES/69/325 | Consolidating gains and accelerating efforts to control and eliminate malaria in developing countries, particularly in Africa, by 2015 and beyond |
| 2016 | A/RES/71/236 | Towards a New International Economic Order |
| 2016 | A/RES/71/237 | International migration and development |
| 2016 | A/RES/71/241 | Second United Nations Decade for the Eradication of Poverty (2008-2017) |
| 2016 | A/RES/71/159 | Global health and foreign policy: health employment and economic growth |
| 2016 | A/RES/70/290 | High-level plenary meeting on addressing large movements of refugees and migrants |
| 2017 | A/RES/72/139 | Global health and foreign policy: addressing the health of the most vulnerable for an inclusive society |
| 2017 | A/RES/72/138 | International Universal Health Coverage Day |
| 2017 | A/RES/72/179 | Protection of migrants |
| 2017 | A/RES/72/235 | Human resources development |
| 2018 | A/RES/73/2 | Political declaration of the third high-level meeting of the General Assembly on the prevention and control of non-communicable diseases |
| 2018 | A/RES/73/195 | Global Compact for Safe, Orderly and Regular Migration |
| 2018 | A/RES/73/241 | International migration and development |
| 2018 | A/RES/73/254 | Towards global partnerships: a principle-based approach to enhanced cooperation between the United Nations and all relevant partners |

Source: Authors, compiled from sources accessed from the Dag Hammarskjold Library General Assembly – Quick Links http://research.un.org/en/docs/ga/quick/regular/ (As at 28 February 2019).

Note
UN reports and studies are listed in References.

*Appendix 1.2*  UN Economic and Social Council (1947–1983)

| Date | Reference | Title |
|------|-----------|-------|
| 1947 | E/RES/85(V) | Protection of migrant and immigrant labour |
| 1947 | E/RES/42(IV) | Migration |
| 1947 | E/RES/41(IV) | Population |
| 1947 | E/RES/43(IV) | Social questions |
| 1948 | E/RES/156(VII) | Migration |
| 1952 | E/RES/434(XIV) | Social activities |
| 1955 | E/CN.4/RES/II/(XI) | Study of discrimination in the matter of emigration, immigration and travel. |
| 1960 | 797 (XXX) | Administrative and technical training |
| 1961 | 817 (XXXI) | Report of the Committee for Industrial Development in its first session |
| 1961 | 838 (XXXII) | Education and training |
| 1962 | 906 (XXXIV) | Education and training |
| 1964 | 1029 (XXXVII) | Training of national technical personnel for the accelerated industrialisation of developing countries |
| 1965 | 1090 (XXXIX) | General review of the development, co-ordination and concentration of the economic, social and human rights programmes and activities of the United Nations, the specialised agencies and the International Atomic Energy Agency as a whole |
| 1967 | 1226 (XLII) | Social questions relating to the extension of health services |
| 1967 | 1274 (XLIII) | Development and utilisation of human resources |
| 1971 | 1573 (L) | Outflow of trained personnel from developing to developed countries |
| 1973 | E/RES/1749(LIV) | Migrant workers |
| 1974 | E/RES/1904(LVII) | Outflow of trained personnel from developing to developed countries. |
| 1975 | 1968 (LIX) | Tripartite World Conference on Employment, Income Distribution, Social Progress and the International Division of Labour |
| 1975 | E/RES/1926(LVIII) | Welfare of migrant workers and their families. |
| 1977 | E/RES/2083(LXII) | Measures to improve the situation and ensure the human rights and dignity of all migrant workers. |
| 1978 | E/RES/1978/22 | Measures to improve the situation and ensure the human rights and dignity of all migrant workers. |
| 1979 | E/CN.4/RES/25/ (XXXV) | Measures to improve the situation and ensure the human rights and dignity of all migrant workers and their families. |
| 1979 | E/RES/1979/52 | Role of qualified national personnel in the social and economic development of developing countries |
| 1980 | E/RES/1980/63 | Role of qualified national personnel in the social and economic development of developing countries |
| 1981 | E/CN.4/ RES/37(XXXVII) | Measures to improve the situation and ensure the human rights and dignity of all migrant workers. |
| 1981 | E/RES/1981/35 | Measures to improve the situation and ensure the human rights and dignity of all migrant workers and their families |
| 1981 | E/RES/1981/21 | Welfare of migrant workers and their families |
| 1981 | E/RES/1981/61 | Global Strategy for Health for All by the Year 2000 |
| 1983 | E/RES/1983/16 | Welfare of migrant workers and their families |

Source: Authors, compiled from sources accessed from https://digitallibrary.un.org/ (As at 28 February 2019).

# Appendix 2

| Date | Reference | Title |
|------|-----------|-------|
| 2006 | WHA59.27 | Strengthening nursing and midwifery |
| 2009 | WHA62.8 | Primary health care, including health system strengthening |
| 2009 | WHA62.10 | Monitoring of the achievement of the health-related Millennium Development Goals |
| 2009 | WHA62.15 | Prevention and control of multidrug-resistant tuberculosis and extensively drug-resistant tuberculosis |
| 2010 | WHA63.16 | WHO Global Code of Practice on the International Recruitment of Health Personnel |
| 2011 | WHA64.6 | Health workforce strengthening |
| 2013 | WHA66.23 | Transforming health workforce education in support of universal health coverage |
| 2014 | WHA67.14 | Health in the post-2015 development agenda |
| 2014 | WHA67.24 | Follow-up of the Recife Political Declaration on Human Resources for Health: renewed commitments towards universal health coverage |
| 2015 | WHA68.11 | WHO Global Code of Practice on the International Recruitment of Health Personnel |
| 2016 | WHA69.11 | Health in the 2030 Agenda for Sustainable Development |
| 2016 | WHA69.19 | Global strategy on human resources for health: workforce 2030 |
| 2016 | WHA69.24 | Strengthening integrated, people-centred health services |
| 2017 | WHA70.6 | Human resources for health and implementation of the outcomes of the United Nations' High-Level Commission on Health Employment and Economic Growth |

Sources: Authors, compiled from sources accessed from http://apps.who.int/gb/or/ and www.who.int/iris (As at 28 February 2019).

# Appendix 3

*Appendix 3* ILO Conventions and Recommendations directly relevant to international health worker-migration and -recruitment (1944–2018), including summary of the key features of up-to-date instruments

| Date | Reference | Title | Relevant features |
|------|-----------|-------|-------------------|
| 1944 | R067 | Income Security Recommendation | Defines guiding principles for income standards in respect of everyone who is employed or self-employed. Identifies social contingencies which social insurance and social assistance schemes should meet. Defines income security as an essential feature of national systems of social security. |
| 1948 | C088 | Employment Service Convention* | |
| 1948 | R086 | Employment Service Recommendation* | |
| 1949 | C096 | Fee-Charging Employment Agencies Convention (Revised)* | |
| 1949 | C097 | Migration for Employment Convention (Revised) | Covers persons who migrate from one country to another with a view to being employed otherwise than on their own account. Includes any person regularly admitted as a migrant for employment. Specifies the minimum conditions under which migration for employment in a regular situation must occur, in recruitment, transit, and arrival. Sets out the need to adopt an active employment policy, to collaborate internationally, and provide information to ILO on national policies, provisions and agreements on migration for employment. Article 6 refers to equal treatment (e.g. in pay, family benefits, social security, taxation and trade union membership) on the basis of non-discrimination in respect of nationality, race, religion or sex. A country shall treat immigrants lawfully within its territories no less favourably than that which it applies to its own nationals. The Convention includes a model employment bilateral agreement and a model contractual agreement. |

| Date | Reference | Title | Relevant features |
|------|-----------|-------|-------------------|
| 1949 | R086 | Migration for Employment Recommendation (Revised) | Elaborates principles and objectives in relation to migration for employment recruitment, placement and employment practices. Article 4 states that countries should 'facilitate the international distribution of manpower [sic] and in particular the movement of manpower [sic] from countries which have a surplus of manpower [sic] to those countries that have a deficiency', having 'due regard to the manpower [sic] situation in the country'. Contains a model agreement on temporary and permanent migration for employment. |
| 1952 | C102 | Social Security (Minimum Standards) Convention, 1952 | Elaborates international minimum standards for social security (income protection and health services). Embeds the principle of equality of treatment of non-national residents: article 68 stipulates that they shall have the same rights as national residents subject to special rules relating to public funds and transitional schemes and to bilateral or multilateral agreements providing for reciprocity between signatory countries. Article 69 sets out the conditions under which access to social security can be suspended, including periods of absence from the country. |
| 1955 | R100 | The Protection of Migrant Workers (Underdeveloped Countries) Recommendation* | |
| 1958 | C111 | Discrimination (Employment and Occupation) Convention | Aims to promote equality of opportunity and treatment in respect of employment and occupation. Covers access to vocational training, employment and to particular occupations, and terms and conditions of employment. Defines discrimination as 'any distinction, exclusion or preference made on the basis of race, colour, sex, religion, political opinion, national extraction or social origin, which has the effect of nullifying or impairing equality of opportunity or treatment in employment or occupation.' It does not mandatorily include distinctions on the basis of nationality. |
| 1958 | R111 | Discrimination (Employment and Occupation) Recommendation | Sets out principles underpinning measures to eliminate discrimination in relation to employment and occupation. |
| 1962 | C117 | Social Policy (Basic Aims and Standards) Convention* | |

| Date | Reference | Title | *Relevant features* |
|------|-----------|-------|---------------------|
| 1962 | C118 | Equality of Treatment (Social Security) Convention | Elaborates equality of treatment of nationals and non-nationals in respect of coverage and right to benefits across all social security schemes in place in the country on the basis of reciprocity. Stipulates that states shall grant equality of treatment to nationals of any state which has ratified the Convention. A signatory country is not obliged to apply equal treatment to the nationals of another country which does not grant equality of treatment in social security to the nationals of the first Member. |
| 1964 | C122 | Employment Policy Convention | Sets out the goal of employment policy as being the pursuit of 'an active policy designed to promote full, productive and freely chosen employment'. This shall be pursued on the basis of equality of opportunity: there shall be 'the fullest possible opportunity for each worker to qualify for, and to use his [sic] skills and endowments in, a job for which he [sic] is well suited, irrespective of race, colour, sex, religion, political opinion, national extraction or social origin.' Employment policy shall take account of the stage and level of economic development and the mutual relationships between employment objectives and other economic and social objectives. |
| 1964 | R122 | Employment Policy Recommendation | Elaborates objectives and general principles of employment policy, including those in relation to different employment measures. 'Industrialised countries should, in their economic policies...take into account the need for increased employment in other countries, in particular in the developing countries' (Article 32). 'International migration of workers for employment which is consistent with the economic needs of the countries of emigration and immigration, including migration from developing countries to industrialised countries, should be facilitated' (article 33), subject to ILO Conventions. |
| 1975 | C142 | Human Resources Development Convention | Concerns the development of 'open, flexible and complementary systems of general, technical and vocational education, educational and vocational guidance and vocational training, whether these activities take place within the system of formal education or outside it'. This shall be on an equal basis and without any discrimination, according to employment needs, opportunities and problems, the stage and level of economic, social and cultural development; and the mutual relationships between human resources development and other economic, social and cultural objectives. |

| Date | Reference | Title | Relevant features |
|------|-----------|-------|-------------------|
| 1975 | C143 | Migrant Workers (Supplementary Provisions) Convention | Sets out principles and standards to protect migrant workers in abusive conditions and to prevent and eliminate such abuses. Obliges countries to declare and pursue a national policy designed to guarantee equality of opportunity and treatment in respect of employment and occupation, of social security, of trade union and cultural rights and of individual and collective freedoms for persons who as migrant workers or as members of their families are lawfully within its territory. Countries may restrict the right to freely chosen employment under certain conditions. Such restrictions are not to affect migrant workers' right to geographical mobility. Encourages recognition of occupational qualifications acquired in another country. |
| 1975 | R151 | Migrant Workers Recommendation | Elaborates standards as regards equality of opportunity and treatment, social policy in regard to migrants and employment and residence. Countries should 'apply a social policy appropriate to national conditions and practice which enables migrant workers and their families to share in advantages enjoyed by its nationals while taking account on the basis of equality of opportunity and treatment' (article 9). The policy 'should be based, in particular, on an examination not only of conditions in the territory of the Member but also of those in the countries of origin of the migrants' (article 10). Elaborates principles relating to the reunification of families, health of migrant workers, social services, and employment and residence. |
| 1977 | C149 | Nursing Personnel Convention | Set in the context of a shortage of qualified nurses and applies to all categories of persons providing nursing care and nursing services. Nurse shortages and sub-optimal utilisation of staff are obstacles to the development of effective health services. Reiterates that nursing personnel are covered by international labour standards on employment and conditions of work, including the right to non-discrimination. Governments shall seek to attract people to the nursing profession and retain them in it by providing education and training appropriate to the exercise of professional functions, employment and working conditions, including career prospects and remuneration which are at least equivalent to those of other workers in the country. National policies shall aim to provide the quantity and quality of nursing care necessary for attaining the highest possible level of population health, and that these shall be co-ordinated with policies relating to other aspects of health care and to other workers in the field of health. Nursing personnel shall participate in the planning of nursing services. |

| Date | Reference | Title | *Relevant features* |
|------|-----------|-------|---------------------|
| 1977 | R157 | Nursing Personnel Recommendation | Elaborates principles underpinning the Convention as well as those guiding international cooperation and international nurse mobility. Promotes exchanges of personnel, ideas and knowledge to improve nursing care. Encourages the harmonisation of education and training, mutual recognition of qualifications acquired abroad, harmonisation of requirements for authorisation to practice, and nursing personnel exchange programmes. Sets out conditions relating to periods of work and/or training abroad. Stipulates that 'where necessary or desirable' nurses they should have the possibility of education and training abroad, as far as possible by way of organised exchange programmes'. Incorporates the principle of conditional and temporary migration, stating that although organised exchange programmes should provide appropriate financial support to the participants, such support may be conditional upon a nurse undertaking to return to their country within a reasonable time and to work there for a specified minimum period in a job corresponding to the newly acquired qualifications, on terms at least equal to those applicable to other nationals. Articles 66 sets out conditions relating to recognition of qualifications and language skills, and provides for equal treatment between foreign and national nurses in relation to employment. Article 67 concerns the conditions under which recruitment of foreign nursing personnel for employment should be authorised: (a) if there is a lack of qualified personnel for the posts to be filled in the country of employment; (b) if there is no shortage of nursing personnel with the qualifications sought in the country of origin. The recruitment of foreign nursing personnel should be undertaken in conformity with the relevant provisions of C097. Nursing personnel employed or in training abroad should be given all necessary facilities when they wish to be repatriated. Foreign nursing personnel shall enjoy equality of treatment with national personnel with regard to social security. Countries may participate in bilateral or multilateral arrangements designed to ensure the maintenance of the acquired rights or rights in course of acquisition of migrant nursing personnel, as well as the provision of benefits abroad. |

| Date | Reference | Title | Relevant features |
|------|-----------|-------|-------------------|
| 1982 | C157 | Maintenance of Social Security Rights Convention | Concerns social security for migrant workers, specifically the maintenance of acquired rights and of rights in course of acquisition. Concerns employees working abroad, even if they reside in another country or if their employer is based in another country than the one in which the employee normally works. Measures taken by governments in this area are on the basis of reciprocity, such that they guarantee benefits corresponding to the benefits provided under the legislation of another Member. |
| 1983 | R167 | Maintenance of Social Security Rights Recommendation | Elaborates the general principles of Convention C157 in relation to different branches of the social security system, including Provident Funds. The Annex incorporates a Model Agreement for the co-ordination of bilateral or multilateral social security instruments. |
| 1984 | R169 | Employment Policy (Supplementary Provisions) Recommendation | Sets out 13 principles, in accordance with the ILO employment principles and labour standards. Section on International Migration and Employment affirms the right to migrate abroad. Encourages policies to promote more and better forms of employment so as to reduce the need to migrate to find employment and ensure that international migration takes place under conditions designed to promote full, productive and freely chosen employment. Article 40 states that 'Members which habitually or repeatedly admit significant numbers of foreign workers with a view to employment should, when such workers come from developing countries, endeavour to co-operate more fully in the development of such countries, by appropriate intensified capital movements, the expansion of trade, the transfer of technical knowledge and assistance in the vocational training of local workers, in order to establish an effective alternative to migration for employment and to assist the countries in question in improving their economic and employment situation.' Article 41 concerns countries which habitually or repeatedly experience significant outflows of their nationals for the purpose of employment abroad should, are to prevent malpractices at the stage of recruitment or departure liable to result in illegal entry to, or stay or employment in, another country. They should also facilitate the voluntary return of their nationals who possess scarce skills, by providing the necessary incentives and enlist the co-operation of the countries employing their nationals as well ILO and other bodies concerned with the matter. All countries should prevent abuse in the recruitment of labour for work abroad, prevent the exploitation of migrant workers, and ensure the full exercise of the rights to freedom of association and to organise and bargain collectively. |

| Date | Reference | Title | Relevant features |
|------|-----------|-------|-------------------|
| | | | All countries should conclude bilateral and multilateral agreements covering issues such as right of entry and stay, the protection of rights resulting from employment, the promotion of education and training opportunities for migrant workers, social security, and assistance to workers and members of their families wishing to return to their country of origin, on the basis of international labour standards. |
| 1997 | C181 | Private Employment Agencies Convention | Principles and standards for the regulation of private employment agencies include equal treatment and non-discrimination on the basis of race, colour, sex, religion, political opinion, national extraction, social origin, disability, age, or any other form of discrimination. Countries shall ensure that migrant workers recruited by or placed in their territory by a private agency are provided with adequate protection in respect of fundamental rights, employment conditions, social security, and from abuses. Private employment agencies shall not charge directly or indirectly, in whole or in part, any fees or costs to workers, except if designated by countries for particular categories of workers. |
| 1997 | R188 | Private Employment Agencies Recommendation | Elaborates standards relating to the regulation of private employment agencies in relation to the protection of workers and the relationship between the public employment service and private employment agencies. Protection includes measures against all forms of unethical practices by private employment agencies, unfair advertising practices and misleading advertisements. Obligations of private employment agencies are set out in terms of their recruitment practices and how their duty to communicate with migrant workers the nature of the position offered and the applicable terms and conditions of employment. |

| Date | Reference | Title | Relevant features |
|------|-----------|-------|-------------------|
| 2004 | R195 | Human Resources Development Recommendation | Encourages countries to formulate, apply and review national human resources development, education, training and lifelong learning policies which are consistent with economic, fiscal and social policies, on the basis of social dialogue. Policies should promote access for people with nationally identified special needs, on the basis of social inclusion and equal opportunity. Section X (International and Technical Cooperation) states that countries should 'develop mechanisms that mitigate the adverse impact on developing countries of the loss of skilled people through migration, including strategies to strengthen the human resources development systems in the countries of origin, recognizing that creating enabling conditions for economic growth, investment, creation of decent jobs and human development will have a positive effect on retaining skilled labour', 'promote recognition and portability of skills, competencies and qualifications nationally and internationally' and 'explore and apply innovative approaches to provide additional resources for human resources development' in relation to indebted developing countries (article 21). |
| 2006 | R198 | Employment Relationship Recommendation | Clarifies duties in situations where the contractual relationship between employer and employee may be unclear in order to guarantee effective protection for workers. Countries should establish specific national mechanisms in order to ensure that employment relationships can be effectively identified within the framework of the transnational provision of services (Article 22). |
| 2012 | R202 | Social Protection Floors Recommendation | Concerns nationally defined sets of basic social security guarantees which secure protection aimed at preventing or alleviating poverty, vulnerability and social exclusion. Provides guidance for establishing, maintaining and implementing guarantees as a fundamental element of their national social security systems. Stipulates aim is to ensure higher levels of social security to as many people as possible, guided by ILO social security standards. |

Source: Authors, compiled from NORMLEX Information system on international labour standards www.ilo.org/dyn/normlex/en (As at 28 February 2019).

Note
Only the features of up-to-date instruments are elaborated.
\* Interim status.

# Appendix 4

## SDG goals and targets pertaining to international health worker-migration and -recruitment

### Goal 1  End Poverty

- Implement nationally appropriate social protection systems and measure for all, including floors, and by 2030 achieve substantial coverage of the poor and the vulnerable
- By 2030, ensure that all men and women, in particular the poor and the vulnerable, have equal rights to economic resources, as well as access to basic services

### Goal 3  Good Health and WellBeing

- By 2030, reduce the global maternal mortality ratio to less than 70 per 100,000 live births
- By 2030, end preventable deaths of newborns and children under five years of age, with all countries aiming to reduce neonatal mortality to at least as low as 12 per 1,000 live births and under-five mortality to at least as low as 25 per 1,000 live births
- By 2030, end the epidemics of AIDS, tuberculosis, malaria and neglected tropical diseases and combat hepatitis, water-borne diseases and other communicable diseases
- By 2030, reduce by one third premature mortality from non-communicable diseases through prevention and treatment and promote mental health and well-being
- Strengthen the prevention and treatment of substance abuse, including narcotic drug abuse and harmful use of alcohol
- By 2020, halve the number of global deaths and injuries from road traffic accidents
- By 2030, ensure universal access to sexual and reproductive health-care services, including for family planning, information and education, and the integration of reproductive health into national strategies and programmes
- Achieve universal health coverage, including financial risk protection, access to quality essential health-care services and access to safe, effective, quality and affordable essential medicines and vaccines for all

- Substantially increase health financing and the recruitment, development, training and retention of the health workforce in developing countries, especially in least developed countries and small island developing States

## Goal 4  Quality education

- By 2030, substantially increase the supply of qualified teachers, including through international cooperation for teacher training in developing countries, especially least developed countries and small island developing states

## Goal 5  Gender Equality

- Ensure universal access to sexual and reproductive health and reproductive rights as agreed in accordance with the Programme of Action of the International Conference on Population and Development and the Beijing Platform for Action and the outcome documents of their review conferences

## Goal 8  Decent Work and Economic Growth

- By 2030, achieve full and productive employment and decent work for all women and men, including for young people and persons with disabilities, and equal pay for work of equal value
- Protect labour rights and promote safe and secure working environments for all workers, including migrant workers, in particular women migrants, and those in precarious employment

## Goal 10  Reduced Inequalities

- By 2030, empower and promote the social, economic and political inclusion of all, irrespective of age, sex, disability, race, ethnicity, origin, religion or economic or other status
- Ensure equal opportunity and reduce inequalities of outcome, including by eliminating discriminatory laws, policies and practices and promoting appropriate legislation, policies and action in this regard
- Adopt policies, especially fiscal, wage and social protection policies, and progressively achieve greater equality
- Facilitate orderly, safe, regular and responsible migration and mobility of people, including through the implementation of planned and well-managed migration policies
- By 2030, reduce to less than 3 per cent the transaction costs of migrant remittances and eliminate remittance corridors with costs higher than 5 per cent

## Goal 16  Peace, Justice and Strong Institutions

- Significantly reduce all forms of violence and related death rates everywhere
- Promote the rule of law at the national and international levels and ensure equal access to justice for all
- Develop effective, accountable and transparent institutions at all levels
- Ensure responsive, inclusive, participatory and representative decision-making at all levels
- Ensure public access to information and protect fundamental freedoms, in accordance with national legislation and international agreements
- Promote and enforce non-discriminatory laws and policies for sustainable development

## Goal 17  Partnerships for the goals

- Enhance international support for implementing effective and targeted capacity-building in developing countries to support national plans to implement all the sustainable development goals, including through North–South, South–South and triangular cooperation
- Enhance policy coherence for sustainable development
- Respect each country's policy space and leadership to establish and implement policies for poverty eradication and sustainable development
- Enhance the global partnership for sustainable development, complemented by multi-stakeholder partnerships that mobilise and share knowledge, expertise, technology and financial resources, to support the achievement of the sustainable development goals in all countries, in particular developing countries
- Encourage and promote effective public, public-private and civil society partnerships, building on the experience and resourcing strategies of partnerships
- By 2020, enhance capacity-building support to developing countries, including for least developed countries and small island developing States, to increase significantly the availability of high-quality, timely and reliable data disaggregated by income, gender, age, race, ethnicity, migratory status, disability, geographic location and other characteristics relevant in national contexts

Source: Authors, compiled from www.un.org/sustainabledevelopment/

# References

Abadalla, F.M., Oar, A.M. and Badr, E.E. (2016) Contribution of Sudanese medical diaspora to the health care delivery system in Sudan: Exploring options and barriers. *Human Resources for Health*, 14(Suppl 1).

Abiiro, G.A. and De Allegri, M. (2015) Universal health coverage from multiple perspectives: a synthesis of conceptual literature and global debates. *BMC international health and human rights*, 15(17).

Abu Sharkh, M. and Gough, I. (2010) Global Welfare Regimes: a Cluster Analysis. *Global Social Policy*, 10(1): 27–58.

Abugala, A. and Badr, B. (2016) Challenges to implementation of the WHO Global Code of Practice on International Recruitment of health personnel: the case of Sudan. *Human Resources for Health*. 14(Suppl 1).

Adams, B. and Martens, J. (2015) *Fit for whose purpose? Private funding and corporate influence in the United Nations.* Bonn/New York: Global Policy Forum.

Addati, L., Cattaneo, U., Esquivel, V. and Valarino, I. (2018) *Care work and care jobs for the future of decent work.* Geneva: ILO.

Adepoju, A. (2007) *Migration in sub-Saharan Africa.* A background paper commissioned by the Nordic Africa Institute for the Swedish Government White Paper on Africa. Retrieved 10 September 2018 from: www.sweden.gov.se/content/1/c6/08/88/66/730473a9.pdf

Adlung, R. and Carzaniga, A. (2001) Health Services under the General Agreement on Trade in Services. *Bulletin of the World Health Organization*, 79(4): 352–364.

Adokli, B.V. (2006) Migration of health workers: Perspectives from Bangladesh, India, Nepal, Pakistan and Sri Lanka. *Regional Health Forum* 10(1): 49–58.

Agunias, D.R. (2011) *Regulating Recruitment Agencies: A Case Study of Filipino and Sri Lankan Migration to Jordan.* Washington, DC: Migration Policy Institute.

Agwu, K. and Llewelyn, M. (2009) Undergraduates in International Health at UCL: Compensation for the brain drain from developing countries. *Lancet*, 373: 1665–1666.

Ahmad, O.B. (2005) Managing medical migration from poor countries. *British Medical Journal*, 331: 43–45.

Al-Janabi, A., Al-Wahdani, B., Ammar, W., Arsenault, C., Asiedu, E.K., Etiebet, M.-A., Forde, I., Gage, A.D., García-Saisó, S., Guanais, F., Hansen, P.M., Hovig, D., Jhalani, M., Kruk, M.E., Maliqi, B., Marikar, K., Matsoso, M.P., Pate, M., Peterson, S., Roder-DeWan, S., Schulze, A., Somers, K., Shiozaki, Y. and Thapa, G. (2018) Bellagio Declaration on high-quality health systems: from a quality moment to a quality movement. *The Lancet Global Health*, 6(11): 1144–1145.

Alliance for Ethical International Recruitment Practices (US) (2011) *Voluntary code of ethical conduct for the recruitment of foreign educated health professionals to the United States.* Washington, DC: AEIRP.

American Association of Colleges of Nursing (2013) *Nursing shortage resources.* Retrieved 27 July 2017 from: www.aacn.nche.edu/media/shortageresource.htm

Antwi, J., and Phillips, D. (2011) *Wages and Health Worker Retention: Evidence from Public Sector Wage Reforms in Ghana.* Accra: Ghana Ministry of Health and the World Bank.

Arunanondchai, J. and Fink, C. (2006) Trade in health services in the ASEAN region, *Health Promotion International* 21(Suppl 1): 59–66.

Asian Development Bank Institute/International Labour Organization/Organization for Economic Cooperation and Development (ADBI/ILO/OECD) (2016) *Labor Migration in Asia: Building Effective Institutions.* ADBI/ILO/OECD.

Association of South-East Asian Nations (ASEAN) (2017) *Building the ASEAN Community Mutual Recognition Agreements in Services. Professionals on the Move.* Retrieved 24 July 2017 from: www.asean.org/storage/images/2015/October/outreach-document/Edited%20MRA%20Services-2.pdf

Awases, M., Gbary, A.R., Nyoni, J. and Chatora, F.C. (2004) *Migration of health professionals in six countries: A synthesis report.* Brazzaville: WHO Regional Office for Africa.

Bach, S. (2004) Migration patterns of physicians and nurses: still the same story? *Bulletin of the World Health Organization,* 82(8): 624–625.

Barnett, M. and Finnemore, M. (2004) *Rules for the World: International Organizations in Global Politics.* Ithaca: Cornell University Press.

Betts, A. (2011) Introduction: Global Migration Governance, in A. Betts (ed.) *Global Migration Governance,* Oxford: Oxford University Press.

Bhagwati, J. (2008) *Termites in the Trade System: how preferential agreements undermine free trade.* Oxford and New York: Oxford University Press.

Bhagwati, J.N. (1976a) *The Brain Drain.* Paper prepared for the Tripartite World Conference on Employment, Income Distribution, Social Progress and the International Division of Labour, ILO, NOEI/D.31, 19–23 January 1976.

Bhagwati, J.N. (1976b) *The brain drain and taxation.* Amsterdam: North Holland Publishing Company.

Bobeva, D. and Garson, J.P. (2004). Overview of bilateral agreements and other forms of labour recruitment. In OECD, (ed.) *Migration for employment: bilateral agreements at a crossroads.* OECD: Paris.

Böhning, W.R. (1977) *Compensating countries of origin for the out-migration of their people.* Working Paper 18E. ILO: Geneva.

Böhning, W.R. (1978) *Elements of a theory of international migration and compensation.* Working Paper 34. ILO: Geneva.

Böhning, W.R. (1982) *Towards a system of recompense for international labour migration,* International Migration for Employment Working Paper 2. ILO: Geneva.

Bourgeault, I.L., Labonté, R., Packer, C., Runnels, V. and Tomblin-Murphy, G. (2016) Knowledge and potential impact of the WHO global code of practice on the international recruitment of health personnel: Does it matter for source and destination country stakeholders? *Human Resources for Health* 14(Suppl 1): 25.

Bretton Woods Project (2017) *GFF falls short on family planning.* At Issue by Taryn Couture. Bretton Woods Project online, January 2017. Retrieved 5 September 2018 from: www.brettonwoodsproject.org/wp-content/uploads/2017/04/At-Issue-GFF-Family-Planning.pdf

Bruckner, T., Liu, J. and Scheffler, R.M. (2016) Demands-based and needs-based forecast for health care workers. In *Human resources for health labor market toolkit*. Washington, DC: World Bank.

Brugha, R., McAleese, S. and Humphries, N. (2015) *A destination and source country for health professional migration*. Dublin: Royal College of Surgeons.

Buchan, J. (2010) Can the WHO Global Code on international recruitment succeed? *British Medical Journal*, 340: 791–793.

Buchan, J. and Dovlo, D. (2004) *International recruitment of health workers to the UK: a report for DFID*. London: DIFID.

Buchan, J., Dhillon, I. and Campbell, J. eds. (2017) *Health employment and economic growth: an evidence base*. Geneva: WHO.

Campbell, J. (2013) Towards universal health coverage: a health workforce fit for purpose and practice. *Bulletin of the World Health Organization*, 91(11), 887–888.

Campbell, J., Dhillon, S. and Siyam, A. (2016) The WHO Global Code: increasing relevance and effectiveness. *Human Resources for Health*, 14 (Suppl 1): 39.

Campbell, J., Dussault, G., Buchan, J., Pozo-Martin, F., Guerra Arias, M., Leone, C., Siyam, A. and Cometto, G. (2013) *A universal truth: no health without a workforce. Forum report.* Third global forum on human resources for health, Recife, Brazil. Geneva: GHWA/WHO.

Chan, M. (2012) *Universal coverage is the ultimate expression of fairness.* Geneva: WHO. Retrieved 6 September 2018 from www.who.int/dg/speeches/2012/wha_20120523/en/index.html#

Chan, M. (2014) *Keynote address to the UN Economic and Social Council. The changing development landscape: what will it mean for specialized agencies in a post–2015 era with focus on sustainable development?* New York, USA, 25 February 2014. Retrieved 6 September 2018 from: www.who.int/dg/speeches/2014/economic-social-council/en/

Chandra, R. (2002) Trade in Health Services. *Bulletin of the World Health Organization*, 80(2): 158–361.

Chen, L.C. and Boufford, J.I. (2005) Fatal flows: Doctors on the move. *New England Journal of Medicine*, 353(17): 1850–1852.

Cheru, F. and Bradford, C. (eds.) (2005) *The Millennium Development Goals: raising the resources to tackle world poverty.* London: Zed Books.

Chikanda, A. (2004) *Skilled health professionals' migration and its impact on health delivery in Zimbabwe.* Centre on Migration, Policy and Society Working Paper No. 4. Oxford: University of Oxford.

Clemens, M.A. (2015) Global Skill Partnerships: a proposal for technical training in a mobile world. *IZA J Labor Policy* 4(2): 1–18.

Clemens, M.A. (2017) *Global Skill Partnerships: a proposal for technical training in a mobile world*, Washington, DC: Centre for Global Development.

Cometto, G., Scheffer, R., Bruckner, T., Liu, J., Maeda, A., Tomblin-Murph, G., Hunter, D. and Campbell, J. (2017) An overview of forecasted trends in the global health labour market in J. Buchan, I.S. Dhillon and J. Campbell, (eds.) *Health Employment and Economic Growth: An Evidence Base*. Geneva, WHO.

Cometto, G. and Witter, S. (2013) Tackling health workforce challenges to universal health coverage: setting targets and measuring progress. *Bull World Health Organ*, 91: 881–885.

Commission of the European Communities (CEC) (2007) *White Paper: Together for Health: A Strategic Approach for the EU*. Brussels: CEC.

Commission of the European Communities (CEC) (2008) *Green Paper on the European Workforce for Health.* COM (2008) 725 final. Brussels: CEC.

Commission of the European Communities (CEC) (2012) *The External Dimension of EU Social Security Coordination.* COM (2012) 153 final. Brussels: CEC.

Commission on Human Security (2003) *Human Security Now: Protecting and Empowering People.* New York: Commission on Human Security.

Commission on International Development (1969) *Partners in Development – Report of the Commission on International Development, Lester B. Pearson (Chairman),* New York, Washington and London: Commission on International Development.

Connell, J. (2010) *Migration and the globalisation of health care: The health worker exodus?* London: Edward Elgar.

d'Oliveira e Sousa, J. (1985) The measurement of human resource flows: Methodology and approach. UNCTAD *Trade and Development – an UNCTAD Review. No. 6.* New York: UNCTAD.

d'Oliveira e Sousa, J. (1989) The Brain Drain Issue in International Negotiations, in R. Appleyard (ed.) *The Impact of International Migration on Developing Countries, Proceedings of a Conference "Migration and Development", Paris, February 1987.* Paris: OECD Development Centre, Committee for International Cooperation in National Research in Demography, and Inter-Governmental Committee for Migration.

Deacon, B. (2007) *Global social governance and policy.* London: Sage.

Deacon, B. (2013) *Global social policy in the making: The foundations of the Social Protection Floor.* Bristol: Policy Press.

Deacon, B. (2014) Global and regional social governance, in N. Yeates (ed.) *Understanding Global Social Policy* (2nd edition). Bristol: The Policy Press.

Deacon, B., Hulse, M. and Stubbs, P. (1997) *Global Social Policy – International Organizations and the Future of Welfare.* London: Sage.

Deacon, M.C., Macovei, L., Van Langenhove, L. and Yeates, N. (eds.) (2009) *World-Regional Social Policy and Global Governance: new research and policy agendas in Africa, Asia, Europe and Latin America.* London: Routledge.

Department of Health, Philippines/ILO (DoH, Philippines/ILO) (2012) Monitoring of the WHO Global Code of Practice on the International Recruitment of Health Personnel. The Philippine Multistakeholder Approach. Manila: ILO. Retrieved June 2018 from www.ilo.org/dyn/migpractice/docs/159/Factsheet.pdf

Department of Health (UK) (DoH, UK) (2004) *Code of practice for NHS employers involved in the international recruitment of health care professionals.* London: Department of Health.

Department of Health and Human Services (US) (2016) *State-Level Projections of Supply and Demand for Primary Care Practitioners: 2013–2025.* Rockville, Maryland: Health Resources and Services Administration, National Center for Health Workforce Analysis. Retrieved 27 July 2018 from: https://bhw.hrsa.gov/sites/default/files/bhw/health-workforce-analysis/research/projections/primary-care-state-projections2013-2025.pdf

Department of Health and Human Services (US) (2017) *National and Regional Supply and Demand Projections of the Nursing Workforce: 2014-2030.* Rockville, Maryland: Health Resources and Services Administration, National Center for Health Workforce Analysis. Retrieved 27 July 2018 from: https://bhw.hrsa.gov/sites/default/files/bhw/nchwa/projections/NCHWA_HRSA_Nursing_Report.pdf

Department of Health/ILO (2012) *Monitoring of the WHO Global Code of Practice on the International Recruitment of Health Personnel.* The Philippine Multi-stakeholder Approach. Manila, ILO.

Department of Labor and Employment (DOLE) (2011) *The Philippine Labor and Employment Plan 2011–2016. Inclusive Growth Through Decent and Productive Work.* Manila: Department of Labor and Employment.

Dhillon, I. (2015) *Assessing the relevance and effectiveness of the WHO Global Code of Practice on the International Recruitment of Health Personnel.* Geneva: WHO.

Dhillon, I. (2016) *International Migration of Health Workers: Advancing Evidence and Governance.* Fourth Global Forum on Human Resources for health, 16 November. Geneva: WHO.

Dhillon, I.S., Clark, M.E. and Kapp, R.H. (2010) *Innovations in Cooperation: A guidebook on bilateral agreements to address health worker migration.* Health worker migration initiative/realizing rights/Global Health development. Washington, DC: Aspen Institute.

Dieleman, J.L., Templin, T., Sadat, N., Reidy, P., Chapin, A., Foreman, K., Haakenstad, A., Evans, T., Murray, C.J. and Kurowski, C. (2016) National spending on health by source for 184 countries between 2013 and 2040, *The Lancet*, 387: 2521–2535.

Directorate for Health and Social Affairs, Norway (2007) *Recruitment of health workers: towards global solidarity.* Oslo: Directorate for Health and Social Affairs.

Dovlo, D. (2007) Migration of nurses from sub-Saharan Africa: A review of issues and challenges, in *Health Services Research*, 42(3) Part 2: 1373–1388.

Dunkley, G. (1997) *The Free Trade Adventure: The WTO, the Uruguay Round and Globalism: A Critique.* London, Zed Books.

Eckenwiler, I.A. (2009) The WHO Code of Practice on the international recruitment of health personnel: we have only just begun. *Developing World Bioethics*, 9: ii–v.

ESTHER (undated) Homepage of the ESTHER Alliance. Retrieved 12 March 2018 from https://esther.eu/

European Public Services Union/European Hospital and Health care Employers' Association (EPSU/HOSPEEM) (2008) *Code of Conduct on ethical cross-border recruitment and retention.* 7 March 2008. Brussels: EPSU/HOSPEEM.

European Public Services Union/European Hospital and Health care Employers' Association (EPSU/HOSPEEM) (2012) Use and implementation of the EPSU-HOSPEEM Code of Conduct on Ethical Cross-Border Recruitment and Retention in the Hospital Sector. Joint Final Report by EPSU and HOSPEEM. Retrieved 28 February 2019 from www.epsu.org/IMG/pdf/Report-Use_Implementation-EPSU-HOSPEEM-CoCECBR_R-adopted-05-09-12.pdf

European Public Services Union/European Hospital and Health care Employers' Association (EPSU/HOSPEEM) (2018) *Employers and trade unions renew commitment to ethical cross-border recruitment and retention policies.* Retrieved 1 September 2018 from: www.epsu.org/article/employers-and-trade-unions-renew-commitment-ethical-cross-border-recruitment-and-retention

European Coalition for Corporate Justice (ECCJ) (2017) *French Corporate Duty of Vigilance Law.* Brussels: ECCJ. Retrieved 10 September 2018 from: http://corporatejustice.org/documents/publications/french-corporate-duty-of-vigilance-law-faq.pdf

European Commission (EC) (2010) *Communication from the Commission to the Council, the European Parliament, the European Economic and Social Committee and the Committee of the Regions: The EU Role in Global Health.* SEC(2010)380 SEC(2010)381 SEC(2010)382. Brussels: European Commission.

European Commission (EC) (2012) *Staff working document on an action plan for the EU health workforce.* Brussels: European Commission.

European Commission (2017) Reflection paper on harnessing globalization. COM(2017) 240 of 10 May 2017. Brussels: European Commission.

European Parliament (2018) *European Parliament resolution on the EU's input to a UN Binding Instrument on transnational corporations and other business enterprises with transnational characteristics with respect to human rights*, (2018/2763(RSP). Brussels: European Parliament.

European Trade Union Confederation (ETUC) (2017) ETUC Resolution for an EU progressive trade and investment policy. Adopted at the Executive Committee Meeting of 13–14 June 2017. Brussels: ETUC.

Every Woman Every Child (2015) *The global strategy for women's, children's and adolescents' health (2016–2030)*. Every Woman Every Child.

Farnsworth, K. (2014) Business and global social policy, in N. Yeates (ed.) *Understanding Global Social Policy* (2nd edition). Bristol: The Policy Press.

Fidler, D.P., Correa, C. and Aginam, O. (2004) *Legal Review of the General Agreement on Trade in Services (GATS) from a Health Policy Perspective*. Geneva: WHO.

Francois, J. and Hoekman, B. (2010) Services Trade and Policy, *Journal of Economic Literature* 48 (September 2010): 642–692.

French, D. and Kotzé, L.J. (eds.) (2018) *Sustainable Development Goals: law, theory and implementation*. Edward Elgar: Cheltenham.

Galvez-Tan, J.Z. (2008) *Framework for the Ethical Recruitment of Nurses, Perspectives from the Philippines*. Academy Health International Exchange. 10 January 2008

Gencianos, G. (2018) *Perspective on Global Skills Partnerships*. Presentation on behalf of PSI. Presentation to meeting of the International Platform on Health Worker Mobility 13–14 September. Geneva: WHO.

Glaser, W. (1978) *The Brain Drain: emigration and return: findings of a UNITAR study multinational comparative survey of professional personnel of developing countries who study abroad*. Oxford: Pergamon Press.

Glinos, I.A. (2014) Going beyond numbers: A typology of health professional mobility inside and outside the European Union. *Policy and Society*, 33(1): 25–37.

Global Forum on Migration and Development (GFMD) (2008) *Report of the first meeting of the Global Forum on Migration and Development*, Belgium, 9–11 July 2007. GFMD.

Global Forum on Migration and Development (GFMD) (2012) *Enhancing the human development of migrants and their contribution to the development of communities and states*. Report of the Proceedings. Sixth meeting of the GFMD, 2012 Summit Meeting Port Louis, Mauritius 19–22 November 2012.

Global Forum on Migration and Development (GFMD) (2013) *Unlocking the potential of migration for inclusive development*. GFMD 2013–2014 Concept paper 30 April 2013.

Global Health Workforce Alliance (GHWA) (2012) *Strategy 2013–2016. Advancing the Health Workforce Agenda within Universal Health Coverage*. Geneva, WHO/GHWA.

Global Health Workforce Alliance (GHWA) (2013) *Global Health Workforce Crisis Key messages – 2013*. Geneva, GHWA.

Global Health Workforce Alliance (GHWA) (2014) *Annual Report 2014*. Geneva: GHWA.

Global Unions/BWI (2018) *The United Nations Agrees on a Global Compact for Safe, Orderly and Regular Migration*. Press Release. Retrieved 20 July 2018 from: www.bwint.org/cms/news-72/press-release-the-united-nations-agrees-on-a-global-compact-for-safe-orderly-and-regular-migration-1121

Gostin, L.O., Friedman, E.A., Ooms, G., Gebauer, T., Gupta, N., Sridhar, D., Wang, C., Røttingen, J.-A. and Sanders, D. (2010) *The Joint Action and Learning Initiative on National and Global Responsibilities for Health*. World Health Report (2010) Background Paper, 53. Geneva: WHO.

Haas, E. (1990) *When Knowledge is Power: three models of change in International Organisations.* Berkeley: University of California Press.

Hardy, J., Shelley, S., Calveley, M., Kubisa, J. and Zahn, R. (2016) Scaling the mobility of health workers in an enlarged Europe: an open political-economy perspective, *European Urban and Regional Studies* 23(4): 798–815.

HSE/Forum of Irish Postgraduate Training Bodies (2014) International Medical Graduate Training Initiative. Adopted by the HSE and The Forum of Irish Postgraduate Medical Training Bodies 15 January 2014. Dublin, HSE and Forum of Irish Postgraduate Training Bodies.

Health Workforce Australia (2012) *Health Workforce 2025 – Doctors, Nurses and Midwives.* Volume 1. Adelaide: Health Workforce Australia.

HealthWorkers4All (2014) *A health worker for everyone, everywhere.* Retrieved 1 March 2019 from www.healthworkers4all.eu/fileadmin/docs/eu/hw4all_papers/hw4all_CTA_-_European_booklet.pdf

HealthWorkers4all (2014) *Call to Action: A Health Worker for Everyone, Everywhere.* Amsterdam: Wemos.

Henderson, G. (1970) *Emigration of Highly Skilled Manpower from Developing Countries,* (UNITAR/RR/3)7. Geneva: UNITAR.

High-Level Commission on Health Employment and Economic Growth (HEEG) (2016) *Working for health and growth: investing in the health workforce.* Report of the High-Level Commission on Health Employment and Economic Growth. Geneva: WHO.

Holden, C. (2014) International trade and welfare, in N. Yeates (ed.) *Understanding Global Social Policy* (2nd edition). Bristol The Policy Press.

Hooper, K. (2018) *Reimagining Skilled Migration Partnerships to Support Development.* Washington, DC: Migration Policy Institute.

Horwitz, A. (1976) The ten-year health plan for the Americas. *Ekistics,* 41(245): 227–229.

Hujo, K. and Piper, N. (eds.) (2010) *South–South migration: Implications for social policy and development.* Basingstoke: Palgrave.

Institute of Policy Studies (Sri Lanka) (2013) Migration Profile – Sri Lanka. Published jointly by Institute of Policy Studies, Ministry of Foreign Employment Promotion and Welfare, International Organization for Migration and Sri Lanka Bureau of Foreign Employment: Colombo.

International Labour Organization (ILO) (1944) *Constitution of the ILO and Declaration concerning the aims and purposes of the International Labour Organisation (Declaration of Philadelphia).* Geneva: ILO.

International Labour Organization (ILO) (1949) *Migration for Employment Convention* (C097). Geneva: ILO.

International Labour Organization (ILO) (1967) *Non-manual workers: problems and prospects.* International Labour Conference, Director-General. Geneva: ILO.

International Labour Organization (ILO) (1975) *Record of Proceedings, International Labour Conference, Sixtieth Session.* Geneva: ILO.

International Labour Organization (ILO) (1976a) *ILO: Declaration of Principles and Programme of Action,* adopted by the Tripartite World Conference on Employment, Income Distribution, Social Progress and the International Division of Labour, Geneva, 4–17 June 1976. Geneva: ILO.

International Labour Organization (ILO) (1976b) ILO World Employment Conference and International Migration of Workers, *The International Migration Review,* 10(3): 389–393.

International Labour Organization (ILO) (1976c) *Report of Proceedings, International Labour Conference, Sixty-first session, Geneva 1975.* Geneva: ILO.

International Labour Organization (ILO) (1977a) *Report of Proceedings, International Labour Conference, Sixty-third Session, Fourteenth Special sitting.* Geneva: ILO.

International Labour Organization (ILO) (1977b) *Nursing Personnel Convention* (C149). Geneva: ILO.

International Labour Organization (ILO) (1977c) *Nursing Personnel Recommendation* (R157). Geneva: ILO.

International Labour Organization (ILO) (1978) *Report of Proceedings, International Labour Conference, Sixty-third session, Geneva 1977.* Geneva: ILO.

International Labour Organization (ILO) (1980) *Migrant Workers. General Survey of the Reports relating to Conventions Nos. 97 and 143 and Recommendations Nos. 86 and 151 concerning Migrant Workers.* Report of the Committee of Experts on the Application of Conventions and Recommendations, International Labour Conference, Sixty-sixth Session. Geneva: ILO.

International Labour Organization (ILO) (1983) *Report of Proceedings, International Labour Conference, Sixty-ninth session.* Geneva: ILO.

International Labour Organization (ILO) (1997b) *Protecting the most vulnerable of today's migrant workers: Tripartite Meeting of Experts on Future ILO Activities in the Field of Migration.* Geneva: ILO.

International Labour Organization (ILO) (1998) *ILO Declaration on Fundamental Principles and Rights at Work.* Geneva: ILO.

International Labour Organization (ILO) (1999) *Migrant Workers. General Survey on the reports on the Migration for Employment Convention (Revised) (No. 97), and Recommendation (Revised) (No. 86), 1949, and the Migrant Workers (Supplementary Provisions) Convention (No. 143), and Recommendation (No. 151), 1975.* Report of the Committee of Experts on the Application of Conventions and Recommendations, International Labour Conference, Eighty-seventh Session. Geneva: ILO.

International Labour Organization (ILO) (2004a) *Towards a fair deal for migrant workers in the global economy.* Report presented to International Labour Conference, Ninety-second Session. Geneva: ILO.

International Labour Organization (ILO) (2004b) *A Fair Globalization: Creating Opportunities for All, World Commission on the Social Dimension of Globalization.* Geneva: ILO.

International Labour Organization (ILO) (2006) *ILO Multilateral Framework on Labour Migration: Non-binding principles and guidelines for a rights-based approach to labour migration.* Geneva: ILO.

International Labour Organization (ILO) (2007) *Guide to private employment agencies. Regulation, monitoring and enforcement.* Geneva: ILO.

International Labour Organization (ILO) (2008) *Declaration on Social Justice for a Fair Globalization*, adopted by the International Labour Conference at its 97th Session, Geneva, 10 June 2008,

International Labour Organization (ILO) (2011) *Equality at work: the continuing challenge.* In *Report of the Director-General. Global Report Under the Follow-up to the ILO Declaration on Fundamental Principles and Rights at Work. Geneva: International Labour Conference, 100th Session, Report I(B).* Geneva: ILO

International Labour Organization (ILO) (2013) *Tripartite Technical Meeting on Labour Migration. Conclusions.* Geneva 4–8 November 2013. Geneva: ILO.

International Labour Organization (ILO) (2014a) *Addressing the Global Health Crisis: Universal Health Protection Policies.* Social Protection Policy Papers, Paper 13. Geneva: ILO.

International Labour Organization (ILO) (2014b) *Fair Migration: Setting an ILO Agenda. International Labour Conference, 103rd Session, 2014.* Report of the Director-General Report I(B). Geneva: ILO.

International Labour Organization (ILO) (2014c) *Recruitment Practices of Employment Agencies Recruiting Migrant Workers.* Geneva: ILO.

International Labour Organization (ILO) (2014d) *World Social Protection Report 2014/15.* Geneva: ILO.

International Labour Organization (ILO) (2016a) *Report for discussion at the Tripartite Meeting of Experts on Fair Recruitment Principles and Operational Guidelines, 5–7 September 2016.* Geneva: ILO.

International Labour Organization (ILO) (2016b) *General principles & operational guidelines for fair recruitment.* Geneva: ILO.

International Labour Organization (ILO) (2016c) *Assessment of labour provisions in trade and investment arrangements*, Studies on Growth with Equity. Geneva: ILO.

International Labour Organization (ILO) (2016d) *Promoting Fair Migration. General Survey concerning the migrant workers instruments.* Report of the Committee of Experts on the Application of Conventions and Recommendations, International Labour Conference, 105th Session. Geneva: ILO.

International Labour Organization (ILO) (2017a) *Inception Report for the Global Commission on the Future of Work.* Geneva: ILO.

International Labour Organization (ILO) (2017b) *Conclusions on improving employment and working conditions in health services.* Tripartite Meeting on Improving Employment and Working Conditions in Health Services. Geneva 24–28 April 2017. Geneva: ILO.

International Labour Organization (ILO) (2017c) *Improving employment and working conditions in health services.* Report for discussion at the Tripartite Meeting on Improving Employment and Working Conditions in Health Services. Geneva, 24–28 April 2017. Geneva: ILO.

International Labour Organization (ILO) (2018a) *Tripartite Meeting of Experts on Defining Recruitment Fees and Related Costs.* Geneva: ILO. Geneva: ILO.

International Labour Organization (ILO) (2018b) *Report VI Social dialogue and tripartism.* International Labour Conference 107th Session, 2018. Geneva: ILO.

International Labour Organization (ILO) (2018c) *Social Dialogue: Recurrent discussion under the ILO Declaration on Social Justice for a Fair Globalization.* Report VI, International Labour Conference, 107th Session. Geneva: ILO.

International Labour Organization (ILO) (2018d) *Ensuring decent working time for the future. General Survey concerning working-time instruments.* Report of the Committee of Experts on the Application of Conventions and Recommendations (articles 19, 22 and 35 of the Constitution) Report III (Part B) International Labour Conference, 107th Session, 2018. Geneva: ILO

International Labour Organization/United Nations Office on Drugs and Crime (ILO/ UNODC) (2015) *Preventing and responding to abusive and fraudulent labour recruitment: A call for action.* Geneva: ILO.

International Labour Organization/Organization for Economic Cooperation and Development/World Health Organization (ILO/OECD/WHO) (2017) *Working for Health.* Geneva: WHO.

International Labour Organization/Organization for Economic Cooperation and Development/World Health Organization (ILO/OECD/WHO) (2018) *Women in the health workforce: Seizing the gender dividend across the sustainable development goals.* EU Infopoint session, Brussels, 7 March 2018. Retrieved 21 December 2018 from www.who.int/hrh/events/2018/women-in-health-workforce/en/

International Organization for Migration (IOM) (2006) *World Migration Report: the costs and benefits of international migration.* Geneva: IOM.

International Organization for Migration (IOM) (2008) *World Migration Report 2008: Managing Labour Mobility in the Evolving Global Economy.* Geneva: IOM.

International Organization for Migration (IOM) and International Organisation of Employers (IOE) (2014) *IOM and IOE Join Forces to Promote Ethical Recruitment of Migrant Workers.* New Release, 14 January 2014. Geneva: IOM and IOE.

International Platform on Health Worker Mobility (2018) Retrieved 1 October 2018 from www.who.int/hrh/migration/int-platform-hw-mobility/en/

International Trade Union Confederation (ITUC) (2011) *Migration: A decent work issue. General Council Resolution,* Elewijt, 17–18 October 2011.

International Trade Union Confederation (ITUC) (2018) *Global Compact on Migration: Recognition of Labour Standards and Unions,* ITUC press release, 17 July 2018. Brussels: ETUC. Retrieved 11 November 2018 from: www.ituc-csi.org/global-compact-on-migration

Irish Aid (2017) *Irish Aid and HSE partner to enhance Ireland's contribution to Global Health.* Press Release. 2 May 2017. Retrieved 20 July 2018 from: www.irishaid.ie/news-publications/press/pressreleasearchive/2017/may/irish-aid-hse-global-health/

Ishikawa, T., Ohba, H., Yokooka, Y., Nakamura, K. and Ogasawara, K. (2013) Forecasting the absolute and relative shortage of physicians in Japan using a system dynamics model approach, *Human Resources for Health* 11(1): 41.

ITUC/IndustriALL/ITF/IUF/PSI/UNI (2018) *ZERO DRAFT of the Legal Binding Instrument to Regulate, in International Human Rights Law, the Activities of Transnational Corporations and Other Business Enterprises (the Binding Treaty). Trade Union Comments.* Brussels: ITUC.

Jamison, D.T., Summers, L.H., Alleyne, G., Arrow, K.J., Berkley, S., Binagwaho, A., Bustreo, F., Evans, D., Feachem, R.G.A., Frenk, J., Ghosh, G., Goldie, S.J., Guo, Y., Gupta, S., Horton, R., Kruk, S., Saxenian, H., Soucat, A., Ulltveit-Moe, K.H. and Yamey, G. (2013) Global health 2035: a world converging within a generation. *The Lancet,* 382: 1898–1955

Japan Institute for Global Health (JIGH) (2017) 'The committee for Asia Health and Human Well-Being Initiative organise their first meeting'. Retrieved 28 November 2018 from http://jigh.org/en/news/local/1747

Joint Civil Society Statement on Business and Human Rights (2011) *Joint Civil Society Statement on the draft Guiding Principles on Business and Human Rights.* 17th Session of the UN Human Rights Council, June 15, 2011. Retrieved 20 July 2018 from www.fidh.org/en/issues/globalisation-human-rights/business-and-human-rights/Joint-Civil-Society-Statement-on,9066

Jones, H. and Pardthaisong, T. (1999) The Impact of Overseas Labour Migration on Rural Thailand: Regional, Community and Individual Dimension. *Journal of Rural Studies* 15(1): 35–47.

Khagram, S. and Levitt, P. (2005) *Towards a Field of Transnational Studies and a Sociological Transnationalism Research Program,* Hauser Center for Non-Profit Organizations, Working Paper No. 24.

Kanithasen, P., Jivakanont, V. and Boonnuch, C. (2011) *AEC 2015: Ambitions, expectations and challenges ASEAN's path towards greater economic and financial integration.* Bangkok: Bank of Thailand.

Keck, M.E. and Sikkink, K. (1998) *Activists Beyond Borders.* Ithaca: Cornell.

Keck, M.E. and Sikkink, K. (1999) Transnational advocacy networks in international and regional politics. *International Journal of Social Science*, 159: 89–101.

Khaliq, A., Broyles, R. and Mwachofi, A. (2009) Global nurse migration: its impact on developing countries and prospects for the future. *World Health and Population*, 10(3): 5–23.

King's Fund/Health Foundation/Nuffield Trust (2018) *The health care workforce in England. Make or break?* London: King's Fund/Health Foundation/Nuffield Trust.

Kofman, E. and Raghuram, P. (2010). The implications of migration for gender and care regimes in the South, in K. Hugo and N. Piper (eds.) *South–South migration: implications for Social Policy and Development.* London: Palgrave: 46–83.

Koivusalo, M. (2014) Global health policies, in Nicola Yeates (ed.) *Understanding Global Social Policy.* (2nd edition) Bristol: The Policy Press.

Koivusalo, M. and Mackintosh, M. (2011) Commercial influence and global non-governmental public action in health and pharmaceutical policies. *International Journal of Health Services.* 41(3): 539–63.

Koivusalo, M. and Ollila, E. (2014) Global health policy, in N. Yeates (ed.) *Understanding Global Social Policy.* (2nd edition) Bristol: The Policy Press.

Kruk, M.E., Gage, A.D., Arsenault, C., Jordan, K., Leslie, H.H., DeWan, S.R., Adevyi, O., Barker, P., Daelmans, B., Doubova, S.V., English, M., Elorrio, E.G., Guanais, F., Gureje, O., Hirschhorn, L.R., Jiang, L., Kelley, E., Lemango, E.T., Liljestrand, J., Malata, A., Marchant, T., Matsoso, M.P., Meara, J.G., Mohanan, M., Ndiaye, Y., Norheim, O.F., Reddy, K.S., Rowe, K.R., Slomon, J.A., Thapa, G., Twum-Danso, N.A.Y. and Pate, M. (2018) High-quality health systems in the Sustainable Development Goals era: time for a revolution. *The Lancet Global Health*, 6(11).

Labonté, R., Blouin, C., Chopra, M., Lee, K., Packer, C., Rowson, M., Schrecker, T., and Woodward, D. (2007) *Towards Health-Equitable Globalisation: Rights, Regulation and Redistribution.* Final Report to the Commission on Social Determinants of Health. Ottawa, Canada: Institute of Population Health, University of Ottawa.

Labonté, R., Sanders, D., Mathole, T., Crush, J., Chikanda, A., Dambisya, Y., Runnels, V., Packer, C., MacKenzie, A., Murphy, G.T. and Bourgeault, I.L. (2015) Health worker migration from South Africa: causes, consequences and policy responses. *Human Resources for Health*, 13: 92.

*The Lancet Global Health* (2015) Health care workers as agents of sustainable development, 3(5): PE249–E250.

*The Lancet* (2016) No health workforce, no global security. 387(10033): 2063.

Langer, A., Meleis, A., Knaul, F.M., Atun, R., Aran, M., Arreola-Ornelas, H., Bhutta, Z.A., Binagwaho, A., Bonita, R., Caglia, J.M., Claeson, M., Davies, J., Donnay, F.A., Gausman, J.M., Glickman, C., Kearns, A.D., Kendall, T., Lozano, R., Seboni, N., Sen, G., Sindhu, S., Temin, M. and Frenk, J. (2015) Women and health: the key for sustainable development. *The Lancet* 386: 1165–210.

Lethbridge, J. (2014) *Financing health care: false profits and the public good.* University of Greenwich, London: PSIRU.

Lidén, J. (2014) The World Health Organization and Global Health Governance: post-1990. *Public Health.* February 2014, 128(2): 141–147.

Little, L. and Buchan, J. (2007) *Nursing self-sufficiency/sustainability in the global context.* Geneva: International Centre on Nurse Migration.

Liua, J.X., Yevgeniy, G., Akiko, M., Bruckner, T. and Scheffler, R. (2016) *Global Health Workforce Labor Market Projections for 2030*. Policy Research Working Paper, No. 7790. Washington, D.C: World Bank.

Lopes, C. (1999) Are structural adjustment programmes an adequate response to globalization? *International Social Science Journal*, 162: 511–519.

Lorenzo, F.M., Galvez-Tan, J., Icamina, K. and Javier, L. (2007) Nurse Migration from a Source Country Perspective, Philippine Country Case Study. *Health Services Research*, 42(3 Pt2) 1406–1418. Retrieved 1 November 2018 from www.ncbi.nlm.nih.gov/pmc/articles/PMC1955369/

Lowell, L.B. and Allan Findlay, A. (2001) *Migration of Highly skilled persons from Developing Countries: impact and policy responses*. Synthesis Report. International Migration Papers 44. ILO: Geneva.

Mackey, T.K. and Liang, B.A. (2013) Rebalancing brain drain: exploring resource reallocation to address health worker migration and promote global health. *Health Policy*; 107: 66–73.

Madhavan, M.C. (1989) Dimensions of skilled migration from developing countries, in R.P. Misra (ed.) *International Division of Labour and Regional Development*. Concept Publishing: New Delhi, India: 203–247.

Mahoney, J. and Rueschemeyer, D. (eds.) (2003) *Comparative Historical Analysis in the Social Sciences*. Cambridge: Cambridge University Press.

MADE Network (2017) *Now and How: TEN ACTS for the Global Compact. A civil society vision for a transformative agenda for human mobility, migration and development*. Retrieved 20 July 2018 from http://madenetwork.org/sites/default/files/Now%20%2B%20How%20TEN%20ACTS%20for%20the%20Global%20Compact-final%20rev%203%20Nov%202017%20%28002%29.pdf

Makulec, A. (2014) *The Effects of the Philippines Bilateral Arrangements with Selected Countries*. Manila: ILO.

Martens, J. (2014) *Corporate Influence on the Business and Human Rights Agenda of the United Nations*. Aachen/Berlin/Bonn/New York: Brot für die Welt/Global Policy Forum/MISEREOR.

Martens, J. and Seitz, K. (2015) *Philanthropic Power and Development Who shapes the agenda?* Aachen/Berlin/Bonn/New York: Brot für die Welt/Global Policy Forum/MISEREOR.

Martin, P. (2005) *Merchants of Labour: Agents of the Evolving Migration Infrastructure*. International Institute for Labour Studies Discussion Paper DP/158/2005. Geneva: International Institute for Labour Studies.

McIntosh, T., Torgerson, R. and Klassen, N. (2007) *The Ethical Recruitment of Internationally Educated Health Professionals: Lessons from Abroad and Options for Canada*. Canadian Policy Research Networks Inc.

Mejia, A. (1978) Migration of Physicians and Nurses: A World Wide Picture. *International Journal of Epidemiology*, 7(3): 207–215.

Mejia, A. (1981) Health manpower migration in the Americas, *Health Policy and Education*, Volume 2, Issue 1, March 1981, Pages 1–31.

Mejia, A., Pizurki, H. and Royston, E. (1979) *Physician and nurse migration: analysis and policy implications*. Geneva: WHO.

Mensah, K., Mackintosh, M. and Henry, L. (2005) *The 'skills drain' of health professionals from the developing world: a framework for policy formulation*. London: Medact.

Meyer, T., Bridgen, P. and Andow, C. (2013) Free Movement? The Impact of Legislation, Benefit Generosity and Wages on the Pensions of European Migrants. *Population, Space and Place*, 19(6): 714–726.

Mills, E.J., Kanters, S., Hagopian, A., Bansback, N., Nachega, J., Alberton, M., Au-Yeung, C.G., Mtambo, A., Bourgeault, I.L., Luboga, S., Hogg, R.S. and Ford, N. (2011) The financial cost of doctors emigrating from sub-Saharan Africa: human capital analysis. *British Medical Journal*, 343.

Moulaert, F., Jessop, B. and Mehmood, A. (2016) Agency, structure, institutions, discourse (ASID) in urban and regional development. *International Journal of Urban Sciences*. Retrieved 3 December 2018 from DOI: 10.1080/12265934.2016.1182054

Munck, R. (2002) *Globalisation and Labour: The New 'Great Transformation'*, London: Zed.

Munck, R. and Waterman, P. (1999) *Labour worldwide in the era of globalization.* Basingstoke: MacMillan.

Muula, A.S., Panulo, B. and Maseko, F.C. (2006) The financial losses from the migration of nurses from Malawi, in *BMC Nursing*, 5(9): 1472–695.

mvoplatform (2018) *Dutch government puts trade objectives above responsible business conduct policies. 12 June 2018.* Retrieved 21 August 2018 from www.mvoplatform.nl/en/dutch-government-puts-trade-objectives-above-responsible-business-conduct-policies

Nepachem, C.C. (2009) *The Impact of the Brain Drain on Health Service Delivery in Zimbabwe: A Response Analysis*. Harare, Zimbabwe: IOM.

Newland, K. (2009) *Circular migration and human development.* Human development research paper 2009/42. New York: UNDP.

Newland, K. (2010) The Governance of International Migration: mechanisms, processes, and institutions. *Global Governance*, 16: 331–343.

Newman, C. (2014) Time to address gender discrimination and inequality in the health workforce. *Human Resources for Health*, 12(25).

O'Brien, P. and Gostin, L. (2011) Health Worker Shortages and Global Justice Health Worker Shortages and Global Justice, Millbank Memorial Fund, 2011. University of Melbourne Legal Studies Research Paper No. 569.

O'Brien, R. (2000) Workers and world order: the tentative transformation of the international union movement. *Review of International Studies*, 26(4): 533–555.

O'Brien, R. (2014) Global labour policy, in N. Yeates (ed.) *Understanding Global Social Policy* (2nd edition). Bristol The Policy Press.

Office of the High Commissioner of Human Rights (OHCHR) (2014) Dataset for International Convention on the Protection of the Rights of All Migrant Workers and Members of their Families. Retrieved 15 September 2018 from http://indicators.ohchr.org/

Orenstein, M.A. (2008) *Privatizing pensions: the transnational campaign for social security reform*. Princeton, N.J: Princeton.

Orenstein, M.A. and Schmitz, H.P. (2006) The New Transnationalism and Comparative Politics. *Comparative Politics*, 38(4): 479–500.

Organization for Economic Cooperation and Development (OECD) (1976) OECD Declaration on International Investment and Multinational Enterprises. Paris: OECD. Retrieved 28 February 2019 from www.oecd.org/daf/inv/investment-policy/oecddeclarationoninternationalinvestmentandmultinationalenterprises.htm

Organization for Economic Cooperation and Development (OECD) (2007) *Immigrant Health Workers in OECD Countries in the Broader Context of Highly Skilled Migration.* International Migration Outlook. Paris: OECD.

Organization for Economic Cooperation and Development (OECD) (2008) *The Looming Crisis in the Health Workforce: How can OECD countries respond?* OECD Health Policy studies. Paris: OECD.

Organization for Economic Cooperation and Development (OECD) (2010) *International Migration of Health Workers: Improving International Cooperation to Address the Global Health Workforce Crisis.* Policy Brief. Paris: OECD.

Organization for Economic Cooperation and Development (OECD) (2015) *International Migration Outlook.* Paris: OECD.

Organization for Economic Cooperation and Development and World Health Organization (OECD/WHO) (2016) *Draft guiding principles for the compilation of a Minimum Data Set for the monitoring of health workforce migration.* Regular national reporting instrument. Part 2: Quantitative information – Minimum Data Sets. OECD/WHO: Paris/Geneva.

Organization for Economic Cooperation and Development, International Labour Organization and World Health Organization (OECD/ILO/WHO) (2017) *Working for Health.* Geneva: WHO.

Organization for Economic Cooperation and Development (OECD) (2018) *What would make Global Skills Partnerships work in practice?* Migration Policy Debates, No. 15, May 2018. Paris: OECD.

Organization for Economic Cooperation and Development/World Health Organization/World Bank Group (OECD/WHO/World Bank) (2018) *Delivering Quality Health Services: A Global Imperative.* Geneva: WHO.

Padarath, A., Chamberlain, C., McCoy, D., Ntuli, A., Rowson, M. and Loewenson, R. (2003) *Health personnel in southern Africa: confronting maldistribution and brain drain.* Equinet Discussion Paper No. 3. Harare, Regional Network for Equity in Health in Southern Africa.

Pagett, C. and Padarath, A. (2007) *A review of codes and protocols for the migration of health workers.* The Regional Network for Equity in Health in east and southern Africa (EQUINET) with the Health Systems Trust. EQUINET Discussion Paper 50.

Paina, L., Ungureanu, M. and Olsavsky, V. (2016) Implementing the Code of Practice on International Recruitment in Romania – Exploring the current state of implementation and what Romania is doing to retain its domestic health workforce. *Human Resources for Health.* 2016; 14(Suppl. 1).

Pan-American Health Organization/World Health Organization (PAHO/WHO) (2002) *Trade in Health Services: Global, Regional, and Country Perspectives.* Washington, DC: PAHO.

Pan-American Health Organization (PAHO) (1966) *Migration of Health Personnel, Scientists, and Engineers.* Latin America Scientific Publications No. 142. Washington, DC: PAHO.

Pierson, P. (2000) Not Just What, but When: timing and sequence in political processes. *Studies in American Political Development,* 14(1): 72–92.

Pillinger, J. (2007) *Feminisation of migration: experiences and opportunities in Ireland.* Dublin: Immigrant Council of Ireland.

Pillinger, J (2010) *Building trade union solidarity and action for workers on the move.* Kenya National Report. Ferney-Voltaire, Public Services International.

Pillinger, J. (2011a) *Quality Health care Workers and Workers on the Move: Ghana National Report.* Ferney-Voltaire: Public Services International.

Pillinger, J. (2011b) *Quality Health care Workers and Workers on the Move: South Africa National Report.* Ferney-Voltaire: Public Services International.

Pillinger, J. (2012) *Quality Health care Workers and Workers on the Move: Australia National Report.* Ferney-Voltaire: Public Services International.

Pillinger, J. (20 13) *Quality Health care Workers and Workers on the Move: Philippines National Report.* Ferney-Voltaire: Public Services International.

Pillinger, J. (2015) *Migration and decent work for public service workers: PSI Nigeria report.* Ferney-Voltaire: Public Services International.

Pittman, P., Davis, C., Shaffer, F., Herrera, C.N. and Bennett, C. (2014) Perceptions of Employment-based Discrimination Among Newly Arrived Foreign-Educated Nurses. *American Journal of Nursing*, 114(1): 26–35.

Plotnikova, E. (2014) The role of bilateral agreements in the regulation of health worker migration, in J. Buchan, M. Wismar, I.A. Glinos and J. Bremner (eds.), *Health professional mobility in a changing Europe: New dynamics, mobile individuals and diverse responses.* Vol. II. Geneva: World Health Organization.

Pomp, R. and Oldman, O. (1977) *Legal and administrative aspects of compensation, taxation and related policy measures: suggestions for an optimal policy mix.* UNCTAD TC/B/C.6/AC.4/7 28 December 1977.

Poppe, A., Wojczewski, S., Taylor, K., Kutalek, R. and Peersman, W. (2016) The views of migrant health workers living in Austria and Belgium on return migration to sub-Saharan Africa. *Human Resources for Health* 14(Suppl. 1).

Poz, M.R., Quain, E.E., O'Neil, M., McCaffery, J., Elzinga, G. and Martineau, T. (2006) Addressing the health workforce crisis: Towards a common approach, *Human Resources for Health* 4: 21.

Pozo-Martin, F., Nove, A., Lopes, S. C., Campbell, J., Buchan, J., Dussault, G., Kunjumen, T., Cometto, G. and Siyam, A. (2017). Health workforce metrics pre- and post-2015: a stimulus to public policy and planning. *Human Resources for Health*, 15(1), 14.

Public Services International (PSI) (2017a) *A better future with public health for all. Manifesto of the PSI Human Right to Health Global Campaign.* Ferney Voltaire, PSI. Retrieved 11 November 2018 from www.world-psi.org/en/manifesto-psi-human-right-health-global-campaign

Public Services International (PSI) (2010) *PSI Policy on labour migration, development and quality public services.* 10th Inter-American Regional Conference (IAMRECON), Cartagena, Colombia, 11–12 September 2010.

Public Services International (PSI) (2012a) *Resolution 25: Labour brokers/employment agencies in the public sector.* The 29th World Congress of Public Services International (PSI), Durban, South Africa, 27–30 November 2012.

Public Services International (PSI) (2012b) *Resolution 37: Ethical International Recruitment.* 29th World Congress of Public Services International (PSI), Durban, South Africa, 27–30 November 2012.

Public Services International (PSI) (2015) *Project on Decent Work and Social Protection for Migrant Workers in the Public Services.* Ferney-Voltaire: PSI.

Public Services International (PSI) (2017b) *Bilateral Agreement Between Germany and the Philippines on the Deployment of Filipino Health Professionals to Germany: Documentation of the Triple Win Project* (unpublished). Ferney-Voltaire: PSI.

Public Services International (PSI) (2018) *Conflict of interest: how corporations that profit from privatisation are helping to write UN standards on PPPs.* November 2018. Ferney-Voltaire: PSI.

Public Services International (undated) *PSI Policy Statement on International Migration with Particular Reference to Health Services.* Ferney-Voltaire: PSI.

Ramaswamy, N.S. and Shah, R. (1973) *Study of the outflow: Mechanics, consequences for developing and developed countries. An international policy to influence net outflow of trained personnel from developing countries.* United Nations Publication ESA/SAT/AC.3/4 October 24, 1973.

Redfoot, D.L. and Houser, A.N. (2005) *We Shall Travel On: Quality of care, economic development, and the international migration of long-term care workers.* Washington, DC: AARP Public Policy Institute.

Reichenbach, L. (ed.) (2007) *Exploring the Gender Dimensions of the Global Health Workforce.* Cambridge: Global Equity Initiative Harvard University.

Reinecke, W. (1998) *Global Public Policy: Governing without government?* Washington, DC: Brookings Institution Press.

Republic of the Philippines and Kingdom of Bahrain (2007) *Bahrain: Memorandum of Agreement between the Government of the Republic of the Philippines and the Government of the Kingdom of Bahrain on Health Services Cooperation.* Retrieved 28 November 2017 from www.poea.gov.ph/laborinfo/bilateralLB/BLA_PH_Bahrain2007.pdf

Republic of Uganda (undated) *Rules and regulations governing the recruitment and employment of Ugandan migrant workers abroad.* Retrieved 14 May 2018 from www.ilo.org/dyn/migpractice/docs/228/Rules

Roffe, P. (1985) Transfer of Technology: UNCTAD's Draft International Code of Conduct. *International Lawyer*, 19(2): 689–707.

Rueschemeyer, D. and Stephens, J. (1997) Comparing Historical Sequences: A powerful tool for causal analysis. *Comparative Social Research*, 17: 55–72.

Ruger, J.P. (2012) Global health governance as shared health governance. *Journal of Epidemiology and Community Health*, 66: 653–661.

Sassen, S. (2000) Women's burden: counter-geographies of globalisation and the feminisation of survival. *Journal of International Affairs*, 53(2): 503–524.

Sauvant, K.P. (2015) The Negotiations of the United Nations Code of Conduct on Transnational Corporations: Experience and Lessons Learned. *Journal of World Investment & Trade* 16: 11–87.

Save the Children. (2015) *A wake-up call: lessons from Ebola for the world's health systems.* London: Save the Children.

Schäferhoff, M., Fewer, S., Kraus, J., Richter, E., Summers, L.H., Sundewall, J., Yamey, G. and Jamison, D.T. (2015) How much donor financing for health is channelled to global versus country-specific aid functions? *The Lancet*, 386 (10011): 2436–2441.

Scheffler, R. and Fulton, B. (2013) Needs-based estimates for the health workforce, in A. Soucat, R. Scheffler and T. Ghebreyesus, (eds.) *The labor market for health workers in Africa: a new look at the crisis.* Washington, DC: World Bank.

Scheffler, R. and Arnold, D. (2018). Projecting shortages and surpluses of doctors and nurses in the OECD: What looms ahead. *Health Economics, Policy and Law*, 14(2): 274–290.

Scheffler, R., Cometto, G., Tulenko, K., Bruckner, T., Liu, J., Keuffel, E.L., Preker, A., Stilwell, B., Brasileiro, J. and Campbell, J. (2016) *Health workforce requirements for universal health coverage and the Sustainable Development Goals.* Background paper No. 1 to the WHO Global Strategy on Human Resources for Health: Workforce 2030. Human Resources for Health Observer Series No. 17. Geneva: WHO.

Scheil-Adlung, X. and Nove, A. (2016) Global estimates of the size of the health workforce contributing to the health economy: the potential for creating decent work in achieving universal health coverage, in: J. Buchan, I. Dhillon and J. Campbell, (eds.) *Health employment and economic growth: an evidence base.* Geneva: WHO.

Scheil-Adlung, X., Behrendt, T. and Wong, L. (2015) Health sector employment: A tracer indicator for universal health coverage in national Social Protection Floors. *Human Resources for Health*, 13(66): 1–8.

Sen, A. (2015) Universal health care: the affordable dream. *Guardian* (London), 6 January 2015.

Shaffer, F.A., Bakhshi, M., Dutka, J.T. and Phillips, J. (2016) Code for ethical international recruitment practices: the CGFNS alliance case study. *Human Resources for Health* 14(Suppl 1): 31.

Shah, R.S. (2010) (ed.) *The International Migration of Health Workers*. Palgrave Macmillan, London.

Sieleunou, I. (2011). Health worker migration and universal health care in Sub-Saharan Africa. *The Pan African Medical Journal*, 10(55).

Sigler, N. (2010) Global Health, Justice and the Brain Drain: A Trade Union Perspective, in R.S. Shah, (ed.) *The International Migration of Health Workers*. Palgrave Macmillan, London.

Siyam, A. and dal Poz, R. (2014) *WHO Migration of Health Workers: The WHO Global Code of Practice and the global economic crisis*. WHO Health Workforce Department, Health Systems and Innovation. Geneva: WHO.

Siyam, A., Zurn, P., Rø, O.C., Gedik, G., Ronquillo, K. and Co, C.J. (2013) Monitoring the implementation of the WHO global code of practice on the international recruitment of health personnel. *Bulletin of the World Health Organization*, 91(11): 816–823.

Skocpol, T. and Pierson, P. (2002) Historical Institutionalism in Contemporary Political Science, in I. Katznelson and H. Milner (eds.) *Political Science: State of the Discipline*. New York: W.W. Norton.

South Centre (2004) Analysis of actual liberalisation versus GATS commitments of quad members: mode 4 and health services. South Centre Analytical Note June, SC/TADP/AN/SV/5.

Southern African Health Ministers (SADC) (2001) Statement by SADC Health Ministers on the Recruitment of Health Personnel by Developed Countries. Pretoria: SADC.

Sri Lanka Bureau of Foreign Employment (undated) *Code of Ethical Conduct for Licensed Foreign Employment Agencies/ Licensees*. Colombo: SLBFE.

Standing, H. (2000) Gender – a Missing Dimension in Human Resource Policy and Planning for Health Reforms. Special Article. *Human Resources Development Journal*, 4(1).

Stenberg, K., Hanssen, O., Edejer, T.-T., Bertram, M., Brindley, C., Meshreky, A., Rosen, J.E., Stover, J., Verboom, P., Sanders, R. and Soucat, A. (2017) Financing transformative health systems towards achievement of the health Sustainable Development Goals: a model for projected resource needs in 67 low-income and middle-income countries. *The Lancet Global Health*, 5(9): 875–887.

Storeng, K. (2014) The GAVI Alliance and the 'Gates approach' to health system strengthening in *Global Public Health*, 9(8): 865–879. Retrieved 14 June 2018 from www.ncbi.nlm.nih.gov/pmc/articles/PMC4166931/pdf/rgph-9-865.pdf

Tankwanchi, A., Vermund, S.H. and Perkins, D.D. (2014) Has the WHO global code of practice on the international recruitment of health personnel been effective? *The Lancet Global Health*, 2(7): 390–391.

Tarrow, S. (1995) The Europeanisation of conflict: reflections from a social movement perspective, *West European Politics*, 18(2): 223–251.

Taylor, A.L. and Dhillon, I.S. (2011) The WHO Global Code of Practice on the International Recruitment of Health Personnel: The Evolution of Global Health Diplomacy. *Global Health Governance*, 5(1); Georgetown Public Law Research Paper No. 11–140; Georgetown Law and Economics Research Paper No. 11–31.

Taylor, A.L. and Dhillon, I.S. (2012). Transformative Diplomacy: Negotiation of the WHO Global Code of Practice on the International Recruitment of Health Personnel, in

E. Rosskam and I. Kickbush, (eds.) *Negotiating and Navigating Global Health Diplomacy* (1st Edition). London: World Scientific Books: 101–128.

Tjadens, F., Weilandt, C. and Eckert, J. (2013) *Mobility of Health Professionals: Health Systems, Work Conditions, Patterns of Health Workers' Mobility and Implications for Policy Makers.* Berlin: Springer-Verlag.

Tomblin-Murphy, G., MacKenzie, A., Waysome, B., Guy-Walker, J., Palmer, R., Rose, A.E., Rigby, J., Labonté, R. and Bourgeault, I.L. (2016) A mixed-methods study of health worker migration from Jamaica. *Human Resources for Health.* 30(14) (Suppl. 1): 36.

Townsend, P. (1993) *The International Analysis of Poverty.* Hemel Hempstead: Harvester Wheatsheaf.

Truong, T.D. (1996) Gender, international migration and social reproduction: implications for theory, policy, research and networking. *Asian and Pacific Migration Journal* 5: 27–52.

United Nations (UN) (1979) *Report of the United Nations Conference on Sciences and Technology for Development,* Vienna 20–31 August 1979 E.79.I.21 and Corrigenda. New York: UN

United Nations Commission for Social Development (UN CfSD) (1967) *Report on the 18th Session, 6–23 March 1968,* E/4324, E/CN.5/416. New York: UN.

United Nations Conference on Science and Technology for Development (UNCSTD) (1979) *Vienna Programme of Action on Science and Technology.* R.240, adopted at UNCSTD Conference, 20 to 31 August 1979.

United Nations Conference on Trade and Development (UNCTAD) (1971a) *The channels and mechanisms for the transfer of technology from developed to developing countries,* TD/B/AC.11/5. New York: UNCTAD.

United Nations Conference on Science and Technology for Development UNCTAD (1971b) Intergovernmental Group on Transfer of Technology, session 1, June 1971. TD/B/365. New York: UNCTAD

United Nations Conference on Science and Technology for Development UNCTAD (1973) Intergovernmental Group on Transfer of Technology, session 2, June 1971. TD/B/424. New York: UNCTAD

United Nations Conference on Science and Technology for Development UNCTAD (1974) Intergovernmental Group on Transfer of Technology, session 3, June 1971. TD/B/520. New York: UNCTAD

United Nations Conference on Trade and Development (UNCTAD) (1975) *The reverse transfer of technology: economic effects of the outflow of trained personnel from developing countries.* New York: UNCTAD.

United Nations Conference on Trade and Development (UNCTAD) (1977) Reverse Transfer of Technology, Resolution 32/192 19 December 1977. New York: UNCTAD.

United Nations Conference on Trade and Development (UNCTAD) (1978a) *Case studies in reverse transfer of technology: a survey of problems and policies in India.* Geneva: UNCTAD

United Nations Conference on Trade and Development (UNCTAD) (1978b) *Case studies in reverse transfer of technology: a survey of problems and policies in Sri Lanka.* Geneva: UNCTAD.

United Nations Conference on Trade and Development (UNCTAD) (1978c) *Developmental aspects of the reverse transfer of technology.* TD/B/C.6/41. New York: UNCTAD.

United Nations Conference on Trade and Development (UNCTAD) (1978d) *Report of the Group of Government Experts on Reverse Transfer of Technology.* TD/B/C.6/28. February/March 1978. New York: UNCTAD

United Nations Conference on Trade and Development (UNCTAD) (1978e) *Reverse Transfer of Technology*, Resolution 33/151 20 December 1978. New York: UNCTAD.

United Nations Conference on Trade and Development (UNCTAD) (1979a) *The reverse transfer of technology: a survey of its main features, causes and policy implications*. UNCTAD TD/B/C.6/47. New York: UNCTAD.

United Nations Conference on Trade and Development (UNCTAD) (1979b) *Technology: Development aspects of the reverse transfer of technology*, TC/239, UNCTAD Secretariat.

United Nations Conference on Trade and Development (UNCTAD) (1979c) *Development aspects of the reverse transfer of technology: an assessment of the results achieved at the fifth session of the United Nations Conference on Trade and Development*. A/34/425, Annex. New York: UNCTAD.

United Nations Conference on Trade and Development (UNCTAD) (1979d) *Reverse transfer of technology: a survey of its main features, causes and policy implications*. Report of the General Secretary. A/34/593. New York: UNCTAD.

United Nations Conference on Trade and Development (UNCTAD) (1979e) *Development aspects of the reverse transfer of technology*. A/C.2/34/L.130, 14 December 1979. New York: UNCTAD.

United Nations Conference on Trade and Development (UNCTAD) (1979f) *Report of the United Nations Conference on Science and Technology for Development. Vienna, 20–31 August 1979*. No. E.79.I.21 and corrigenda. New York: UNCTAD.

United Nations Conference on Trade and Development (UNCTAD) (1981) *Proceedings of the United Nations Conference on Trade and Development, Fifth Session, Manila, 7 May–3 June 1979 Volume I, Report and Annexes*. New York: UNCTAD.

United Nations Conference on Trade and Development (UNCTAD) (1982) *Report of the Intergovernmental Group of Experts on the Feasibility of Measuring Human Resource Flows. Geneva, 30 August–6 September 1982*. TD/B/C.6/AC.8/2, Annexes I and II. Geneva: UNCTAD.

United Nations Conference on Trade and Development (UNCTAD) (1983a) *Report of the Meeting of Governmental Experts on the reverse transfer of technology. September*. UNCTAD: Geneva.

United Nations Conference on Trade and Development (UNCTAD) (1983b) *Towards an integrated approach to international skill exchange: proposals for policy and action on reverse transfer of technology*. TD/B/AC.35/2. UNCTAD: Geneva.

United Nations Conference on Trade and Development (UNCTAD) (1983c) *Consideration of Recommendations on Policies and Concrete Measures with a view to mitigating the adverse consequences for the developing countries of the reverse transfer of technology, including the proposal for the establishment of an international labour compensatory facility*. TD/B/AC.35/2. 17 June. UNCTAD: Geneva.

United Nations Conference on Trade and Development (UNCTAD) (1984a) *Preliminary Outline of a Set of Guidelines on the Reverse Transfer of Technology*. TD/B/AC.35/12 and Corr.1. New York: UNCTAD.

United Nations Conference on Trade and Development (UNCTAD) (1984b) *Proposals on Concrete Measures to Mitigate the Adverse Impact of Reverse Transfer of Technology on Developing Countries, Note by the UNCTAD Secretariat*. TD/B/AC.35/6. Geneva: UNCTAD.

United Nations Conference on Trade and Development (UNCTAD) (1985a) *Report of the Third Meeting of Government Experts on the Reverse Transfer of Technology, held at Geneva, 20th August–4th September 1985*. TD/B/1973-TD/B/AC.35/14. Geneva: UNCTAD.

United Nations Conference on Trade and Development (UNCTAD) (1985b) *Trade and Development Board.* TC/B/L/778, 11 November 1985. New York: UNCTAD.

United Nations Conference on Trade and Development (UNCTAD) (1985c) *The history of UNCTAD 1964–1984.* New York: UNCTAD.

United Nations Conference on Trade and Development (UNCTAD) (1986) *Report of the Trade and Development Board Vol. II (31st Session), General Assembly Official Records, 40th Session.* Suppl. No. 15 (A/40/15). New York: UNCTAD.

United Nations Conference on Trade and Development (UNCTAD) (1987) *Trends and current situation on reverse transfer of technology.* Paper prepared for the Fourth meeting of Governmental Experts on the reverse transfer of technology, 31 August, Geneva. Geneva: UNCTAD.

United Nations Conference on Trade and Development (UNCTAD) (2001) *Transfer of Technology.* UNCTAD Series on issues in international investment agreements. New York and Geneva: UNCTAD.

United Nations Conference on Trade and Development (UNCTAD) (2014) *Transfer of Technology and knowledge sharing for development. Science, technology and innovation issues for developing countries.* UNCTAD Current Studies on Science, Technology and Innovation, No. 8.

United Nations Conference on Trade and Development (UNCTAD) (2017) *World Investment Report 2017: Investment and the digital economy.* UNCTAD: Geneva.

United Nations Development Programme (UNDP) (2012a) *Evaluation of UNDP Partnership with Global Funds and Philanthropic Foundations.* New York: UNDP.

United Nations Development Programme (UNDP) (2012b) *Management response to the evaluation of UNDP partnerships with global funds and philanthropic foundations.* (DP/2012/24). New York: UNDP.

United Nations Development Programme (UNDP/Foundation Center/Rockefeller Philanthropy Advisors/Conrad N. Hilton Foundation/MasterCard Foundation/Ford Foundation) (2014) *A Post-2015 Partnership Platform for Philanthropy.* Background. New York: UNDP.

United Nations Economic and Social Committee (UN ECOSOC) (1964) Training of National Technical Personnel for Accelerated Industrialisation of Developing Countries. Report of the Secretary-General. 37th Session, E/3901, E/3901/Corr.1, E/3901/Corr.2, E/3901/Add.1, E/3901/Add.1/Corr.1, E/3901/Add.2, E/3901/Add.2/Corr.1, E/3901/Add.2/Corr.2. 3 June 1964. New York: ECOSOC.

UNESCAP (2017) *Regional road map for implementing the 2030 Agenda for Sustainable Development in Asia and the Pacific.* ESCAP, Fourth Asia-Pacific Forum on Sustainable Development, Bangkok, March. Retrieved 14 July 2017 from www.unescap.org/sites/default/files/pre-ods/B1700338_Report%20No.%202_Rev.%201_E_replaced%2031%20Mar%2017.pdf.

United Nations Educational, Scientific and Cultural Organisation (UNESCO) (1962) *Recommendation concerning technical education adopted in 1962 by the General Conference of UNESCO.* Paris: UNESCO.

United Nations Educational, Scientific and Cultural Organisation (UNESCO) (1966) *Records of the General Conference.* Paris: UNESCO.

United Nations Educational, Scientific and Cultural Organisation (UNESCO) (1968a) *The problem of emigration of scientists and technologists: General appraisal of the phenomenon.* Preliminary Report prepared at the request of the Advisory Committee of the Economic and Social Council on the Application of Science and Technology to Development, SC/WS/57, 29 February 1968, Paris.

United Nations Educational, Scientific and Cultural Organisation (UNESCO) (1968b) *Records of the General Conference*. Paris: UNESCO.

United Nations Educational, Scientific and Cultural Organisation (UNESCO) (1968) *Resolutions and Decisions Adopted by the Executive Board at its 78th Session, Paris 13 May–21 June 1968*. 78 EX/Decisions. Paris: UNESCO: 28.

United Nations Educational, Scientific and Cultural Organisation (UNESCO) (1971) *Scientists Abroad: a study of the international movement of persons in Science and Technology*. UNESCO: Paris.

United Nations Educational, Scientific and Cultural Organisation (UNESCO) (1972) *Records of the General Conference*. Paris: UNESCO.

United Nations Educational, Scientific and Cultural Organisation (UNESCO) (1974) *Emigration of Talent. Report of the Director-General, 98 EX/29, 20 September 1974*. Paris: UNESCO.

United Nations Educational, Scientific and Cultural Organisation (UNESCO) (1984) Brain Drain or the Migration of Talent and Skills, in the UN Department of Economic and Social Affairs, Population Distribution, Migration and Development: 427–441. New York: UNESCO.

United Nations Educational, Scientific and Cultural Organisation (UNESCO) (1987) *The brain drain problem: its causes, consequences, remedies and the role of UNESCO in this regard*. 127 EX/SP/RAP.2, 27 August 1987. UNESCO: Paris.

United Nations Educational, Scientific and Cultural Organisation (UNESCO) (1998) *World declaration on higher education for the twenty-first century: Vision and action*. World Conference on Higher Education. Paris: UNESCO.

United Nations General Assembly (UNGA) (1969) *Declaration on Social Progress and Development*. Proclaimed by General Assembly resolution 2542 (XXIV) of 11 December 1969. New York: UNGA.

United Nations General Assembly (UNGA) (1970) *International Development Strategy for the Second United Nations Development Decade*, UN General Assembly Resolution 2626 (XXV), 24 October 1970, paragraph 43. New York: UNGA.

United Nations General Assembly (UNGA) (1974a) *Declaration on the Establishment of a New International Economic Order*. A/RES/3201 (S-VI). New York: UNGA.

United Nations General Assembly (UNGA) (1974b) *Programme of Action on the Establishment of a New International Economic Order*. A/RES/3202 (S-VI). New York: UNGA.

United Nations General Assembly (UNGA) (2012) *Global health and foreign policy*. Sixty-seventh session, A/67/L.36. New York: UNGA.

United Nations General Assembly (UNGA) (2015) *Transforming our world: the 2030 Agenda for Sustainable Development*, A/RES/70/17/35. New York: UNGA.

United Nations General Assembly (UNGA) (2016) *Global health and foreign policy: health employment and economic growth*. Resolution adopted by the General Assembly on 15 December 2016. New York: UNGA.

United Nations General Assembly (UNGA) (2018) *Global Compact for Safe, Orderly and Regular Migration*. New York: UNGA.

United Nations Human Rights Council (UNHRC) (2008) *Protect, Respect and Remedy: a Framework for Business and Human Rights*. Report of the Special Representative of the Secretary-General on the issue of human rights and transnational corporations and other business enterprises, John Ruggie. Geneva: UNHRC.

United Nations Human Rights Council (UNHRC) (2011) *Report of the Special Representative of the Secretary-General on the issue of human rights and transnational corporations and other business enterprises, John Ruggie. Guiding Principles on Business and Human Rights: Implementing the United Nations "Protect, Respect and Remedy" Framework.* Geneva: UNHRC.

United Nations Human Rights Council (UNHRC) (2013) *Summary of discussions of the Forum on Business and Human Rights, prepared by the Chairperson, Makarim Wibisono.* Human Rights Council Forum on Business and Human Rights Second session 2–4 December 2013, A/HRC/FBHR/2013/4. Geneva: UNHRC.

United Nations Human Rights Council (UNHRC) (2017a) *2017 United Nations Forum on Business and Human Rights,* Geneva, 27–29 November. Geneva: UNHRC.

United Nations Human Rights Council (UNHRC) (2017b) Elements for the draft legally binding instrument on transnational corporations and other business enterprises with respect to human rights. Chairmanship of the OEIGWG established by HRC Res. A/HRC/RES/26/9. Geneva: UNHRC.

United Nations Human Rights Council (UNHRC) (2018a) *Report of the Working Group on the issue of human rights and transnational corporations and other business enterprises,* 02/05/2018, A/HRC/38/48. Geneva: UNHRC. Geneva: UNHRC.

United Nations Human Rights Council (UNHRC) (2018b) *Corporate human rights due diligence: emerging practices, challenges and ways forward.* Summary of the report of the Working Group on Business and Human Rights to the General Assembly, October 2018 (A/73/163), Geneva: UNHRC.

United Nations Research Institute for Social Development (UNRISD) (2016) *Policy Innovations for Transformative Change: UNRISD Flagship Report 2016.* Geneva: UNRISD.

United Nations Secretary-General (UNSG) (1967) Development and Utilisation of Human Resources in Developing Countries, Report by the Secretary-General, E/4353/Add.l (3 May 1967), E/4353-E (8 May 1967), E/4353/Add.l/Corr.l (5 June 1967).

United Nations Secretary-General (UNSG) (1964) Training of National Technical Personnel for Accelerated Industrialisation of Developing Countries, Report by the Secretary-General, E/3901, E/3901/Add.1, E/3901/Add.2., 3 June 1964, UN New York: ECOSOC.

United Nations Secretary-General (UNSG) (1968) *Outflow of trained personnel from developing countries to developed countries,* A7294. New York: UNSG.

United Nations Secretary-General (UNSG) (1972) *Outflow of Trained Personnel from Developing to Developed Countries,* Report of the Secretary-General, E/C.8/21. New York: UN.

United Nations Secretary-General (UNSG) (1980) *Establishment of an international labour compensatory facility.* Report of the Secretary-General A/35/198 (3 October 1980). New York: UN.

United Nations Secretary-General (UNSG) (1982) *Report on establishment of an international labour compensatory facility.* A/36/483. Proceedings of the General Assembly, 36th session 1981–1982. New York: UN.

United Nations Secretary-General (UNSG) (2013) *Report of the Secretary-General on enhanced cooperation between the United Nations and all relevant partners, in particular the private sector.* A/68/326. New York: UN.

United States Department of Health, Education and Welfare (US DHEW) (1975) *International Migration of Physicians and Nurses: An annotated bibliography.* DHEW Publication No. (HRA) 75–28. Public Health Service, Health Resources Administration. Washington, DC: US DHEW.

UN Women (2017) *Turning Promises into Action: Gender Equality in the 2030 Agenda.* Summary Report. New York: UN Women.

Van de Pas, R., Mans, L., de Ponte, G. and Dambisya, Y. (2016) The Code of Practice and its enduring relevance in Europe and East and Southern Africa. *Human Resources for Health*, 2016. 14 (Suppl. 1).

Wickramasekara, P. (2002) Asian Labour Migration. Issues and Challenges in an Era of Globalization. ILO International Migration Papers #57, International Migration programme, Geneva.

Wickramasekara, P. (2008) Globalisation, international labour migration, and the rights of migrant workers. *Third World Quarterly* 29(7): 1247–1264.

Wickramasekara, P. (2010) International migration and employment in the post-reforms economy of Sri Lanka. Geneva: ILO.

Wickramasekara, P. (2011) *Circular Migration: A triple win or a dead end?* Global Union Research Network Discussions Papers No. 15. Geneva: ILO.

Wickramasekara, P. (2014) *Assessment of the impact of migration of health professionals on the labour market and health sector performance in destination countries. A report prepared for the EU–ILO project on Decent work across borders: a pilot project for migrant health professionals and skilled workers.* Manila: ILO Country Office for the Philippines.

Wickramasekara, P. (2015) *Bilateral agreements and memoranda of understanding on migration of low-skilled workers: a review.* International Migration Papers No. 120. ILO: Geneva.

Wickramasekara, P. and Ruhunage, L.K. (2018) *Good practices and provisions in multilateral and bilateral labour agreements and memoranda of understanding.* ILO Country Office for Bangladesh.

Willets, A. and Martineau, T. (2004) *Ethical international recruitment of health professionals: will codes of practice protect developing country health systems?* Liverpool: Liverpool School of Tropical Medicine

Wismar, M., Maier, C.B., Glinos, I.A., Dussault, G. and Figueras, J. (eds.). (2011). *Health professional mobility and health systems: Evidence from 17 European countries.* Observatory studies series 23. Geneva: WHO.

West Asia–North Africa Institute (WANA) (2015) The case for establishing an international labour compensatory facility. Amman: WANA Institute.

WONCA (2002) (International Council of Nurses and World Organization of National Colleges, Academies and Academic Associations of General Practitioners/Family Physicians) *A Code of Practice for the International Recruitment of Health care Professionals: The Melbourne Manifesto.* Melbourne: WHA/WONCA.

World Bank (2004) *Doing business in 2004: Understanding regulation.* Washington, DC: World Bank.

World Bank (2015) *Global Financing Facility in Support of Every Woman Every Child: Business Plan.* Washington, DC: World Bank.

World Bank (2017) *World Development Indicators.* Washington, DC: World Bank.

World Employment Federation (formerly CIETT) (2016) *Code of Conduct.* Brussels: World Employment Federation.

World Health Assembly (WHA) (1961a) *Declaration concerning the Granting of Independence to Colonial Countries and Peoples and the Tasks of the World Health Organization* (WHA14.58). Geneva: WHO.

World Health Assembly (1961b) *Fourteenth World Health Assembly, New Delhi, 7–24 February 1961: part II: plenary meetings: verbatim records: committees: minutes and reports.* World Health Organization. Retrieved June 2018 from http://apps.who.int/iris/handle/10665/85738

World Health Assembly (WHA) (1968) *Study of the Criteria for assessing the Equivalence of Medical Degrees in Different Countries* (WHA21.35). Geneva: WHO.

World Health Assembly (WHA) (1969a) *Study of the Criteria for assessing the Equivalence of Medical Degrees in Different Countries* (WHA22.42). Geneva: WHO.

World Health Assembly (WHA) (1969b) *Training of Medical Personnel and the "Brain Drain"* (WHA22.51). Geneva: WHO.

World Health Assembly (WHA) (1969c) *Second United Nations Development Decade* (WHA22.55). Geneva: WHO.

World Health Assembly (1971) *Twenty-fourth World Health Assembly, Geneva, 4–20 May 1971: Part II: plenary meetings: verbatim records: committees: summary records and reports.* Geneva: WHO. Retrieved June 2018 from www.who.int/iris/handle/10665/85835

World Health Assembly (WHA) (1972) *Training of National Health personnel* (WHA25.42). Geneva: WHO.

World Health Assembly (1975) *Twenty-eighth World Health Assembly, Geneva, 13–30 May 1975: part II: verbatim records of plenary meetings: summary records and reports of committees.* Geneva: WHO. Retrieved June 2018 from www.who.int/iris/handle/10665/86023

World Health Assembly (1976a) *Twenty-ninth World Health Assembly, Geneva, 3–21 May 1976: part II: verbatim records of plenary meetings: summary records and reports of committees.* World Health Organization. Retrieved June 2018 from www.who.int/iris/handle/10665/86030

World Health Assembly (WHA) (1976b) *Health manpower development* (WHA29.72). Geneva: WHO.

World Health Assembly (1977a) *Thirtieth World Health Assembly, Geneva, 2–19 May 1977: part II: verbatim records of plenary meetings: summary records and reports of committees.* Geneva: WHO. Retrieved June 2018 from www.who.int/iris/handle/10665/86037.

World Health Assembly (WHA) (1977b) *The role of nursing/midwifery personnel in primary health care teams* (WHA30.48). Geneva: WHO.

World Health Assembly (1978a) *Thirty-first World Health Assembly, Geneva, 8–24 May 1978: part II: verbatim records of plenary meetings: summary records and reports of committees* Geneva: WHO. Retrieved June 2018 from www.who.int/iris/handle/10665/86044

World Health Assembly (WHA) (1978b) *Health conditions of the Arab population in the occupied Arab territories including Palestine* (WHA31.38). Geneva: WHO

World Health Assembly (WHA) (1979) *Formulating strategies for health for all by the year 2000: guiding principles and essential issues. Annex 2.* Geneva: WHO.

World Health Assembly (1983a) *Thirty-sixth World Health Assembly, Geneva, 2–16 May 1983: verbatim records of plenary meetings, reports of committees.* Geneva: WHO. Retrieved June 2018 from www.who.int/iris/handle/10665/159887

World Health Assembly (WHA) (1983b) *The role of nursing/midwifery personnel in the strategy of health for all* (WHA36.11). Geneva: WHO.

World Health Assembly (1986) *Thirty-ninth World Health Assembly, Geneva, 5–16 May 1986: verbatim records of plenary meetings, reports of committees.* World Health Organization. Retrieved June 2018 from www.who.int/iris/handle/10665/162253

World Health Assembly (1988) *Forty-first World Health Assembly, Geneva, 2–13 May 1988: verbatim records of plenary meetings, reports of committees.* Geneva: WHO. Retrieved June 2018 from www.who.int/iris/handle/10665/164198

World Health Assembly (WHA) (1989)ﾠ*Forty-second World Health Assembly, Geneva, 8–19 May 1989: verbatim records of plenary meetings, reports of committees.* Geneva: WHO. Retrieved June 2018 from www.who.int/iris/handle/10665/171212

World Health Assembly (WHA) (1991)ﾠ*Forty-fourth World Health Assembly, Geneva, 6–16 May 1991: summary records of committees.* Geneva: WHO. Retrieved June 2018 from www.who.int/iris/handle/10665/173863

World Health Assembly (WHA) (1992)ﾠ*Forty-fifth World Health Assembly, Geneva, 4–14 May 1992: summary records of committees.* Geneva: WHO. Retrieved June 2018 from www.who.int/iris/handle/10665/175632

World Health Assembly (WHA) (1993)ﾠ*Forty-sixth World Health Assembly, Geneva, 3–14 May 1993: summary records and reports of committees.* Geneva: WHO. Retrieved June 2018 from www.who.int/iris/handle/10665/176279

World Health Assembly (WHA) (1996)ﾠ*Forty-ninth World Health Assembly, Geneva, 20–25 May 1996: summary records and reports of committees.* Geneva: WHO. Retrieved June 2018 from www.who.int/iris/handle/10665/178944

World Health Assembly (WHA) (1997) *Strengthening health systems in developing countries* (WHA50.27) Geneva: WHO.

World Health Assembly (WHA) (1998) *Non-communicable disease prevention and control* (WHA51.18) Geneva: WHO.

World Health Assembly (WHA) (1999) *Strengthening health systems in developing countries* (WHA52.23) Geneva: WHO.

World Health Assembly (WHA) (2001) *Strengthening nursing and midwifery* (WHA54.12) Geneva: WHO.

World Health Assembly (WHA) (2004) *International migration of health personnel: a challenge for health systems in developing countries* (WHA57.19) Geneva: WHO.

World Health Assembly (WHA) (2005) *Sustainable health financing, universal coverage and social health insurance* (WHA58.33). Geneva: WHO.

World Health Assembly (WHA) (2006a) *Rapid scaling up of health workforce production* (WHA59.23). Geneva: WHO.

World Health Assembly (WHA) (2006b) *International migration of health personnel: a challenge for health systems in developing countries* (WHA59.18). Geneva: WHO.

World Health Assembly (WHA) (2006c) *International trade and health* (WHA59.26) Geneva: WHO.

World Health Assembly (WHA) (2006d)ﾠ *Fifty-ninth World Health Assembly, Geneva, 22–27 May 2006: summary records of Committees, reports of Committees.* World Health Organization. Retrieved June 2018 from http://apps.who.int/gb/ebwha/pdf_files/WHA59-REC3/A59_REC3-en.pdf.

World Health Assembly (WHA) (2010) *WHO Global Code of Practice on the International Recruitment of Health Personnel* (WHA63.16) Geneva: WHO.

World Health Assembly (WHA) (2013) A 66/25. *The health workforce: advances in responding to shortages and migration, and in preparing for emerging needs.* Report by the Secretariat. In: Sixty-sixth World Health Assembly, 20 28 May 2013, Geneva: WHO. Retrieved June 2018 from http://apps.who.int/gb/ebwha/pdf_files/WHA66/A66_25-en.pdf

World Health Assembly (WHA) (2013) *WHA66/2013/REC/3, summary record of the fifth meeting of Committee B of the Sixty-sixth World Health Assembly,* document A66/25. Geneva: WHO.

World Health Assembly (WHA) (2016) *Global strategy on human resources for health: workforce 2030* (WHA69.19) Geneva: WHO.

World Health Organization (WHO) (1946) *Constitution of WHO, Official Records of the World Health Organisation*, 2, 100. Geneva: WHO.

World Health Organization (WHO) (1958) The First Ten Years of the World Health Organization. Geneva: WHO.

World Health Organization (WHO) (1959) *First report on the world health situation 1954–1956.* Official Records of the World Health Organization, No. 94, Geneva: WHO.

World Health Organization (WHO) (1962) *Second report on the world health situation 1957–1960.* World Health Assembly, A15/P8&B/3 Part I 13 April 1962, Geneva: WHO.

World Health Organization (WHO) (1967) *Third report on the world health situation 1961–1964.* Official Records of the World Health Organization, No. 155, Geneva: WHO.

World Health Organization (WHO) (1968) *The Second Ten Years of the World Health Organization: 1958–1967.* Geneva: WHO.

World Health Organization (WHO) (1972) *Training of national health personnel. Progress report by the Director-General (A25/7).* Geneva: WHO.

World Health Organization (WHO) (1978) Declaration of Alma-Ata. International Conference on Primary Health care, Alma-Ata, USSR, 6–12 September 1978, Geneva: WHO.

World Health Organization (WHO) (1979) *Formulating strategies for health for all by the year 2000: guiding principles and essential issues, document of the Executive Board of the World Health Organization.* Geneva: WHO.

World Health Organization (WHO) (1981) *Global Strategy Health for All by the Year 2000.* Geneva: WHO.

World Health Organization (WHO) (1982) *Nursing and midwifery workforce strategy.* Geneva: WHO.

World Health Organization (WHO) (1992) *The Work of WHO 1990–1991 Biennial Report of the Director-General to the World Health Assembly and to the United Nations.* Geneva: WHO.

World Health Organization (WHO) (1993) Proposed programme budget for the financial period 1994–1995: programme support costs, WHO Executive Board, EB91/5 18 January 1993. Geneva: WHO.

World Health Organization (WHO) (2005) International trade and health. Report by the Secretariat. Executive Board, EB116/4 116th Session 28 April 2005

World Health Organization (WHO) (2006a) *Working Together for Health.* The World Health Report 2006. Geneva: WHO.

World Health Organization (WHO) (2006b) *International trade and health.* Item 11.10 of the Agenda (Documents EB117/2006/REC/1, resolution EB117.R5, and A59/15). Geneva: WHO.

World Health Organization (WHO) (2006c) *International migration of health personnel: a challenge for health systems in developing countries.* A59/18, 4 May 2006. Geneva: WHO.

World Health Organization (WHO) (2008) *The third ten years of the World Health Organization: 1968–1978.* Geneva: WHO.

World Health Organization (WHO) (2009a) *International recruitment of health personnel: draft global code of practice.* Report by the Secretariat. WHO Executive Board 126th Session 3 December 2009. Geneva: WHO.

World Health Organization (WHO) (2009b) *A World Health Organization code of practice on the international recruitment of health personnel: Background paper.* Health

Systems and Services Cluster (HSS) Department of Human Resources for Health (HRH) Health Workforce Migration and Retention Team (HMR). Geneva: WHO.

World Health Organization (WHO) (2010a) *WHO Global Code of Practice on the International Recruitment of Health Personnel.* Geneva: WHO.

World Health Organization (WHO) (2010b) *International recruitment of health personnel: draft global code of practice.* Report by the Secretariat, Sixty-Third World Health Assembly Provisional Agenda 11.5 (2010) (WHA A63/8). Geneva: WHO.

World Health Organization (WHO) (2010c) *Health Systems Financing: The path to universal coverage.* World health report. Geneva: WHO.

World Health Organization (WHO) (2011a) *Public hearing on the draft guidelines for monitoring the implementation of the WHO Global Code of Practice on the International Recruitment of Health Personnel,* 21 March to 17 April 2011. Geneva: WHO.

World Health Organization (WHO) (2011b) *The Abuja Declaration: Ten years on.* Geneva: WHO.

World Health Organization (WHO) (2011c) *Strengthening health systems in developing countries.* (WHA54.13). Geneva: WHO.

World Health Organization (WHO) (2011d) *The fourth ten years of the World Health Organization: 1978–1987.* Geneva: WHO.

World Health Organization (WHO) (2012) *WHO Country Assessment Tool on the uses and sources for human resources for health (HRH) data.* Geneva: WHO.

World Health Organization (WHO) (2013a) A 66/25. *The health workforce: advances in responding to shortages and migration, and in preparing for emerging needs.* Report by the Secretariat. In: Sixty-sixth World Health Assembly, 20–28 May 2013. Geneva: WHO.

World Health Organization (WHO) (2013b) *WHO policy dialogue on international health workforce mobility and recruitment challenges technical report.* Amsterdam: WHO.

World Health Organization (WHO) (2014) *Migration of Health Workers: WHO Code of Practice and the global economic crisis.* Geneva: WHO.

World Health Organization (WHO) (2015a) *Report of the Expert Advisory Group on the Relevance and Effectiveness of the WHO Global Code of Practice on the International Recruitment of Health Personnel (2010).* Report by the Director-General. Sixty-Eighth World Health Assembly, A68/32 Add.1 Agenda item 17.2. Geneva: WHO.

World Health Organization (WHO) (2015b) *WHO leadership statement on the Ebola response and WHO reforms* (online). Retrieved 10 June 2018 from: www.who.int/csr/disease/ebola/joint-statement-ebola/en/

World Health Organization (WHO) (2015c) *Tracking universal health coverage: first global monitoring report.* Geneva: WHO.

World Health Organization (WHO) (2016a*) WHO Global Code of Practice on the International Recruitment of Health Personnel: second round of national reporting. Report by the Secretariat.* Sixty-ninth World Health Assembly A69/37, April 2016. Geneva: WHO.

World Health Organization (WHO) (2016b) *Framework on integrated, people-centred health services. Report by the Secretariat.* Sixty-ninth World Health Assembly A69/39, 15 April 2016. Geneva: WHO.

World Health Organization (WHO) (2016c) *Global strategy on human resources for health: workforce 2030.* Sixty-ninth World Health Assembly. Resolution WHA69.19 Agenda item 16.1 28 May 2016. Geneva: WHO.

World Health Organization (WHO) (2016d) *Framework of engagement with non-State actors.* Sixty-ninth World Health Assembly WHA69.10 Agenda item 11.3 28 May 2016. Geneva: WHO.

World Health Organization (WHO) (2016e) *World Health Statistics 2016: Monitoring health for the SDGs.* Geneva: WHO. Retrieved 20 June 2018 from: www.human-resources-health.com/content/13/1/66

World Health Organization (WHO) (2016f) *World health statistics 2016: monitoring health for the Sustainable Development Goals.* Geneva: WHO.

World Health Organization (WHO) (2017a) *Health Workforce Migration and the WHO Global Code of Practice on the International Recruitment of Health Personnel.* Geneva: WHO.

World Health Organization (WHO) (2017b) *Dublin Declaration on Human Resources for Health: Building the Health Workforce of the Future.* Fourth Global Forum on Human Resources for Health, Dublin. Geneva: WHO

World Health Organization (WHO) (2017c) *International Health Worker Migration: A High-Level Dialogue.* Fourth Global Forum on Human Resources for Health. Dublin. Geneva: WHO.

World Health Organization (WHO) (2018a) *Working for Health. Five-Year Action Plan for Health Employment and Inclusive Economic Growth (2017–2021).* Geneva: WHO.

World Health Organization (WHO) (2018b) *WHO Global Code of Practice on the International Recruitment of Health Personnel Independent Stakeholders Reporting Instrument.* Geneva: WHO.

World Health Organization (WHO) (2018c) *Draft thirteenth general programme of work 2019–2023: promote health, keep the world safe, serve the vulnerable.* Geneva: WHO.

World Health Organization (WHO) (2018d) *Global Health Workforce Statistics Database.* Geneva: World Health Organisation. Retrieved from www.who.int/hrh/statistics/TechnicalNotes.pdf

World Health Organization (WHO) (undated) National Reporting Instrument (NRI) reports database. WHO: Geneva www.who.int/hrh/migration/code/code-nri/reports/en/.

World Health Organization Regional Office for Africa (WHO-AFRO) (2002) *Human Resources Development for Health: Accelerating Implementation of the Regional Strategy.* 52nd Session of the WHO Regional Committee for Africa, Harare, Zimbabwe. 8–12 October 2002. Brazzaville, Congo: WHO Regional Office for Africa.

World Health Organization (WHO) and GHWA (2015) *Relevance and effectiveness of the WHO Global Code in Ireland: processes and achievements.* Policy Brief B. Geneva: WHO.

World Health Organization, OECD, and International Bank for Reconstruction and Development/The World Bank (WHO/OECD/World Bank) (2018) *Delivering quality health services: A global imperative for universal health coverage.* Geneva/Paris/Washington, DC: WHO/OECD/World Bank.

World Health Organization (WHO) and World Bank (2015) *Tracking universal health coverage: first global monitoring report.* Geneva/Washington, DC: WHO/World Bank.

World Health Organization (WHO) Global Health Observatory (2017) *Global Health Observatory Dataset.* Retrieved June 2018 from www.who.int/gho/en/

World Health Organization (WHO) Regional Office for Europe (2008) *Recruitment and retention of health workers: Policy options towards global solidarity.* WHO: Copenhagen.

World Health Organization (WHO)/Western Pacific (2007) *Pacific Code of Practice for Recruitment of Health Workers and Compendium.* Endorsed at the Seventh Meeting of Ministers of Health for Pacific Island Countries in Port Vila, Vanuatu, 12 to 15 March 2007.

World Health Organization Reporting Instrument (2015) *Reports database*, World Health Organization, Geneva. Retrieved 25 July 2017 from www.who.int/hrh/migration/code/code_nri/reports

World Health Organization-Europe (WHO-Europe) (2012) *Implementing the WHO Global Code of Practice on the International Recruitment of Health Personnel in the European Region: A Policy Brief.* Draft prepared by Professor Gilles Dussault, Professor Galina Perfilieva and Mr Jakob Pethick, for Regional Technical Committee 63, Malta, Technical Briefing 2.

World Health Organization/Global Health Workforce Alliance (WHO/GHWA) (2008) *The Kampala declaration and agenda for global action: Health workers for all and all for health workers.* Geneva: WHO.

World Health Organization/Global Health Workforce Alliance (WHO/GHWA) (2013) *Global Forum on Human Resources for Health*, Recife, Brazil, (10–13 November 2013). Geneva: WHO.

World Health Organization/Global Health Workforce Alliance (WHO/GHWA) (2014) *Follow-up of the Recife Political Declaration on Human Resources for Health: renewed commitments towards universal health coverage.* Sixty-Seventh World Health Assembly, WHA67.24 Agenda item 15.8, 24 May 2014. Geneva: WHO/GHWA.

World Health Organization/Global Health Workforce Network/Women in Global Health (WHO/GHWN/WGH) (2018) *Working paper on Gender & Equity in the Health and Social Care Workforce.* Consultative Draft Report. Geneva: WHO.

World Health Organization/Organization for Economic Cooperation and Development (WHO/OECD) (2010) *International migration of health workers. Improving international cooperation to address the global health workforce crisis.* Paris: OECD.

World Health Organization/World Intellectual Property Organization/World Trade Organization (WHO/WIPO/WTO) (2012) *Promoting access to medical technologies and innovation: Intersections between public health, intellectual property and trade.* Geneva: WTO.

World Health Organization/World Trade Organization (WHO/WTO) (2002) *WTO agreements and public health: a joint study by the WHO and the WTO secretariat.* Geneva: WHO/WTO.

World Trade Organization (WTO) (2009) *Presence of Natural Persons (Mode 4). Background Note by the Secretariat.* S/C/W/31. September 2009. Geneva: WTO.

Yagi, N., Mackey, T.K., Liang, B.A. and Gerit, L. (2014) Japan–Philippines Economic Partnership Agreement (JPEPA): analysis of a failed nurse migration policy. *International Journal of Nursing Studies* 51(2): 243–250.

Yeates, N. (2001) *Globalisation and Social Policy.* London: Sage.

Yeates, N. (2002) Globalization and Social Policy: from global neoliberal hegemony to global political pluralism. *Global Social Policy*, 2(1): 69–91.

Yeates, N. (2004a) A dialogue with 'global care chain' analysis: nurse migration in the Irish context. *Feminist Review*, 77: 79–95.

Yeates, N. (2004b) Global care chains: critical reflections and lines of enquiry. *International Feminist Journal of Politics*, 6(3): 369–391.

Yeates, N. (2005a) The General Agreement on Trade in Services (GATS): What's in it for social security? *International Social Security Review*, 58(1): 3–22.

Yeates, N. (2005b) *Global care chains: A critical introduction* (Global Migration Perspectives No. 44). Geneva: Global Commission on International Migration.

Yeates, N. (2007) The global and supra-national dimensions of the welfare mix, in M. Powell (ed.) *Understanding the Mixed Economy of Welfare.* The Policy Press, Bristol.

Yeates, N. (2008) Here to stay? Migrant health workers in Ireland, in J. Connell (ed.) *The International Migration of Health Workers*, London: Routledge.

Yeates, N. (2009a) Production for export: the role of the state in the development and operation of global care chains. *Population, Space and Place*, 15(2): 175–187.

Yeates, N. (2009b) *Globalising Care Economies and Migrant Workers: Explorations in global care chains*. Palgrave: Basingstoke.

Yeates, N. (2010) The Globalization of Nurse Migration: Policy Issues and Responses. *International Labour Review*, 149: 423–440.

Yeates, N. (2011) Ireland's contributions to the global nursing and health crises, in B. Fanning and R. Munck (eds.) *Globalization, migration and social transformation: Ireland in Europe and the World*. Farnham: Ashgate.

Yeates, N. (2012) Global care chains: state of the art review and future directions, *Global Networks: a journal of transnational affairs*, 12(2): 135–154.

Yeates, N. (2014a) The Socialisation of Regionalism and the Regionalisation of Social Policy: contexts, imperatives and challenges, in A. Kaasch and P. Stubbs (eds.) *Transformations in Global and Regional Social Policies*. Basingstoke: Palgrave

Yeates, N. (2014b). Global care chains: Bringing in transnational reproductive laborer households, in W.A. Dunaway (ed.), *Gendered Commodity Chains*. Stanford, CA: Stanford University Press: 175–189.

Yeates, N. (2017) *Beyond the Nation State: How can regional social policy contribute to achieving the Sustainable Development Goals?* UNRISD Issue Brief no. 5. UNRISD: Geneva.

Yeates, N. (2018a) *Global approaches to social policy: a survey of analytical methods*, United Nations Research Institute for Social Development Thematic Paper, New Directions in Social Policy Series. WP 2018–2. Geneva: UNRISD.

Yeates, N. (2018b) Social security in global context, in J. Millar and R. Sainsbury (eds.) *Understanding Social Security*. 3rd edition. Bristol: The Policy Press.

Yeates, N. and Deacon, B. (2010) Globalisation, regional integration and social policy, in B. Deacon, M.C. Macovei, L. van Langenhove and N. Yeates (eds.) *World-Regional Social Policy and Global Governance: new research and policy agendas in Africa, Asia, Europe and Latin America*. London: Routledge.

Yeates, N., Macovei, M. and van Langenhove, L. (2010) 'The evolving context of world-regional social policy: bilateralism and trans-regionalism', in B. Deacon, L. van Langenhove, M. Macovei and N. Yeates (eds.) *World-regional social policy and global governance: new research and policy agendas in Africa, Asia, Europe and Latin America*. London: Routledge

Yeates, N. and Pillinger, J. (2013) *Human resources for health migration: Global policy responses, initiatives, and emerging issues*. Milton Keynes: The Open University/ University of Ottawa.

Yeates, N. and Pillinger, J. (2018) International health care worker migration in Asia Pacific: international policy responses. *Asia Pacific Viewpoint*. 59(1): 92–106.

Yeates, N., Macovei, M., and van Langenhove, L. (2010) The evolving context of world-regional social policy: bilateralism and trans-regionalism, in B. Deacon, L. van Langenhove, M. Macovei and N. Yeates (eds.) *World-regional social policy and global governance: new research and policy agendas in Africa, Asia, Europe and Latin America*. London: Routledge: 191–212

Youde, J. (2012) *Global health governance*. Cambridge: Polity Press.

Zhao, F., Squires, N., Weakliam, D., Van Lerberghe, W., Soucat, A., Toure, K., Shakarishvili, G., Quain, E. and Maeda, A. (2013) Investing in human resources for health: The need for a paradigm shift. *Bull World Health Organ*, 91(11): 799–799A.

# Index